KU-544-150

Epidemics

Pathways to Sustainability Series

This book series addresses core challenges around linking science and technology and environmental sustainability with poverty reduction and social justice. It is based on the work of the Social, Technological and Environmental Pathways to Sustainability (STEPS) Centre, a major investment of the UK Economic and Social Research Council (ESRC). The STEPS Centre brings together researchers at the Institute of Development Studies (IDS) and SPRU (Science and Technology Policy Research) at the University of Sussex with a set of partner institutions in Africa, Asia and Latin America.

Series Editors:
Melissa Leach, Ian Scoones and Andy Stirling
STEPS Centre at the University of Sussex

Editorial Advisory Board:
Steve Bass, Wiebe E. Bijker, Victor Galaz, Wenzel Geissler, Katherine Homewood, Sheila Jasanoff, Colin McInnes, Suman Sahai, Andrew Scott

Titles include:
Dynamic Sustainabilities
Technology, Environment, Social Justice
Melissa Leach, Ian Scoones and Andy Stirling

Avian Influenza
Science, Policy and Politics
Edited by Ian Scoones

Rice Biofortification
Lessons for Global Science and Development
Sally Brooks

Epidemics
Science, Governance and Social Justice
Edited by Sarah Dry and Melissa Leach

'This book is of particular interest for those who feel there is a need to change the ways we think and go about the protection of human health, in particular where it comes to invasive intruders lurking in the animal world. Pandemic threats and emerging diseases are invariably the result of human choices and actions. Collectively we create new niches for new diseases. Food and agriculture brings a growing number of influenza viruses. A set of global factors is at work to explain why pathogens flare-up at the animal–human–environment interface. Disease agents invade new areas, turn more aggressive or start infecting novel host species. Humans are not the sole victim; plants and animals are also affected by invasive species. It is clear that a business-as-usual approach will not hold back the tide of novel threats. The veterinary and medical professions will continue to try to nip the problem in the bud and prevent escalation. Yet emergency response is only part of the storyline and it alone will not solve the problem. Addressing the root causes of disease emergence concerns the public at large. Healthy animal agriculture and natural resource management are among the require-ments to counter disease flare-up. This clearly places people rather than health authorities at the centre stage. As it is convincingly argued in this book, novel diseases – and responses to them – should not be viewed in isolation. Instead they need to be considered and addressed jointly with the challenges of socio-economic development, sustainable agriculture, rural development, and the protection of the environment. Health is the domain of all of us.'

Jan Slingenbergh, Head, Animal Health Emergency Prevention System, Animal Health Service, Food and Agriculture Organization, UN

'How best can our agents of government use good science to shape a better future for us? What boundaries and controls do we need to prevent the scientific agendas growing uncontrollably, metastasizing and taking over the other cherished aspects of our lives? These, I believe, are the most important questions of our time – encompassing the issues of global warming, AIDS, maternal deaths, nuclear disarmament, macro-economic stability, satellite and phone-tapping espionage. This book addresses them through specific cases of unexpected infectious diseases: epidemics – one of the most emotive, frightening and chal-lenging emergencies, during which the usual rules and laws of the land may be suspended and extreme measures may be taken, for example, slaughter of the pigs of Egypt, invol-untary detention without trial or charge, known euphemistically as quarantine. During an epidemic our response to the biological reality of a life-threatening infection comes into conflict with our individual rights and autonomy. The outcome of the conflict may easily be influenced by powerful political actors, and could become a tool to enforce a political agenda separate and distinct from the biological problem. In this book you can read the stories of how this has happened, and perhaps recognize a better way.'

Professor Samuel J. McConkey, Head, Department of International Health and Tropical Medicine, Royal College of Surgeons in Ireland

'The book is highly informative, original, and its trans-disciplinary approach is quite appropriate. It broadens our knowledge horizon about epidemics, and should be of equal interest to epidemiologists, public health specialists, social scientists, policy analysts, ethi-cists and postgraduate students in international health. It should become compulsory reading for civil servants and policy makers involved in drawing up health policies on epidemic p

LIVERPOOL JMU LIBRARY

3 1111 01461 7961

Philippe (ion Unit on Humanitarian Stakes and Practi ntières, Switzerland

Epidemics

Science, Governance and Social Justice

Edited by
Sarah Dry and Melissa Leach

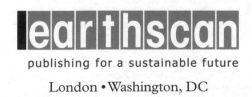

publishing for a sustainable future

London • Washington, DC

First published in 2010 by Earthscan

Copyright © Sarah Dry and Melissa Leach, 2010

All rights reserved. No part of this publication may be reproduced, stored in a retrieval system, or transmitted, in any form or by any means, electronic, mechanical, photocopying, recording or otherwise, except as expressly permitted by law, without the prior, written permission of the publisher.

Earthscan Ltd, Dunstan House, 14a St Cross Street, London EC1N 8XA, UK
Earthscan LLC, 1616 P Street, NW, Washington, DC 20036, USA
Earthscan publishes in association with the International Institute for Environment and Development

For more information on Earthscan publications, see www.earthscan.co.uk or write to earthinfo@earthscan.co.uk

ISBN: 978-1-84971-101-2 hardback
ISBN: 978-1-84971-102-9 paperback

Typeset by Composition and Design Services
Cover design by Susanne Harris

A catalogue record for this book is available from the British Library

Library of Congress Cataloging-in-Publication Data

Epidemics: science, governance, and social justice/edited by Sarah Dry and Melissa Leach.
    p. cm.
  Includes bibliographical references and index.
    ISBN 978-1-84971-101-2 (hardback) – ISBN 978-1-84971-102-9 (pbk.) 1. Epidemics.
2. Epidemics–Social aspects. 3. Epidemics–Political aspects. I. Dry, Sarah, 1974- II. Leach, Melissa.
  RA651.E617 2010
  614.4–dc22   2009051968

At Earthscan we strive to minimize our environmental impacts and carbon footprint through reducing waste, recycling and offsetting our CO_2 emissions, including those created through publication of this book. For more details of our environmental policy, see www.earthscan.co.uk.

Printed and bound in the UK by CPI Antony Rowe
The paper used is FSC certified.

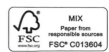

Contents

List of Contributors

Editors

Sarah Dry is a Research Officer at the STEPS Centre, Institute of Development Studies, where she focuses on epidemics. Her research interests include Victorian meteorology and government science, the history of 20th century medicine and global health policy. She received her PhD in History of Science from Cambridge University and has held an ESRC Postdoctoral Fellowship at the Centre for Analysis of Risk and Regulation, London School of Economics.

Melissa Leach is a Professorial Fellow at the Institute of Development Studies and Director of the STEPS Centre. She is a social anthropologist specializing in environmental, health and science–society issues, with long research experience in West Africa. Her research interests include social and institutional dimensions of environmental and technological change, and issues of knowledge, power and citizen engagement.

Authors

Gerald Bloom is a physician and health systems analyst. He is a Fellow at the Institute of Development Studies, where he convenes the health and disease domain of the STEPS Centre. He has particular interests in health system transition in rapidly changing contexts.

Jerker Edström is a Fellow at the Institute of Development Studies, where he leads the HIV and Development programme. Prior to joining IDS he worked for the International HIV/AIDS Alliance, and has many years of research and practical experience with HIV programming in Africa and Asia.

Barry S. Hewlett is Professor of Anthropology at Washington State University, Vancouver. He received a PhD from the University of California, Santa Barbara in 1987 and has had appointments at Southern Oregon University, Tulane University and Oregon State University. He has conducted research in central Africa since 1973 and is the author of *Intimate Fathers: The Nature and Context of Aka Pygmy Paternal Infant Care, Hunter-Gatherer Childhoods* (edited with Michael Lamb), *Ebola, Culture and Politics* (with Bonnie Hewlett) and 'Human behavior and cultural context in disease control', Special Issue of *Tropical Medicine and International Health* (edited with Joan Koss-Chioino).

Hayley MacGregor is a Fellow at the Institute of Development Studies. She is a medical doctor and social anthropologist whose areas of research include mental health, social protection and disability, human rights discourses and health citizenship, the regulation of and responses to medical technologies, and the effects of global health funding on local responses to HIV and AIDS in southern Africa.

Erik Millstone is a Professor based at Science and Technology Policy Research (SPRU), University of Sussex. He co-convenes the STEPS Centre's Food and Agriculture domain. He originally trained as a physicist and philosopher, but now works on science and public health policy. His interests include public and environmental health protection policies, the interactions between scientific and policy considerations in both risk assessment and risk management, BSE, GM crops and obesity policy.

Paul Nightingale is a Deputy Director of SPRU, Science and Technology Policy Research, University of Sussex. He is a visting Professor of Corporate Strategy at Cass Business School (City University) and an Associate Fellow of the Open University's Innovation, Knowledge and Development centre. He is currently a UK editor of *Industrial and Corporate Change*, and was previously editor of *Research Policy*. He has published widely on innovation in bio-pharmaceuticals, financial services, capital goods use in service firms, financing of biotechnology, biosecurity, and the nature and use of knowledge.

Ian Scoones is a Professorial Fellow at the Institute of Development Studies, and Co-Director of the STEPS Centre. He originally trained as an ecologist but his research over many years has linked natural and social sciences, focusing on relationships between science and technology, local knowledge and livelihoods and the politics of agricultural, environment and development policy processes.

Mariz Tadros is a Fellow at the Institute of Development Studies. She obtained her doctorate degree from the International Development Centre, Queen Elizabeth House at the University of Oxford in 2004, and her MA in 1999 from the American University in Cairo (AUC). She has worked as an assistant professor of political science at the American University in Cairo. She also worked for many years as a journalist for *Al-Ahram Weekly*, an English language newspaper covering women's rights, NGOs, human rights and poverty-related issues. Her research interests include aid for civil society promotion of democratization, gender and development in the Middle East, NGOs and civil society in the Arab world, and Islamist politics in Egypt and the region.

Preface and Acknowledgements

The challenge of responding effectively to epidemic diseases is upon us. With recent outbreaks of haemorrhagic fevers, SARS, H1N1 and avian influenza capturing public and policy attention, and the prediction of more emerging and re-emerging infectious diseases to come, there is a pressing need to take action. But what is the best form for such action to take? Too often, responses to epidemic diseases are focused on short-term, emergency measures that may fail to address the underlying drivers of outbreaks. Acute outbreaks are privileged while chronic diseases may be neglected. Eradication may be attempted when control and management would be more appropriate. In light of the complexity of both disease and political dynamics, how can policy-makers, health practitioners and citizens contribute to generating sustainable responses to epidemic diseases that benefit the health and well-being of all? This book aims to answer these questions by revealing the implicit assumptions that shape epidemic policy and exploring the alternative perspectives that are often left out of responses.

In a series of case studies, we focus on how different policy-makers, scientists and local populations construct narratives – accounts of the causes and appropriate responses to outbreaks – about epidemics at the global, national and local level. Our case studies cover a broad historical, geographical and biological range, including avian influenza, SARS, obesity, H1N1 influenza, HIV/AIDS, tuberculosis and haemorrhagic fevers. This allows us to analyse how the category of epidemic disease itself is constructed in different settings, with some diseases traversing the boundary between endemic and epidemic multiple times. Our cases reveal the power of dominant narratives about epidemics to shape policy in intended as well as unintended ways, along with the contributions that neglected understandings of health and disease in a given community may make to effective responses. Better policy responses, our cases suggest, can be achieved by paying more attention to the full range of health problems in a given setting and by thinking deeply about the interaction between long-term and short-term drivers in the complex interplay between humans, animals and microbes.

This book forms part of the Pathways to Sustainability series and draws on the thinking and discussion that has occurred at the STEPS Centre during its first three years. The STEPS Centre is committed to exploring the challenges of building pathways that link technology and the environment with improved livelihoods and social justice, especially for people currently living in poverty. Epidemics epitomize these complex dynamics. This book is a product of research and reflection on these dynamics by members of the Epidemics group using the STEPS Centre's pathways approach.

We are grateful to all our colleagues in the STEPS Centre, as well as members of the Knowledge, Technology and Society Team at the Institute of Development Studies, for providing a stimulating and responsive environment in which to develop these ideas. Nearly all of our contributors presented their work and received feedback during a workshop on Epidemics held at the STEPS Centre in December 2008. We would like to acknowledge the contribution of the participants of that seminar: Uli Beisel, Ruth Branston, Philippe Calain, Stefan Elbe, Isabel Fletcher, Paul Gully, Monica Janowski, Henry Lucas, Maria McPhillips, Sandra Mounier-Jack, Jan Slingenbergh and Annie Wilkinson. We would also like to thank the following individuals, who have reviewed or commented on some part of the manuscript: Philippe Calain, Wenzel Geissler, Colin McInnes and Melanie Newport. Finally, our grateful thanks are due to Harriet Le Bris for supporting the process of editing and production.

List of Acronyms and Abbreviations

AIDS	Acquired Immune Deficiency Syndrome
ALP	AIDS Law Project
ANCS	Alliance National Contre le Sida à Sénegal
APE	Association for the Protection of the Environment
ARASA	AIDS and Rights Alliance for Southern Africa
ARV	antiretroviral
ARVs	antiretroviral drugs
ASRU	AIDS and Society Research Unit
ATICC	AIDS Training and Counselling Centre
BCG	Bacillus Calmette-Guerin
BMI	body mass index
BSE	Bovine Spongiform Encephalopathy
CDC	Centers for Disease Control (US)
CMC	Crisis Management Centre
DDT	dichlorodiphenyltrichloroethane
DHS	Demographic and Health Surveys
DOTS	Directly Observed Treatment, Short Course
DRC	Democratic Republic of Congo
DRS	Global Project on Drug Resistance Surveillance
EID	emerging infectious disease
EMPRES	Emergency Prevention
ESRC	Economic and Social Research Council
EU	European Union
FAO	Food and Agriculture Organization of the United Nations
FBO	faith based organization
FDF	Food and Drink Federation
FPP	Frontiers' Prevention Project
GAVI	Global Alliance for Vaccines and Immunization
GDP	gross domestic product
GFATM	Global Fund to Fight AIDS, Tuberculosis and Malaria
GHI	global health initiative
GIDEON	Global Infectious Diseases Epidemiology Online Network
GLEWS	Global Early Warning System for Major Animal Diseases
GMA	Grocery Manufacturers of America

GOARN   Global Outbreak Alert and Response Network
GPA   Global Programme on AIDS
GPEI   Global Polio Eradication Initiative
GPHIN   Global Public Health Information Network
GRID   gay-related immune deficiency
HAART   highly active antiretroviral therapy
HAT   harmonized assessment tool
HHS   US Department of Health and Human Services
HIV   human immunodeficiency virus
HPAI   highly pathogenic avian influenza
HSRC   Human Sciences Research Council
ICT   information and communication technology
IDS   Institute of Development Studies
IDU   injecting drug users
IHR   International Health Regulations (WHO)
IUATLD   International Union Against Tuberculosis and Lung Disease
MDR-TB   multidrug-resistant tuberculosis
MSF   Médecins Sans Frontières
MSM   men who have sex with men
NAPWA   National Association of People with AIDS
NCMS   new cooperative medical system
NDP   National Democratic Party
NGO   non-governmental organization
NIH   National Institutes of Health
NSWP   Global Network of Sex Work Projects
OECD   Organisation for Economic Co-operation and Development
OFFLU   OIE/FAO network of experts on animal influenza
OIE   World Organization for Animal Health
PEPFAR   President's Emergency Plan for AIDS Relief
PHEIC   public health emergency of international concern
PICT   provider-initiated counselling and testing
SANAC   South Africa National AIDS Council
SARS   Severe Acute Respiratory Syndrome
SHOC   Strategic Health Operations Centre
SPRU   Science and Technology Policy Research
STEPS   Social, Technological and Environmental Pathways to
           Sustainability
SW   sex worker
TAC   Treatment Action Campaign
TB   tuberculosis
UNAIDS   Joint United Nations Programme on HIV/AIDS
UNDP   United Nations Development Programme

UNICEF	United Nations Children's Fund
UNSIC	UN System Influenza Coordination
WHO	World Health Organization
XDR-TB	extensively drug-resistant tuberculosis

Chapter 1

Epidemic Narratives

Melissa Leach and Sarah Dry

In June 2009, the World Health Organization (WHO) officially declared that the world was experiencing a global pandemic of H1N1 influenza. An initial outbreak of a new virus in Mexico (termed 'swine' flu because of its early identification in pigs and mix of pig, avian and human genetic material) had jumped to humans and was now sweeping the world, hastened by travel and rapid transmission on our interconnected and crowded planet. Soon after the emergence of the virus, the WHO had called the outbreak an 'extreme expression of the need for global solidarity' (WHO, 2009). Pandemic preparedness plans, put into place in many industrialized countries in response to the earlier threat of H5N1 avian influenza, were mobilized at scale. Yet by July, it was clear that the battle to halt the epidemic had been lost. With thousands of new cases being reported every day and scientists predicting a huge rise as the winter flu season kicked in, some governments, such as the UK and US, switched strategy from containment to damage limitation, through a mix of public hygiene campaigns and the handing out of stockpiled antiviral drugs such as Tamiflu to reported cases.

Swine flu may be the latest epidemic outbreak to be hitting the headlines, but it is, of course, not the first and it will not be the last. Current global health policy is dominated by a preoccupation with infectious diseases and in particular with so called 'emerging' or 're-emerging' infectious diseases that threaten to 'break out' of established patterns of prevalence or virulence into new areas and new victims (Kickbusch, 2003; Foresight, 2006; Knobler et al, 2006). Such episodes are variously described as outbreaks, epidemics or pandemics depending on their severity, temporal or geographic reach, or their ability to capture our attention (or frighten us). Of the many risks currently facing the international community, the 'most feared security threat' is that a highly infectious and virulent form of human influenza will develop, causing a global pandemic potentially worse than the epidemic that killed so many in 1918–1919 (WHO, 2007a, p45). But the complete list of significant global health risks that have the potential to become epidemic is long and includes multidrug-resistant tuberculosis, malaria, newly emerging and highly infectious viral diseases such as Ebola, Marburg and Nipah, and a growing worldwide resistance to frontline antibiotics. Addressing such diseases ranks high on almost any league table of global health policy (Lee, 2000, 2003a; Saker et al, 2004).

Epidemics can be defined as an increase, over and above what would normally be expected during a particular period of time, in cases of disease within a community or region. Earlier epidemics serve as a sharp reminder of the power of infectious disease to wreak havoc on lives, economy and society. Estimates of the numbers killed in the influenza epidemic of 1918–1919 range from 20 to 100 million. In today's world of mobile people and microbes, the power of infectious diseases has been massively magnified: swine flu has illustrated the capacity for outbreaks to become global pandemics with unprecedented rapidity.

The image of swine flu as a disease emerging 'out of Central America' and going global also evokes earlier events and fears, whether the emergence of Severe Acute Respiratory Syndrome (SARS) 'out of Asia' in 2003, or the emergence of human immunodeficiency virus (HIV) and Ebola 'out of Africa' in the 1980s and 1990s. Such fears contrast sharply with 20th century post-war optimism that infectious disease would soon be conquered with a potent mix of sanitary hygiene, vector control (notably through the use of dichlorodiphenyltrichloroethane (DDT)), vaccines and antibiotics. Notwithstanding what today seem the outsize ambitions of such post-war responses, several disturbing trends of the past 20 years threaten to undermine the successful control of infectious diseases that has been achieved in industrialized nations (Barrett et al, 1998). Firstly, there is a clear increase in the rate at which new diseases (such as H1N1 influenza, SARS, Bovine Spongiform Encephalopathy (BSE) and H5N1 avian influenza) are emerging. At the same time, established diseases, such as malaria, are shifting into new geographical niches as climate change broadens the zones in which vector species (such as mosquitoes) can survive. Finally, newly resistant disease strains, such as drug-resistant malaria, HIV and tuberculosis (TB), represent a growing class of re-emerging infectious diseases, which were once considered tractable but now threaten populations anew.

Of these trends, the swine flu outbreak highlights in particular the threat to humans from zoonosis, the process whereby new diseases somehow manage to 'jump' from an animal species to infect human beings. A sharp rise in such zoonotic diseases in the past 20 years is one of the most startling of the findings indicating a growing threat from infectious diseases. Humans and microbes have been evolving together over hundreds of thousands of years, and some new diseases that make their way into human hosts are to be expected. But things are changing more rapidly than such evolutionary processes would suggest. One important study indicates that all new infectious diseases of human beings to emerge in the past 20 years have had an animal source, and that more than 60 per cent of emerging infectious disease events since 1940 have involved zoonoses (Jones et al, 2008; see also Woolhouse, 2008). Such data may point to a dangerous 'phase' shift in the balance between humans and their pathogens, caused by dramatic shifts in population and climate over a relatively short time frame (Wolfe et al, 2005, 2007). Recent research reveals multiple causes for this increase, including increased human and domestic animal populations, migration, increased human/animal encounters, habitat disturbance, climate change, deforestation, wars, loss of social cohesion and natural disasters (Morens et al, 2004). Scientists, it is argued, must therefore be poised to discover and identify emerging diseases before they have a chance to spread. 'Virus-hunting' needs investment and profile (Wolfe, 2009a). And infrastructures and resources for surveillance, preparedness, rapid containment and protection through public health measures need to be put in place across the globe.

There is good reason to fear the effects of emerging diseases and the epidemics they can cause. Despite the successes of industrialized nations, the current global burden of infectious disease remains enormous: roughly one-quarter of annual global deaths can be attributed to infectious diseases (Morens et al, 2004; WHO, 2004a). A disproportionate amount of this burden sits squarely on the shoulders of the world's poorest people, as would any future burden associated with emerging infectious diseases. This is no coincidence. The conditions of poverty, such as overcrowding, lack of sanitation and forced migration, are precisely those which encourage the transmission and persistence of infectious disease. The combination of the massive current burden of infectious disease with the possibility of more bad news ahead (with the added potential for climate change to worsen the global health situation) has mobilized the global health community (Haines et al, 2006; WHO, 2008a). In recent years, an infusion of new cash and new initiatives – such as the Global Fund to Fight AIDS, TB and Malaria, the Bill and Melinda Gates Foundation global health program, the Millennium Development Goals (especially numbers four, five and six) and the recent revisions in the WHO's International Health Regulations (Dry, this volume) – have transformed the global health policy landscape. The result is that infectious diseases, and the epidemics they can cause, are at the top of the global health agenda.

However, the resulting appearance of a consensus about the risks of global outbreaks hides a set of assumptions – about the nature of the threat and the best way to address it – that may be counter-productive to the goal both of reducing the global burden of infectious disease (in epidemic and endemic forms) and, more broadly, to the goal of creating a more equitable and just world for the long term. By being more critical about the nature of our understanding of epidemic disease at the global, national and local

levels, we can better equip ourselves to deal with disease in all its manifestations, as it affects the world's poorest as well as those with access to the best
preventive and curative medicine available.

What follows, therefore, is an attempt to make explicit some of the implicit
assumptions that shape scientific and policy perspectives on and responses
to epidemics, and global health more generally, today. Indeed in many
respects, the story of swine flu as it unfolded during 2009 is a prime example
of what Wald (2008) has termed 'the outbreak narrative': '[this] begins with
the identification of an emerging infection, includes discussion of the global
networks throughout which it travels, and chronicles the epidemiological
work that ends with its containment' (Wald, 2008, p2). It is versions of such
a narrative – in the case of swine flu and other recent epidemics – that have
underpinned the mobilization of vast scientific and policy resources and
infrastructures. These are aimed at protecting and re-establishing what is
increasingly portrayed as global health security, defined by the WHO as a
set of actions which 'minimize vulnerability to acute public health events
that endanger the collective health of populations living across geographical
regions and international boundaries' (WHO, 2007a). Such understandings
of epidemic outbreaks and emergent diseases, albeit with particular nuances,
are now well established in media and public discourse, and in the arguments and strategies of international agencies and many governments.

Yet the outbreak narrative is not the only story to be told about the
2009 events around 'swine flu'. Behind the headlines, and emanating from
people, places and perspectives not so prominent in the glare of global
policy concern, are a range of other accounts. These include the story from
Mexico, of a much longer-established pig influenza, and of the political
economy of highly industrialized, intensive pork production methods
and worker conditions which may have enabled its spread and species
jump. They also include the case of Egypt, where politicians jumped on
the WHO's early labelling of the disease as 'swine flu' to call for a mass
culling of Cairo's pig population (Tadros, this volume). Alternative stories
also encompass a view of H1N1 as a relatively mild influenza, with much
in common with regular seasonal influenzas, and, like these, manageable
through routine health care and available drugs – and unlikely to kill if these
are used. But while such a narrative was, by late 2009, becoming part of the
mainstream in many industrialized countries endowed with effective health
systems, others were voicing fears about a different spectre for other parts
of the world: the devastating impact that a 'mild' disease in the industrialized world could have if it emerged, at scale, into places and populations
that lacked effective, accessible health care – such as many parts of Africa.

These alternative stories about swine flu highlight how the particular
'outbreak narrative' discussed above is just one among many. How an epidemic

is defined, in space and time, in terms of populations, institutions and interventions, depends on who gets to do the defining. There is always more than one way to tell a story, or 'frame' a particular issue. Within alternative narratives, the dynamics of a given disease, what counts as a problem, and to whom, can vary greatly. This extends to the very notion of an epidemic: whether disease incidence is 'unusual' or expected clearly depends on the place, timescale and vantage point from which it is looked at. From a perspective focused on disease-specific interventions and biomedical control, epidemics are implicitly linked with the goal of disease eradication. From another perspective, the same diseases could be seen as part of the historical, geographical and social landscape, something to be accommodated when possible and occasionally suffered when not. Equally, the notion of 'emergent' disease clearly depends on perspective: what appears to populations of industrialized nations as an emergent disease from an 'other' place, affecting them for the first time, may actually have been long-established, and lived with, there – as it seems may be the case for 'Mexican swine flu'. But while a sensitivity to narrative reveals a diversity of such framings, it also demonstrates their relative authority or dominance. In this sense, not all stories are created equal.

In such ways, narratives – in constructing disease issues in particular ways – frequently also construct people and populations, labelling and making moral judgements about them. Thus colonial assumptions about the backward, insanitary customs and lifestyles of poorer African and Asian populations that motivated often coercive public health campaigns in the early 20th century (e.g. Vaughan, 1991; Manderson, 1996) find their contemporary counterpart in narratives that identify livelihood and lifestyle practices with the spread of disease. Such labelling often accompanies accusation. Some of these linkages explored in the following chapters include: African forest bushmeat hunters and Ebola; Asian poultry farmers and avian flu; people engaged in risky sexual behaviour and HIV; Christian garbage collectors and H1N1; and urban slum-dwellers and SARS (on the politics of disease and accusation, see Farmer, 1992, 1999a, 2003).

In these ways, narratives about disease are also deeply intertwined with issues of power and social justice. The perspective from which a disease is understood, who is threatened, who is blamed, and who is called upon to change their ways can have profound implications for what is done, and who gains or who loses. The view of avian flu as a threat to global populations requiring large-scale culling of poultry, and a view of the same disease as a local problem that must be lived with, have very different implications for the lives and livelihoods of backyard poultry farmers in places like Indonesia and Thailand and those of the inhabitants of industrialized nations.

A central proposition of this book, then, is that disease and epidemics are constructed through different narratives that justify and shape different pathways of response. Narratives, in this sense, are not just stories; they are stories with purposes and consequences. Narratives about epidemics matter because they shape the pathways by which certain responses – of institutions, healthcare practitioners, the media and individuals – are justified and come to be dominant, with profound practical and material implications for how 'successful' responses are, gauged in which terms, and for whom.

Current concern with epidemics can be seen as another instalment in a long-running debate over how global health funds should be invested. Classically, this debate has been argued in terms of disease-specific programmes on the one hand, and primary health care-oriented interventions, on the other. The 30th anniversary of the famous International Conference on Primary Health Care at Alma-Ata in 1978, which represented an apogee of the health systems approach, has led to some renewed soul searching in the international community. The recent publication of the WHO's annual report, titled *Primary Health Care: Now More Than Ever*, may indicate an attempt by that agency to swing the pendulum back to a focus on health systems strengthening, a year after its 2007 report, *A Safer Future: Global Public Health Security in the 21st Century*, on the increased security risks associated with disease outbreaks and epidemics (WHO, 2007a, 2008a). The big difference today is that the players in this drama have changed significantly, with civil society organizations playing a much more prominent role, and charities, the 'new global philanthropy' and public–private partnerships like the Global Fund and Gates Foundation investing far more money than the WHO or most individual nations can.

An approach to thinking about epidemics in terms of narratives and pathways thus provides a distinctive window onto some highly pressing practical and policy challenges. Understanding how epidemics and pandemics emerge and how they might be tackled have become major preoccupations. Yet, we argue, current approaches are often restricted by implicit assumptions that provide only narrow, partial perspectives on the dynamics and experiences associated with epidemics. Important, multi-scale interactions between disease, ecology, society and politics are often inadequately addressed. Not incidentally, the perspectives of people living with disease are also often neglected. How effective will different responses be, given rapid changes in viral, social and political dynamics at a staggering range of scales, from the microscopic to the truly global? How will responses cope with the inevitable uncertainty and surprise? How will responses themselves feed back to shape the dynamics of disease? And who will gain or lose in the process? These are critical questions, and addressing them is vital to building pathways of disease response that are both effective responses to fast-changing conditions and socially just. Our central argument in this book is that doing so effectively requires a better understanding and appreciation of the multiplicity of epidemic narratives, and their links with actual and potential pathways of response. At the same time, we suggest that responses that take into account neglected perspectives, and neglected people, will be better for all of us because they will be more likely to address both the long-term and short-term drivers of outbreaks.

This requires bringing to light alternative narratives which may give voice to important yet neglected perspectives and priorities, including those of marginalized people and places. And it requires addressing the social, political and institutional processes through which narratives and pathways arise and are reproduced, and through which some come to dominate. As we argue, meeting contemporary disease challenges requires far greater attention to such social and governance processes, including the relationships between knowledge and power. It requires both an opening-up to acknowledge multiple narratives and pathways, and astute reflection on the potential priorities, trade-offs and complementarities between these in particular disease and social settings.

Focal diseases

Diseases that are novel and threatening to those living in industrialized nations – such as SARS, Ebola and emerging influenzas – have garnered a disproportionate share of policy and media attention in recent years. HIV/AIDS, understood as an exceptional disease requiring an exceptional response, has attracted resources that dwarf the budgets devoted to other health issues in many African and Asian settings. Yet the fact remains that lower-profile diseases cause far greater damage to lives and livelihoods, especially amongst poorer populations: 750,000 children a year in Africa die from malaria, until recently a neglected disease, and an estimated one in five of all child deaths globally is due to diarrhoeal diseases (WHO, 2008b; Wardlaw et al, 2009). Such diseases and their impacts warrant far greater research, policy and public attention.

This book, therefore, is organized around a paradox. While we argue that disease-specific policies and an epidemic focus tend to obscure narratives emphasizing long-term factors in the causes of epidemics and experiences of multiple, interacting health problems, we have nonetheless organized our book into case studies of particular epidemic diseases. One reason for this is that our contributors' expertise tends to lie within individual disease categories (a fact which itself reflects deep structuring tendencies within health and development studies). More to the point, by taking the bull by the horns in this way, we are also able to show, in some cases, how dominant certain narratives have become. The flipside of this is that having outlined such dominant approaches, our contributors can indicate more strongly what is left out of such accounts. What is left out, as the following chapters show, is often the chronic, the endemic and the entrenched: the flipside of the exciting, if unnerving image of a fast-moving, interconnected globe that animates many outbreak narratives. As the following chapters indicate, each disease is subject to a range of understandings, or narratives, with more on-the-ground complexity than a global outbreak narrative can capture.

The book is made up of case studies of seven diseases: haemorrhagic fevers (Ebola and Lassa), SARS, HIV/AIDS, Highly Pathogenic Avian Influenza (HPAI), tuberculosis (TB), obesity and H1N1 (or swine) influenza. These offer an important set of commonalities and contrasts in relation to our core concerns. All have, as we show, been understood as presenting epidemics – at least by some people and institutions, at some times. Several have starred in headline-dominating global outbreak narratives – including Ebola, SARS, HIV/AIDS, H1N1 and HPAI. These five infectious diseases have also been understood as newly emergent – at least in some analyses. In TB, we have a different kind of case – an 'old' and endemic disease that is now re-emerging in new, drug-resistant forms. This is similar to malaria, a case which we do not include, but which is also an old, endemic disease now raising new concerns, as it threatens to make inroads into new areas made hospitable to mosquito vectors by climate change and as drug resistance even to Artemisinin therapies emerges. In obesity, we are looking at a 'lifestyle' disease, akin to heart disease, cancer or tobacco-related afflictions, rather than an infectious or communicable one. Yet obesity rates have risen with the speed of a classic epidemic. Taken as a group, this range of cases enables us to test the concept of epidemic quite strongly, viewing it from many different angles and beginning to dismantle its significant parts. We see that some diseases with similar biological, ecological or epidemiological profiles are addressed very differently, while others which share fewer of these characteristics can nonetheless be grouped together in an analysis of responses.

These cases also highlight how disease definitions and characterizations can shift over time. They show how diseases come to be seen as epidemic, when they do, and how diseases may cross the boundary between epidemic and endemic multiple times. Each case study works to show how defining a disease as epidemic has implications for the most vulnerable members of a given population. HIV/AIDS, for instance, has been variously understood as a global pandemic, as a series of localized epidemics with distinct characteristics (Piot et al, 2009) and – most recently – as a chronic disease amenable to long-term therapy. Ebola, may look like a new, emerging disease from the perspective of populations of industrialized countries who feel threatened by it, but for many Central African forest people who have lived with the disease for generations it is more endemic than epidemic. In short, whether a disease is considered old or new, endemic or epidemic depends on the perspective from which it is viewed. The cases we have chosen highlight these shifting definitions, and the social and institutional processes which underlie them and flow from them.

A pathways approach to epidemics

What, more precisely, do we mean by a narratives and pathways approach to epidemics, and how does the book develop it? In the following sections, we elaborate some key features (see also Leach et al, 2010a and b). We combine a recognition of highly complex social-ecological-disease dynamics with a constructivist view of how these come to be known and elaborated in policy and practice. We highlight how, in certain cases, key narratives come to be overwhelmingly dominant in terms of what policies get implemented, while in others, superficial consensus masks a varied group of self-interested actors, with little practical effect. Diversity of narratives, we argue, is a key feature of the policy landscape for some diseases. At the same time, we recognize that there can be important gaps between the strength of the rhetoric used to convey a given narrative, and the practical, or material, effects of such an account, in terms of actual policy implementation. Put another way, while some narratives translate into pathways, others do not. Some remain merely rhetorical; others remain marginalized or even hidden. We introduce political and institutional issues important to considering why narratives take particular forms, which come to dominate, when and how; and whether and how they become linked with particular pathways of disease and response. And we consider the question of interplay between different narratives in particular settings.

Complex dynamics

Humans and bugs have evolved together over hundreds of thousands of years; epidemics have always been a part of this shared history. A complex mixture of underlying conditions and precipitating events – biological, ecological, epidemiological and social – contribute to their emergence. Today technological interventions such as drugs, vaccines and other public health measures also contribute to the course an epidemic takes. Epidemics are thus part of complex, dynamic systems in which social, ecological and technological processes are inter-coupled (Bloom et al, 2007; Leach et al, 2010).

Appreciation of this is, we suggest, an essential starting point to understanding and dealing with epidemics. This requires broadening our perspective beyond the confines of particular disciplines, linking the medical and epidemiological perspectives which have tended to dominate analysis with insights from other fields, from disease ecology and environmental studies to anthropology, history, and science and technology studies. Our overall approach in this book is based on a commitment to integrating insights across disciplines, complementing recent social science work on global health, epidemics and emerging diseases (Castro and Singer, 2004; Nichter, 2008; Janes and Corbett, 2009; Kaufmann, 2009; Singer, 2009). The contributors bring a diversity of social science backgrounds, in some instances combined with training in medicine or ecology and on-the-ground development work, thus offering a range of perspectives within a broadly shared agenda.

Although mindful of the dangers of counterposing a dynamic present to a more static, stable past, it does appear that the acceleration of a range of biological, social, ecological and technological processes during the last half-century has contributed to contemporary epidemic challenges. These processes include the evolutionary dynamics of pathogens, as viruses and vectors exploit niches that become available through environmental, demographic and livelihood changes. There is growing evidence of the capacity of pathogens to rapidly evolve, challenging linear views of the relationship between human and disease ecology. HIV, for example, can generate more than 10^9 virions per day. Its mutation rate is around 10^{-5} mutations per nucleotide per cycle of replication, some 10,000,000 times the rate for human DNA. Each affected person hosts a vast and genetically highly diverse virus population, posing immense targeting problems for the immune system and any conceivable drug treatment.

There are more people – and more domesticated animals such as poultry, pigs and cattle – in the world than ever before and they are moving around at unprecedented rates. Both this growth and this mobility affect disease dynamics in complex and often unexpected ways. Much attention has focused on the more than 2 billion air journeys a year that make the isolation of a disease outbreak an increasingly formidable task (OAG Review, 2006). But in some countries internal rural–urban migration is equally important. For example, 80–100 million Chinese constitute the so-called 'floating population', who work in the more prosperous urban areas and typically return to their family homes in poor, and possibly relatively isolated, rural areas at least once each year to celebrate the Spring Festival. Similarly, according to conventional epidemiological models, bigger and more mobile populations increase the likely number of individuals infected by a given disease, and the probability that new pathogens or new strains of existing pathogens will arise via spontaneous genetic mutation within those human hosts. But the assumptions built into such models do not always reflect how specific social and cultural factors can significantly affect contact rates and disease transmission dynamics. Contact rates across population members can differ greatly: 'super-spreaders', individuals with very high contact rates, can have a big impact on the course of an epidemic (Lloyd-Smith et al, 2005). As work on HIV/AIDS has shown so clearly, these social and cultural factors apply at all scales, from the most intimate aspects of bodily comportment and behaviour, to intra-household, community and wider societal norms and practices (Edström, this volume).

Human–animal demography also affects zoonosis, the process whereby disease passes to humans from other species. A relatively recent editorial in the *Lancet* (2004, p257) states that 'all new infectious diseases of human beings to emerge in the past 20 years have had an animal source'. Given the huge reservoir of known and unknown pathogens in animal species, the number of such diseases has been predicted to increase (WHO, 2004a). Both wild and domestic animals are implicated in zoonosis. Thus, for example, the HIV-1 virus is assumed to have evolved from a very similar virus found in the wild chimpanzee species *Pan troglodytes troglodytes* (Gao et al,1999), while a variety of haemorrhagic fevers in African forest settings are associated with wild animal reservoirs in rats and bats. Domestic animal examples include the recent H1N1 'swine flu', while it has been argued that 'integrated pig-duck agriculture, an extremely efficient food produc-tion system traditionally practiced in certain parts of China, puts these two species in contact and provides a natural laboratory for making new influenza recombinants' (Morse, 1995, p11). While the wild populations of most species have been tending to decline in numbers, growth in domestic livestock populations has been rapid, mirroring that in the human popula-tions that consume them or their products. In China, meat production has been increasing at a rate of nearly 8 per cent per year for the past 25 years, with much of this increase occurring at the level of the 100 million peasant household-run farms, which still account for nearly half of all livestock production in the country despite a rapid growth in industrial scale farming operations (Li, 2009, p222).

The emergence and transmission of zoonoses are, then, also shaped by changing food production and livelihood systems that alter the intensity of contact between domestic animals and between people and animals. Where wildlife disease reservoirs and vectors are involved, environmental and land-use changes that affect human contact with these become key. Attention has focused, in particular, on the environmental impacts resulting either from the 'invasion' of areas that have previously been sparsely inhabited or from radical changes in land use. For example, Greger (2007) associ-ated the emergence and spread of zoonotic haemorrhagic fevers in South America with the clearance of forests for crop or livestock cultivation over the second half of the 20th century. Lassa fever and Rift Valley Fever have been linked to deforestation and population shifts in Africa (Morse, 1995).

Here the contributing political-economic dynamics have varied from dam construction to diamond mining and logging. For instance, as roads have been driven into isolated and remote areas, increases in population and commercial activity to support logging operations have resulted in an upsurge in demand for bushmeat, wild animals killed, butchered and sold locally for food. It is now widely believed that this practice may have been responsible for the initial transmission of the HIV virus to humans and that the transmission of a range of retroviruses is 'a regular phenomenon and a cause for concern' (Wolfe at al, 2004, p932). Climate change, it is argued, is likely to bring further influences to ecosystem and land-use patterns with major implications for disease emergence (Patz et al, 2005). The force of these interacting social, ecological and microbial processes has been termed 'socioemergence', to indicate the inextricable linkages between supposedly social and natural realms (Hardin, forthcoming).

At different moments in history, technologies such as vaccines, drugs and even controversial chemicals such as DDT, have given hope for disease control and even eradication (achieved triumphantly, and so far uniquely, in 1977 for smallpox). By insinuating themselves into the complex dynamics of epidemics, these tools can also lead to new disease patterns, some of which are relatively benign while others pose serious new risks, such as drug resistance. The emergence of multidrug-resistant TB (MDR-TB) is a case in point. Evidence of growing malarial resistance to Artemisinin therapy is another; in this case recommended combination therapies, designed to avoid resistance, have proved very difficult to implement in fragmented, pluralized health systems and social conditions in parts of Africa and Southeast Asia. In Thailand and Cambodia, for example, the continued use of mono-therapies appears to have enabled resistance to emerge (Dondorp et al, 2009).

Thus the outbreak, spread and impact of epidemics relate to how pathogens interact with a complex of social, technological and environmental processes. These processes are highly interdependent and often context-specific. They are characterized by non-linear patterns of changes across time and space – including those that have the potential to turn small-scale local epidemics into large-scale global problems. Epidemics implicate a diversity of spatial scales – from the individual diseased body to the globe – as well as temporal ones, as short-term outbreaks interact with longer-term predisposing conditions, stresses and drivers. Some disease drivers and effects involve short-term shocks – as in an ecosystem 'switch' that triggers a sudden epidemic outbreak – while others involve longer-term trends and stresses. And disease responses themselves can feed back to shape these dynamics. We suggest that recognizing such complex dynamics is a necessary starting point for understanding and dealing with epidemics.

This complex interaction of multiple dynamics – biological, demographic, ecological, economic, social, political and cultural – operating at different scales and at different speeds results in deep uncertainties, and often ignorance, about likely outcomes and their consequences. It has been observed that all recent pandemic threats have taken the world by surprise. While it is often implied that this is because of lack of knowledge, poor scientific understanding and inadequate surveillance systems that can be rectified by more knowledge, more science and more surveillance, we suggest that such complex dynamics make uncertainty and surprise inevitable. Building disease surveillance and response systems that are resilient in the face of such uncertainties is a major challenge.

Framing and narratives

Crucially, though, different people and groups in society tend to understand and experience these dynamics in very different ways. The scientific perspectives of epidemiologists or ecologists, or the analyses of social scientists, offer only some amongst multiple ways of thinking about and representing disease drivers, impacts and why they matter. Other understandings may be linked to different policy networks, field practitioners, government spokespeople, international agencies or non-governmental organizations (NGOs), or to networks or epistemic communities (Haas, 1992) that connect them. Different understandings again may emerge from the experiences, knowledge and perceptions of people living with diseases on a daily basis, or as related to the influence of media, religious or other groupings. How epidemic problems are understood also relates to location, wealth, livelihood, gender and other factors that shape people's vulnerability both to disease, and to the effects of particular kinds of response. All accounts are thus in some senses partial and positioned (Haraway, 1988) – a point which also applies to the brief outline and exemplification of complex dynamics in the previous section. Reflexively, we must acknowledge that this could have been written in other ways, shining light on the issues from different angles.

It is such different ways of understanding disease dynamics, and their links to responses, that we explore in this book through the ideas of framing and narratives. By framing (Leach et al, 2010) we mean that system boundaries are always open to multiple forms of interpretation. Depending on which actors (working within which institutions and political contexts) are doing the framing, different forms of knowledge, different entities and, indeed, different problems, will be considered relevant. Those which are framed outside can become effectively invisible when approaches and solutions are considered.

Recognizing diverse framings in this way complements those traditions of work in medical anthropology and sociology that have long appreciated the significance of diverse worldviews about health. Whether discussed in terms of medical or therapeutic pluralism (Kleinman, 1988; Johannessen and Lázár, 2006) or diverse cultural models (Hewlett and Hewlett, 2008), it is well established that such understandings can encompass not just bodily and social dimensions of disease, but also their wider political dimensions (Williams and Calnan, 1996; Rose, 2006; Leach and Fairhead, 2007). Yet much of this work stops short at identifying competing worldviews and their social and political origins; their implications for policy and action are more rarely spelled out. In contrast, we are interested specifically in how perspectives and worldviews come to inform and justify particular sorts of action and pathways of intervention and response.

This is where narratives come into play. Particular framings often become part of narratives about a problem or issue; simple stories with beginnings defining a problem, middles elaborating its consequences and ends outlining the solutions (Roe, 1991). Importantly, narratives justify and often become interlocked with particular institutional approaches to addressing health problems, and particular kinds of intervention; they become part and parcel of epidemics governance. Today, such governance arrangements are themselves increasingly complex and multi-scale, encompassing international agencies and global public–private partnerships, governmental and private sector institutions, and a variety of civil society and patients' groups.

For instance, in the case of pandemic threats, various versions of an 'outbreak narrative' tend to dominate. These run along the lines that 'the global threat of a pandemic and its consequences for massive mortalities and economic costs require substantial investments in surveillance, drug stockpiling and intervention in areas of the world where outbreaks originate, in order to protect us all'. This focuses on a particular framing of 'the system' and goals (global, aimed at protecting/reducing mortality amongst global populations), a particular interpretation of disease dynamics (sudden emergence, fast-changing, far-reaching spread) and a particular version of response (universalized emergency-oriented at-source control, aimed at eradication). Such a narrative has been typical of both the human health and veterinary international responses to HPAI and haemorrhagic fevers, for example, and has underlain at least some of the response to swine flu. This narrative calls upon particular kinds of knowledge and expertise – notably formal science and epidemiology – in diagnosing and solving the problem. This in turn has given rise to the plethora of initiatives and associated institutional arrangements focused on early warning, risk assessment, intensive surveillance, outbreak monitoring, pandemic preparedness planning, rapid response teams, contingency plans and so on.

There is nothing inherently 'wrong' with this narrative (both in terms of problem diagnosis and solutions), and there are many merits to the sort of response infrastructure that has been built. Yet in practice, there are several problematic tendencies. First, selective narratives can omit crucial factors and elements of dynamics that may be essential to effective and resilient responses, amidst the complexities of epidemics. Second, diverse narratives can undermine each other, in ways that may lead to practical problems in implementation. Third (and in some degree of tension with the second tendency), in practice a few narratives tend to dominate, to the exclusion of others. Not surprisingly, these tend to be the narratives of powerful actors and institutions. In dominating, they may obscure alternative narratives that may provide valuable, complementary solutions.

Such alternative narratives may well be less coherent and explicit than those associated with powerful health governance arrangements. There are many alternatives to the emergency-response, 'outbreak' narrative. They include more localized, developmental models, which focus on active intervention in a particular setting to reduce disease risk and exposure. They include narratives about the longer-term changes in environment, social conditions or health systems that underlie the emergence of particular outbreaks, linked to arguments and strategies to address these. They include narratives that give far more weight to 'indigenous' cultural models of disease causation, associated with particular logics and practices as to how transmission risks might be reduced. They also include stories where suffering, from disease and marginalization, is part of a way of life, which, if not necessarily celebrated, is necessarily accommodated and integrated into the identity of a particular group. This variety of story-telling about illness and health brings with it a salutary diversity of understandings and responses. Taken together, all these narratives can help us to question our assumptions when it comes to the 'right' or 'best' way to tackle the serious challenges of disease in all its manifestations.

Narratives interplay in ways shaped by politics and power. Not all lead to response pathways. Some may remain marginalized or even hidden. The interactions between different narratives and the practices linked to them may involve convergence, complementarity, contestation, overt clashes, hard choices and trade-offs, or even a drama of dominance and resistance – as sometimes occurred, for instance, where local people refused or resisted top-down public health campaigns that failed to meet their concerns (e.g. Yahya, 2006; Leach and Fairhead, 2007). How such interactions unfold clearly depends very much on context – of disease, of place, and of social and political setting. It also depends on histories and memories of past disease and intervention experiences. What is clear is that such interactions may, in turn, feed back to shape the dynamics of response, forcing a

modification of pathways. For instance, local resistance to top-down imposition of health technologies may force approaches to be adapted. Emergent
drug resistance – unanticipated in an internationally sponsored roll-out,
but plausible within narratives giving more weight to the uncertain consequences of pharmaceutical–microbial–market interactions in weakly regulated health systems – might derail the best-laid epidemic response plan,
forcing new strategies. Or, over time, initially contested narratives might
come to converge, enabling new, more inclusive pathways.

It is these shifting narratives and pathways around epidemics, their interactions in today's complex world of health governance, and the implications for dealing with epidemics and related challenges that are the central
concerns of this book. How might the challenges posed by emerging and
re-emerging diseases in a context of endemic poverty and illness, population growth and climate change be understood and met in ways that
address both short-term and long-term needs of all the people of the world,
including the very poorest? This is an ambitious question that brooks no
tidy answers. The chapters that follow provide a sense of solutions that are
available if we make ourselves both more critical of and more receptive to
the narratives that shape our responses.

Epidemic narratives and pathways in cases and contexts

As we have discussed, epidemic narratives and response pathways are deeply
interlocked with processes of governance. Chapter Two sets the scene for
those to follow by linking a set of dominant narratives about epidemics and
infectious disease with what is often called the architecture, or organizational landscape, of global health policy. In particular, this chapter explores
the effect of landmark revisions in the WHO's International Health Regulations that entail significant changes for the way epidemics are governed
at a global scale, embracing unofficial sources of information for the first
time. Issues of coordination, integration and harmonization have accordingly come to the fore as the amount of data – and global health actors – has
increased exponentially. The chapter analyses how this new organizational
and informational landscape and the framing of epidemic disease interact.
Centrally, it explores what effect that interaction has on the ability of
the global health community to respond to disease threats of all kinds. It
suggests that neither organizational complexity or 'openness' nor rigid lines
of command-and-control can ensure resilience in the face of unpredictable risks. Instead, methods are needed to encourage feedback and integration between competing narratives of health and disease. Yet the character

of these narratives, and the challenges of their interaction, vary greatly according to disease and context – as the next seven chapters explore.

Haemorrhagic fevers, the topic of Chapter Three, have come to exemplify popular ideas about highly contagious and often gruesome illnesses that emerge 'out of Africa'. Associated with wildlife vectors in forested environments, viral haemorrhagic fevers such as Ebola, Marburg and Lassa fever were the subjects of outbreak narratives in the 1990s, justifying rapid and sometimes draconian international policy responses and control measures. Leach and Hewlett contrast these first global outbreak narratives and the cultural models that inform them, with three other narratives that highlight outbreaks as deadly local disease events, as matters best managed with local cultural practices, and as requiring longer-term insights from both ecology and social science approaches. The chapter shows how each of these narratives highlights different temporal and spatial scales, validating different kinds of knowledge, and assigning cause, blame and vulnerability differently. Each suggests different pathways of response, involving different combinations of actors. Discussing the institutional and power relations that have shaped their interaction, the chapter concludes by addressing both the potentials and the challenges of integrating them.

In Chapter Four, Bloom turns to SARS, which has achieved iconic status as a potentially disastrous outbreak that was successfully controlled by a coordinated public health response. SARS emerged in southern China in late 2002 and by August 2003 had caused 8422 cases and 916 deaths in 32 countries. After a short delay, the governments of affected countries and the international community mobilized a major response, which successfully contained the outbreak. Once the epidemic was controlled, its influence lived on in the form of competing narratives and their influence on the direction of development of national and international health systems. This chapter outlines three versions of the narrative about '*a big epidemic that might have been*', addressing the preoccupations and interests of the international health community (and especially the WHO), the Chinese Ministry of Health and other policy actors in China and, finally, the growth of a partnership between China and the international health community in matters of health governance. This chapter illustrates the high political cost to a national government of being seen to have responded inadequately to a new disease. It also provides an example of an effective multilateral response to a global challenge, when powerful forces in the US favoured unilateralism. This chapter outlines how particular narratives about SARS influenced both the reform of China's health system and the global response to potential epidemics.

The next two chapters, by contrast, explore a major pandemic which, for a variety of reasons, was not successfully controlled at the outset – HIV/AIDS. The overarching story of HIV/AIDS tracks some major shifts, from emergent zoonotic disease, to 1980s epidemic, to global pandemic, and finally to what some now characterize as a chronic, manageable disease. With this 'older' status providing an interesting counterpoint to other cases, the chapter by Edström tracks how such epidemiological shifts have co-evolved with contested perspectives on the social causes and consequences of AIDS, and what to do about it. Authored by a scholar who was personally involved with AIDS policy and grassroots activism throughout much of this period, the chapter ties a taxonomy of different narratives and approaches around HIV/AIDS to an overall historical account. This demonstrates how attitudes and approaches – in assigning agency and responsibility, prioritizing and targeting prevention and treatment, and locating the disease as an exception or a part of broader health and social systems – have shifted over time. In particular, the chapter explores how different narratives emphasize issues of risk and threat, justice and vulnerability in different ways. Yet these approaches operate in parallel as well as in series, generating a picture of a series of contested narratives, linked with different (though sometimes overlapping) sets of actors and institutions. The chapter reflects on the challenges of balancing the importance of both individual choices and agency, with larger-scale processes of population mixing, mobility, inequality and change.

The next chapter explores in particular the role of exceptionalist thinking in shaping HIV/AIDS narratives in specific settings in South Africa where the disease is said to have become 'hyperendemic'. In particular, it considers how practical is it to concentrate on counselling and individual patients' rights in relation to HIV testing when rates of infection are so high and resources so scarce in these hyperendemic regions. MacGregor examines the durability of the exceptionalist narrative in relation to HIV/AIDS at the same time as she reveals how rhetoric can be simply that, with practical action often diverging significantly from official procedure. Two case studies illuminate the complexity of on-the-ground interventions. The first focuses on the vexed issue of social assistance for people with HIV, and whether the disease should be defined as a disability even if people remain healthy, revealing the limitations of simple binary definitions such as chronic versus infectious disease. The second case study explores the changing roles of lay counsellors in the testing and management of HIV, demonstrating further how changes in the prevalence of the disease, and the resources available to fight it, make it impractical to meet minimum 'requirements' for informed consent. Whose interests, MacGregor asks, does the exceptionalist narrative serve? And which other perspectives on this complex hyperendemic situation are not being heard?

Different ways of representing and responding to risk and uncertainty are a feature of epidemic narratives. The next chapter picks up on this particular theme through the case of avian influenza. Scoones examines the role of risk and uncertainty in three overlapping 'outbreak' narratives that have framed the international response. First, a strong narrative links veterinary concerns with agriculture and livelihood issues, where responses have centred on veterinary control measures and industry 'restructuring' to increase biosecurity and reduce risk. Second, there is a human public health narrative. Here a combination of drugs, vaccines and risk-reducing behaviour change dominate the response. Finally, there is a narrative focused on pandemic preparedness, where responses focus on civil contingency planning, business continuity approaches and containment strategies. Each outbreak narrative is associated with particular professional, disciplinary, procedural and institutional parameters that define the way incomplete knowledge about the future – and so notions of risk and uncertainty – is approached. Across these narratives, surveillance is a common theme, and is defined and designed in particular ways, informed by these outbreak narratives. Using Stirling's framework for exploring incertitude, the chapter argues that these narratives make potentially dangerous assumptions about the applicability and reliability of a risk-based surveillance-based approach to managing epidemics. The chapter concludes with a set of challenges for the recasting of surveillance for emerging infectious diseases that take on board these lessons from the international response to avian influenza.

Chapter Eight focuses on tuberculosis, and the recent emergence of strains of MDR-TB. It thus addresses a disease which is both 'old', with a long latency period and also increasingly an element of the 'outbreak' oriented approach to global health. Nightingale considers the transformation of tuberculosis as a result of the interaction of social, microbial, ecological and technological processes. Following a discussion of early perspectives on tuberculosis and its shift from being framed as a threatening epidemic to a more controllable disease, the chapter gives sustained analytical attention to the more recent history of tuberculosis, including the co-emergence of HIV and MDR-TB in the 1980s. In relation to MDR-TB, Nightingale discusses the rise of three narratives that are shaping responses. In the first, MDR-TB is understood as a potential national security threat, with marginalized groups such as infected Russian prisoners posing risks to global populations on their release. In the second, structural problems in health care globally that allow drug supplies to dwindle and treatment programmes, such as Directly Observed Treatment, Short Course (DOTS), to falter are to blame for the growth in infection rates. According to this narrative, focused technical solutions, backed up with sufficient funds and decisive government intervention, represent the best pathway to success. Finally, a 'structural violence' and rights-based narrative draws attention to issues of social justice, emphasizing context-specific interventions rather than generic top-down approaches. Throughout, Nightingale considers the relationships between poverty/inequality and pathogen evolution and, as with the chapters on HIV/AIDS, their varying emphasis on vulnerability versus rights in relation to marginalized groups (such as prisoners and the homeless).

Obesity, the subject of Chapter Nine, has been a feature of many societies in many eras, but has only recently emerged as a key public health policy issue. Certain politicians and policy-makers have called obesity a 'lifestyle' disease of industrialized societies and a modern 'epidemic'. Millstone therefore draws into the book's comparative frame what has been labelled an epidemic of a non-infectious disease, and moreover one emerging primarily out of North America and Europe rather than the less industrialized world. Many of the disagreements about appropriate responses to the obesity epidemic focus on the attribution of responsibility – both for causation and for remediation. Positions taken in those debates vary across time, cultures and interests, and they are compounded by macro-social changes and culturally diverse perspectives. One important axis in the debate is marked by two competing framings: one that attributes responsibility for rising rates of obesity to individual choices and actions versus a contrary perspective that locates responsibility in features of the social and economic environment. A second axis concerns competing views on the potential role for governments: one narrative suggests that governments might have to intervene actively and extensively, while a contrary view argues that governments should play only a very limited or vanishingly slight role. As the chapter explores, these competing narratives have been put forward by different groups of actors – from scholars and activists to governments and the food industry. Issues of political economy are key in explaining the interactions between them, and the relative power of the response pathways associated with them at any given time.

Our final case study explores the dramatic response to the novel influenza virus H1N1, commonly referred to as swine flu, in Egypt. Tadros reveals how global outbreak narratives play out in national settings, with surprising consequences. In response to the perceived threat to its human population, in June 2009 the Egyptian government implemented a mass culling of all the nation's pigs following the declaration of an imminent global pandemic. These pigs were owned by Zabaleen, garbage collectors who were also members of the country's Christian minority. The Zabaleen used the pigs to sort and dispose of huge amounts of the nation's organic waste, supporting an informal but effective system of neighbourhood recycling and garbage disposal. Once the pigs were killed, garbage collection in the city effectively ground to a halt, leading to piles of rubbish accumulating in the streets; the phantom threat of swine flu being contracted from pigs was replaced by the real threat of illness caused by rotting waste. This chapter explores the nature of the mainstream narrative, propounded by members of the government and the mainstream media, that supported this severe response. In this dominant narrative, both religious justifications (about the inappropriateness of keeping pigs in a Muslim country) and scientific arguments for the cull were put forward. Tadros also reveals the neglected accounts of the Zabaleen about the effects of the cull on their lives and livelihoods, which were severely curtailed by the loss of the pigs.

In our concluding chapter we integrate the seven disease clusters considered in the book (haemorrhagic fevers, SARS, avian influenza, HIV/AIDS, TB, obesity, and H1N1 influenza) into a comparative frame, explore cross-cutting themes, and draw out implications for the governance of epidemics and epidemic threats, now and in the future. By drawing these diverse cases together, we are able to offer a new set of reflections on the science, politics, governance and implications for social justice of epidemic responses. Approaches to dealing with epidemics, with endemic disease situations, and with the broadest questions of primary health need, we argue, to be more unified. While the language of integration and harmonization has become prominent in global health policy circles, we suggest that so far not enough practical action has been taken to create responses that take into account the broad effects of illness and diseases on lives and livelihoods across the globe. Such an analysis is meaningful and necessary both because it is more socially just, and also because it is more likely to respond successfully to the complex multi-scale interactions that shape disease dynamics. Long-term changes and the lives and livelihoods of the poor matter even in situations where powerful policy narratives emphasize epidemic 'shocks' and top-down, rapid response. These alternative perspectives, we argue, need to move from the marginal into a mainstream where they too can shape pathways of disease response. By highlighting implications for researchers, national and international institutions, we aim to facilitate reflection on how the construction and implementation of responses might become more effective and sustainable for all the world's population.

Chapter 2

New Rules for Health? Epidemics and the International Health Regulations

Sarah Dry

Introduction

In issues of disease and policy, scale matters. The chapters that make up the bulk of this volume are filled with detail about how individual diseases are understood and addressed in local and national settings. This chapter takes on the so-called 'view from nowhere' (Nagel, 1989), analysing how epidemics and infectious disease have come to constitute a large part of global health policy. In doing so, I try to show how such 'global' policy, often referred to as if it were a disembodied and somewhat autonomous set of practices, is produced by a particular set of actors operating under contingent circumstances as well as structured political and institutional relations. While the other chapters in this volume describe narratives that shape policy for individual diseases, this chapter attempts to contextualize these accounts by relating a more generalized narrative about epidemics and infectious disease to what is often called the architecture, or organizational landscape, of global health policy.

This dominant narrative frames epidemics as novel, global and fast moving, while de-emphasizing underlying, often long-term changes (such as changing patterns of migration or livestock management) that may help account for the growth in emerging infectious diseases. Global health architecture refers to a diverse network of national, international and non-governmental organizations that contribute to health policy at the global scale. Prominent among them are agencies such as the WHO, partnerships such as the Global Fund to Fight AIDS, Tuberculosis and Malaria, and philanthropic organizations such as the Rockefeller and Gates foundations. Recent changes in the organizational landscape of global health have created new power relations, as well as uncertainty about which organizations, if any, are 'in control' of global health policy. Issues of coordination, integration and harmonization have accordingly come to the fore. This chapter will analyse how this new organizational landscape and the framing of epidemic disease interact. Centrally, it will explore what effect that interaction has on the ability of the global health community to respond to disease threats of all kinds, and, in particular, how surveillance has come to be defined. This has two analytic dividends. On the one hand, uncovering the relationships between dominant narratives and the complex organizational structures of global health reveals how alternative ideas and narratives about disease and health become neglected, or invisible. On the other hand, by joining an analysis of narratives with one of organizational structures, this paper seeks to demonstrate how we might address policy blind spots, by paying attention to the key role of formal versus informal knowledge.

Globalization and infectious disease policy

Globalization has become so ubiquitous a language to describe contemporary events that it has slipped into cliché and near invisibility. The discourse of globalization is also foundational to the most dominant strand of the epidemic narrative. In the field of global health, sensitivity to global relations has come to be labelled with a strikingly ambiguous phrase: global health security (Chen et al, 2003; McInness and Lee, 2006; Aldis, 2008). Referring both to the health and well-being of individuals and the protection of states from economic and social disorder, policy responses informed by concerns about global health security are characterized by an extreme sensitivity to the flow of disease across national borders. But while phrases such as 'disease knows no borders' are routinely used to justify policy responses, the mobility of certain disease organisms lies in stark contrast to the entrenched poverty, inequality and political instability that are ultimately responsible for most of the global burden of disease. This troubling tension runs through the heart of globalization discourse more generally. Much talk of globalization, with its metaphors of interconnectedness and assumptions about the fast and efficient transfer of goods, capital and people, obscures the fact that while some things travel quickly and easily, others, to put it crudely, do not. To be sure, ever-steeper gradients of inequality are a well-recognized feature of globalization, but the inherent tensions in the discourse of globalization – between an interconnected world and one of sharp divisions in wealth and health – are not always made clear. Frequently, the language of change and networks, of flow, speed and connectivity, trumps the language of structures, of rootedness, embeddedness and entrenchment. While the former discourse points to unity, the latter draws our attention, ultimately, to inequality. Both discourses – of flow and rootedness – capture certain aspects of the phenomenon of globalization. But these aspects, or realities, are experienced by sharply divided sets of people.

Epidemics are increasingly seen to be a symptom of globalization in its guise of interconnectivity, while critics of global health policy often point to long-term, structural causes of inequality (Farmer, 1999a; Kim et al, 2005). By paying attention to the so-called 'global' risks of epidemics, such critics suggest, we may turn to certain kinds of interventions that are not those best suited to addressing the root (as opposed to the intermediate) causes of the problem. By focusing on such shared 'global' risks as pandemic flu, global health policies run the risk of neglecting the underlying structural deficiencies that produce the conditions from which epidemics emerge. Such approaches to supposedly 'shared' global threats may in fact address the concerns of the wealthiest and most influential populations of the globe, while tending to ignore specific local vulnerabilities which are themselves linked to this global inequality. As a result, the current dominant narrative around global health security and 'shared' global risks may have in fact narrowed the set of policy options that are considered appropriate, while alternative visions of global health have been sidelined. As a result, supposedly 'broad' or 'comprehensive' approaches to the global risk of epidemics are, paradoxically, often more narrowly conceived than are many projects oriented to local or regional contexts and concerns.

Overlapping with these issues of spatial scale are questions of time: global health policy around epidemics privileges acute outbreak events that occur on a daily or weekly basis as opposed to chronic factors, such as changes in land use and host and vector population, which occur over years or decades, and which account for broader trends. In a sense, this difference in temporal frame reflects different modes of causal explanation. An acute model might explain the appearance of a cluster of new cases of extensively drug-resistant tuberculosis (XDR-TB) with a narrative about a person with tuberculosis who is unsuccessfully treated with antibiotics and develops a drug-resistant strain of the bacillus, sickens further, and exposes others in a matter of weeks, if not days. Chronic accounts might explain an epidemic (still XDR-TB, for example) in terms of an increase, over months or years, in the population of the overcrowded slums of a major metropolis, where clean water and sanitation are lacking, broad-spectrum antibiotics may be purchased informally, and a large percentage of the population is immuno-compromised because they are also suffering from HIV/AIDS. Currently, the emphasis is on short-term factors, with long-term indicators often left out of policy decision-making altogether. What is really needed are analytic and policy tools for combining both types of factor into a shared model of disease and health, in order to get beyond long-lived and often ideologically freighted debates about primary health versus disease-specific programming.

Indeed, how we speak of (and understand) the global risk of epidemics today testifies to a history of encounters between the powerful and the vulnerable that stretches back centuries (King, 2002). Neither epidemics, nor our understanding of them as presenting novel risks, nor the tendency to divide factors into sharply opposing dyads, are new. What I have described as opposing discourses of global public health – acute versus chronic – can also be understood as twin strands in the history of 19th and 20th century medicine and public health. What used to be called sanitary hygiene is the 19th century progenitor of public health initiatives that take into account factors such as the environment, housing and poverty. The social reformers of Victorian Britain fought to improve the living and working conditions of the urban poor as a way of curtailing the spread of epidemic diseases such as cholera, typhoid and typhus. On the other hand and in the same time period, proponents of the germ theory of disease pictured microbes travelling with alarming speed and specificity. They argued that targeted interventions into acute disease outbreaks, based on vaccination and control of pathogens, rather than social and environmental changes, were the key to addressing epidemic disease (Porter and Porter, 1988). With the development of the professional discipline of tropical medicine in the late 19th century, these divisions became more sharply defined and became associated, in Britain, with the Liverpool and London Schools of Tropical Medicine respectively. Activity in Liverpool focused on prevention (largely sanitary measures and the elimination of disease vectors such as mosquitoes, flies and rats), while in London the focus was on creating a new scientific sub-discipline at the confluence of medicine and parasitology. Work in the field would be based on reductionist research, with the goal of discovering vaccine and drug-based cures to epidemic diseases (Chernin, 1988). Today's vocabulary of acute versus chronic, vertical versus horizontal, and community health versus disease-specific interventions draws on, rather than replaces, these older categories.

Both broad formulations of disease explain some aspects of an epidemic – neither is fully 'right' nor 'wrong'. But the formulation of epidemics policy on the global scale, using global language, has largely adopted a 'fast-twitch' approach to a problem that most agree has plenty of 'slow-twitch' causes: epidemics-oriented policy has become a policy of rapid response rather than long-term commitment. It often takes the form of highly focused emergency programmes (eradication efforts and national immunization days are classic examples) dependent on sensitive surveillance systems that are 'tuned' to daily or weekly events, rather than long-term programmes that respond to longer-wave feedback about environmental and social factors and may be more sustainable. Such changes include transformations in agriculture and land use brought about both by social and natural factors (population growth, migration and urbanization; climate change, deforestation); poor population health (caused by malnutrition and existing diseases such as HIV and TB); the evolution of pathogens; international trade; contamination of water and food sources; and hospitals and medical treatment (antibiotic resistance) (Morse, 1995; Weiss and McMichael, 2004; Haines et al, 2006). There is also a deeper irony here, because 'fast-twitch' information may be the best way to learn about long-wave change. Rapidly evolving infectious agents are like canaries in a coal mine or polar bears on melting ice caps: changes in their behaviour reflect a range of more complex and long-term changes in the environment and in the behaviour of their human hosts (Morens et al, 2004).

Embedded in the framing of epidemics as acute events is the potential for international spread, for the transformation of a local concern into a global one. Policing the border between the local and the global, in semantic, political and epidemiological terms, thus becomes ever more important. Rather than borders dropping out of such approaches, they become definitional. Although the language of global and local has been used by many scholars seeking to redress the power imbalances that bedevil development policy, the terminology is problematic. The distinction between global and local is ultimately a false one. It can be argued that every place is local, including such global paragons as the WHO and the UN and, as the examples above suggest, 'local' places increasingly contribute to global dialogues (Kickbusch, 1999). This insight applies equally to the distinction between national and global health policy; globalization has not elided this distinction but created new fault lines between shared global goods and questions of national sovereignty and security. Along with more anthropology of non-Western peoples, then, perhaps what is really needed is a fuller understanding of how knowledge circulates at multiple levels and in multiple forms (for one example of such a project, see the Pro-Poor HPAI Risk Reduction study, www.hpai-research.net), as well as studies of how global ideas become reinterpreted in different local settings, and vice versa (such as, for example, many of the case studies in this volume provide). By revealing how variegated the global actually is, such studies will further demonstrate the discursive power of 'global' language to summon into existence an imaginary consensus on health policy (on the fragmentary nature of one WHO-led intervention, see Bhattacharya, 2006; on the 'tacit globalism' of contemporary vaccine policy, see Blume and Zanders, 2006).

One way to introduce complexity into thinking about epidemics is to draw on recent scholarship (in a range of fields including ecology and management studies) on dynamic systems, which operate in non-linear, inherently uncertain ways with which purely quantitative risk management tools may be unable to cope (Jasanoff, 2005; Scoones et al, 2007; Leach et al, 2010). When such tools are nonetheless still retained and applied, the result can be a dangerous rigidity. Such an unwillingness to recognize the limits to knowledge or to entertain alternative ways of understanding precludes the discovery of alternate means of understanding, and thus managing, the system. Only by 'opening up' such processes of knowledge making, and revealing the deep uncertainties and complexities inherent in the system itself can policies be formulated that respond realistically to a dynamic system as it undergoes dramatic changes. In tandem with the recognition of the internal uncertainty of the system, such a process also recognizes the diversity of social perspectives, or framings, of that system. As a result, an iterative process of deliberation and learning can be built into policy processes. This provides a means of responding to uncertain systems as they change over time, rather than pursuing an unachievable ideal equilibrium state. The challenge is to develop methods for constant re-evaluation and reflection which themselves do not become routinized and narrow (Stirling, 2008).

These ideas about dynamic systems can be usefully applied to global health, which has become increasingly complex, in social, environmental, biological and technological terms. As already mentioned, in recent years the world of global health policy has changed dramatically, with an influx of new money and an efflorescence of new partnerships. This change has engendered what Kickbusch has dubbed a 'policy paradox': at the same time that global public health policy frame has narrowed to focus on infectious disease, the political response has widened outwards from the WHO to encompass a new and far more complex political 'ecosystem' populated by a diverse range of actors, including health activists, NGOs, global philanthropists and the private sector (Kickbusch, 2003). What was formerly known as 'international' health governance, coordinated centrally by international bodies like the WHO at the nation-state level, has been replaced by a networked and 'global' health governance, characterized by mixed networks and coalitions of actors that include NGOs, activists, philanthropists and new multi-partner initiatives like the Global Fund (Lee et al, 2002; Lee, 2003b; Brown et al, 2006).

The big story then is not just emerging infectious disease but emerging policy actors and networks that are transforming the health policy world. How are these two phenomena – the changing landscape of global health governance and the changing landscape of infectious disease – interacting? Some argue that Kickbusch's policy paradox may not be so paradoxical after all – that it is precisely the 'unstructured plurality' of the new global health governance that has allowed global health to become so prominent on the world stage. Global public health has risen in importance, they argue, *because* of the lack of central governance in this field, not in spite of it (Bartlett et al, 2006; Fidler, 2007).

But a further set of questions must be asked: how have these changes in governance affected not just the focus of health policy on infectious diseases but the *kind* of infectious disease policy that has been emerging? And what is the effect of an epidemics-dominated health policy on the health, liveli-hoods and well-being of the world's poorest and most vulnerable people? In contrast to those who identify an increasing decentralization in global health governance, some analysts claim that the WHO is increasingly powerful. Davies, for example, identifies an increase in the mediating power of the WHO but argues that this rise in influence is only possible because of support from Western states. Such states see the WHO as a politically convenient proxy, enabling them to forward policies it would not be seemly for individual states to promote. Under the banner of 'global' health, argues Davies, essentially protectionist policies aimed at keeping pathogens out of Western states can be safely labelled 'shared' objectives (Davies, 2008).

Having just noted the profusion of policy-makers and the complex relations between such actors, what does it mean to speak of a 'dominant' policy framework? The profusion of actors makes certain kinds of interven-tions much harder to achieve and others more likely to be attempted. In such a situation, focused programmes, which are ideally disease-specific, time-limited and have narrowly defined and easily measurable outcomes, get prioritized. One-off disease eradication or control programmes, versus ongoing health systems strengthening, become the implicit model for, and often explicit aim of, health interventions.

Both the fragmentation (or, to use a positive term, networked aspects) of global health governance and the novel dangers of infectious diseases are 'caused' by globalization, which creates new networks and connections at the same time as it (necessarily) destroys old structures. This circular rela-tionship between the production and management of risks at a global scale is a key dimension of what theorists have identified as 'reflexive modernity' (Beck et al, 1994). In the case of the pathogen environment, pre-existing relationships between humans, animals, infectious agents and the natural world have been destroyed as populations become increasingly mobile, occupying new social and ecological niches, and thus creating more oppor-tunities for new pathogens to emerge, or for existing pathogens to advance. In the case of the policy world, the vision of a simple command-and-control structure of international health (whether it ever existed in reality is a separate question) has been replaced by a floating 'global assemblage' of incompletely networked policy actors and forms of knowledge (Ong and Collier, 2005). At the same time, health has become explicitly geopolitical: the governance of health has become a concern not simply for individual states but for international relations.

Globalization in the guise of global health security has, to a certain extent, engendered the new networked architecture of global health policy (Fidler, 2007). This is not necessarily a bad thing for responding to both epidemics and long-term health challenges. It could be argued that it might result in a useful redundancy or plurality at the level of policy that is a form of insurance against the unpredictable system shocks that we fear. Fragmentary systems may also be resilient systems. They might allow some of the multi-scale and multi-disciplinary connections – from emergency-oriented actors at WHO to health workers engaged in health systems strengthening on the ground – that could help dissolve the misleading divisions between chronic and epidemic, or global and local.

It becomes important to ask, therefore, how policy-makers might encourage 'useful' chaos at the level of policy while avoiding both wasteful redundancies and a kind of passive 'groupthink'. This is an especially salient question because the decentralization in the field of global health governance has led to calls for integration, harmonization and coordination (Muraskin, 2004; Lee and Fidler, 2007). New alliances that seek to join a diverse set of actors into a unified approach include the Global Alliance for Vaccines and Immunization (GAVI), and the Global Fund to Fight AIDS, Tuberculosis and Malaria. Such 'global assemblages' are responses to the perceived need to coordinate action in order to avoid redundancy, wastefulness or conflict. The language of integration, like that of globalization, assumes an equal sharing of both the risks and benefits of such harmonization. But integration is never neutral. The people who set the terms of such efforts determine how success is measured in a way that may not be that different from those who would design stand-alone interventions.

This is not to say that the best hope for equity or resilience lies simply in an unregulated 'free market' policy landscape. An uncoordinated policy landscape is not necessarily a diverse policy landscape. For many reasons, multiple actors may behave in very similar ways when faced with a chaotic and uncoordinated environment. As Davies suggests, for example, Western governments may support the WHO in its 'securitization' of infectious disease policy for reasons of national self-interest that nonetheless take the guise of global responsibility (Davies, 2008). The struggle to 'succeed' in a disordered environment may force organizations, or states, to adopt very similar strategies – highly focused, time-limited interventions with easily measurable outcomes – in order to reduce their risk of failure as defined by their own metrics. To what extent then, is the networked architecture of policy made up of qualitatively different approaches to health issues? Or does the plurality of institutional actors mask a homogeneous set of approaches based on shared assumptions and similar survival strategies? How diverse are our narratives about epidemics and health policy at the global level?

Surveillance and the new International Health Regulations

Epidemic surveillance systems provide a good case study with which to try to answer these questions. Star players in global outbreak narratives, such systems provide a semblance of global control in the light of fragmented on-the-ground programmes, and seek to 'fill the gap' created by the various paradoxes of globalization. For while global systems create opportunities for productive linkages, this interconnectivity also creates opportunities for systemic meltdown, such as pandemic flu. Similarly, the new decentralized systems of global health governance create the risk of both resource-draining redundancy in programmes and unseen gaps in interventions that may leave key areas unaddressed. By looking at surveillance systems, we can get a sense of how coordinated (or uncoordinated) responses are, and how diverse.

Surveillance has always been central to attempts to control epidemic disease. In recent years, however, this historical commitment to detection and monitoring has taken on a new aspect. Surveillance has received renewed and enthusiastic attention from a range of actors who argue that it is precisely because national health systems are failing that we need a better global surveillance network. In 2005, a dramatic shift in the way epidemic surveillance is conceived at a global level occurred with the revisions of the WHO's International Health Regulations (IHR) (Fidler, 2005; World Health Assembly, 2005; Baker and Fidler, 2006). When they were first introduced in 1969, the IHR were intended to stop epidemic disease from spreading beyond national borders. Six diseases – cholera, plague, relapsing fever, smallpox, typhus and yellow fever – were designated as legally notifiable under the regulations. WHO member states did not uniformly comply with these regulations, nor were they given any guidelines or funding to aid them in doing so. From 1996 to 2005, the regulations were revised and the resulting new regulations, IHR 2005, were implemented in June 2007. These new regulations make surveillance the centrepiece of what the WHO calls 'global public health security.' As the WHO explains:

> *A more secure world that is ready and prepared to respond collectively in the face of threats to global health security requires global partnerships that bring together all countries and stakeholders in all relevant sectors, gather the best technical support and mobilize the necessary resources for effective and timely implementation of IHR (2005). This calls for national core capacity in disease detection and international collaboration for public health emergencies of international concern. While many of these partnerships are already in place, there are serious gaps,*

> *particularly in the health systems of many countries, which weaken the consistency of global health collaboration. In order to compensate for these gaps, an effective global system of epidemic alert and response was initiated by WHO in 1996.* (WHO, 2007a, pp12–13)

This new focus on surveillance has the goal of implementing rapid responses to episodes at their sources. The fixation, under IHR 1969, on international borders and a limited set of diseases has given way to a concern to pinpoint at their source 'all events which may constitute a public health emergency of international concern' (or PHEIC) within 24 hours of detection (World Health Assembly, 2005, Article 6.1). Such events are not limited to naturally arising infectious diseases, and may include both deliberate and accidental releases of hazardous materials, including biological, chemical and radioactive materials. Under earlier IHR, the focus of concern – halting the spread of infection at the border – was spatial. Under IHR 2005, the focus – pinpointing events within 24 hours of detection – is now temporal. This has resulted in a redefinition of surveillance on the world stage. Surveillance, which can include long-term demographic measurements and community-led programmes, has instead come to mean rapid-response-oriented early warning systems that feed into a global network of laboratories and control centres overseen by the WHO.

This narrowed definition of surveillance has significant ramifications both for the ability of local administrators and health personnel to gain valuable knowledge about health and disease as well as for our ability to respond to fast-changing global health needs in the face of highly complex and unpredictable dynamics. Attempts to separate acute from chronic conditions – and manage them differently – may in fact compound problems of both types. One example can be found in the recent rise in co-infection of patients with HIV and XDR-TB (see Nightingale, this volume). In response to the identification of an outbreak of XDR-TB in 2005–2006 among a group of patients in the KwaZulu-Natal province of South Africa, the WHO instituted a Global Task Force on XDR-TB to determine whether the event should count as a PHEIC under the new IHR. The Task Force ruled that because the epidemic did not pose an immediate threat of international spread and, more significantly, because the IHR 'are really intended for outbreaks of acute disease, rather than the "acute-on-chronic" situation of MDR-TB and XDR-TB' (WHO, 2007b) that the outbreak did not qualify as a PHEIC. This interpretation of the IHR has been contested by scholars who claim that it misrepresents the content of the regulations (Calain and Fidler, 2007). The episode nonetheless reveals how embedded assumptions about 'acute' versus 'chronic' or even 'acute-on-chronic' events may lead to dangerous sidelining of threats that are urgent and potentially wide reaching.

The language of integration and harmonization is often used to counter claims of lack of coordination or wasteful redundancy, but recognizing the limited definition of epidemic surveillance today demonstrates how much more substantial such calls for integration could be. To be sure, integrating existing infectious disease surveillance systems that are oriented to identifying rapidly developing outbreaks with the potential for wide geographical spread is essential. But integration can go further. For example, registration systems, which keep track of births, deaths and marriages, are essential both for managing infectious diseases prone to epidemic outbreaks and in creating the conditions necessary for improved primary health. The WHO is sponsoring a programme based on these principles called the Health Metrics Network. It aims to strengthen health information systems in developing countries, with the goal of providing better and timelier information on disease prevalence for use in local as well as global settings (Szreter and Woolcock, 2004; Szreter, 2006; Abou Zahr et al, 2007; Mahapatra et al, 2007; Setel et al, 2007; WHO, 2008c). An older proposal labelled 'surveillance for equity' aimed to harness the technology and infrastructure of health surveillance and vital statistics to enable people on the ground to identify where interventions are most needed, in local terms, and act accordingly (Taylor, 1992).

Projects such as the Health Metrics Network recognize and make explicit the link between knowledge about a population (its vital and epidemiological statistics) and the rights and status afforded to individuals within that community. The intended beneficiaries of such statistical reform extend far beyond centralized bastions of control and associated 'technocratic' interventions. Ideally, they are created 'principally for the liberty and the use of private individuals, and not to serve the purposes of commercial organizations or states' (Szreter, 2006). As an added dividend, while such projects can be tools for local empowerment, they also broaden our knowledge of how social and natural factors conspire to create the conditions from which epidemics arise, making them critical elements of a global health programme. Such research impels us to ask, more broadly than the work on integration mentioned above: what impact do global systems of surveillance have on global inequality?

Unofficial information and formal decision-making

At the same time that the revised IHR have helped to define epidemic surveillance in terms of rapid response early warning systems, they have also led to a sea change in the way that official and unofficial sources of information are treated by the WHO. A key element of the new IHR and, by the WHO's own account, a 'revolutionary departure' from previous international regulations, is the acknowledgement that 'non-state sources of information about outbreaks will often pre-empt official notifications'. In this way, an emphasis on identifying (and thus possibly preventing the spread of) outbreaks as quickly as possible is linked with a project to extend surveillance across a much broader field (WHO, 2007a) This 'revolutionary departure' formally acknowledges the fact that electronic communication via the internet and cell phones renders hopeless any attempt to conceal outbreaks (see Bloom, this volume). It also represents a sea change in the agency's attitude towards surveillance, indicating a new desire to cast a much wider net to gather 'infectious disease intelligence' (Heymann and Rodier, 2001).[1] Such a change has been welcomed by some analysts. Fidler argues that 'new information technology and their global dissemination', such as GOARN, have 'transformed not only the technological context but also the political and economic realities of infectious disease reporting', making it more 'dynamic, flexible and forward-looking' by empowering non-state actors to contribute on a more equal footing (Fidler, 2005, p362). By all accounts, the new regulations have already led to substantial changes in the make-up of infectious disease reporting. Initial reports indicate that over two-thirds of the information on outbreaks that reaches the WHO outbreak verification team is based on unofficial information provided by NGOs, health professionals and the general public, with only one-third coming from WHO and national health agencies (Grein et al, 2000). This has ramifications for how much control local populations have over disease information and responses, as well as how the global system operates, which may not be clear cut. There is potentially new scope for participatory surveillance that draws on the local knowledge and conceptual frameworks of those experiencing disease (Groce and Reeve, 1996). A successful initiative to eradicate rinderpest in Sudan in the 1990s using these techniques has led to more recent attempts to control H5N1 avian influenza in Indonesia (Jost et al, 2007; Normile, 2007; Lawson and Mariner, 2008). However, as is the case with the rapid response element of the IHR, the new approach to unofficial information may have a negative bearing on the overall ability of the system to respond to unexpected events.

As the WHO acknowledges, both the changing reality of communication and the resulting shift in the official stance on notification have significant ramifications for how global public health is managed (Heymann and Rodier, 1998, 2001; Grein et al, 2000). As information about disease outbreaks travels both more quickly and more freely, mechanisms for evaluating the nature and significance of such information must also change. One important challenge is that of distinguishing 'real' events from the surrounding noise of random variation, error, rumour and possible deliberate obfuscation.

Such 'noise' or 'chatter' has always mattered to epidemiological surveillance. What is new is the changed stance of the WHO and other international health organizations in relation to that noise. In the past, a formal distinction between 'official' and 'unofficial' channels of information provided a means of triaging information. While superficially crude – only official information was officially acknowledged – such a procedure may in practice have allowed for a surprising degree of subtlety and flexibility. In any case, it kept attention focused on creating and maintaining channels of official information that were as robust and reliable as possible. The downside of such a focus is a dangerous rigidity; the upside is trustworthiness and stability.

To adapt to the new IHR, the WHO has developed another formal process for evaluating the significance of outbreak information from both formal and informal sources. This process occurs under the rubric of the Global Outbreak Alert and Response Network (GOARN), launched in 2000 (Grein et al, 2000; Heymann and Rodier, 2001). GOARN represents a formalization of a set of procedures spanning detection, verification, alert and response that have long formed the basis of any global response to an outbreak. Central to this process is an outbreak verification team based in Geneva. This team meets regularly to evaluate outbreak reports culled from a variety of official and unofficial sources, which include national institutes of public health, WHO offices and other agencies in the UN system; NGOs; newspapers, television, and radio; and electronic discussion groups and internet postings. Most of the latter are identified in the first instance by the Global Public Health Information Network (GPHIN), an online trawling programme that tracks over 600 published information sources, including major newspapers, wire services and biomedical journals. If a given outbreak report has the potential to be a PHEIC, the outbreak verification team contacts people in the relevant WHO regional offices, who themselves then attempt to confirm reports from health authorities on the ground in the affected location. On the basis of initial reports of possible PHEICs, an email is sent directly to partners and to a wider audience via the outbreak verification list, a weekly email letter distributed to 800 subscribers, which include WHO staff worldwide, other UN agencies, national health authorities, and non-governmental programmes. The outbreak verification list includes information on unconfirmed reports and is limited to subscribers. Once an outbreak report has been verified by communication with those in the field, verified outbreak reports are often also posted on the WHO Disease Outbreak News portion of the WHO website but only after they have been officially confirmed.

During this process, the boundaries between public and private are routinely crossed but they are not permeable in all directions. Outbreak verification depends on the *input* of outbreak reports from a wide and unregulated public sphere. Like other user-generated content, such as Wikipedia and the blogosphere, this is part of its strength. But those reports are still verified largely by using the WHO formal channels of governance, through regional offices and country health authorities. Similarly, though NGOs may also be contacted at this point, there is no official procedure for attempting to use wiki-like tools, such as citizen or volunteer assessment of outbreak reports, to verify outbreaks. More significantly, there is no attempt to provide local communities with epidemiological information for their own use in managing public health on a daily basis, in the absence of a confirmed outbreak. In other words, there is no attempt to make the wealth of information collected under the auspices of GOARN work for local communities during the vast majority of the time when the locale is not subject to emergency control actions.

Instead, the outbreak verification team is responsible for transforming 'raw intelligence gleaned from all formal and informal sources ... into meaningful intelligence' (Heymann and Rodier, 2001). The dissemination of outbreak reports *outwards* occurs along carefully delineated lines. Only 800 subscribers get the outbreak verification report, which thus remains more or less private until a report is 'officially confirmed' at which point it is spread widely via the WHO Outbreak News (the most frequently consulted portion of the WHO's website) and the Weekly Epidemiological Record. Of course, one of the key reasons why the dissemination of outbreak reports must be carried out carefully is that the WHO must avoid the danger of spreading mass panic or, alternately, of becoming a 'boy who cried wolf', with a subsequent public failure to respond in the event of a real emergency. Nonetheless, the imbalance in the breadth of the inputs versus the closedness of the outputs of this system reflects and reinforces assumptions about who should rightly govern responses to epidemics. The result is a shift towards official centralized control and away from locally managed processes. In a sense, this is unavoidable. The WHO, and its associated programmes, are by definition institutions of focused control. What is instructive is the agency's stance towards the relative authority of different kinds of knowledge within the official system. In this respect, the title of a WHO-authored paper on GOARN is instructive. 'Rumours of disease in the global village' seeks to frame the WHO's programme as simply an exceptional (for which read 'global') version of 'local' and 'traditional' responses to disease (Grein et al, 2000). But is this simply pandering or does it represent a serious attempt by the WHO to revise its own self-understanding?

With the opening-up, under IHR 2005, of new kinds of global health surveillance, the distinction between unofficial and official sources of information has not fallen out of global health surveillance under the WHO but rather become more delicate and more involved. Much rhetoric about the irrelevance of national boundaries to disease pathogens notwithstanding, national boundaries may become more, rather than less, important with respect to both surveillance and response. Today, national boundaries may be less important geographically as points of epidemiological control (as they were under the old IHR 1969), but nations, and their sovereignty, have become arguably more important as infectious diseases continue to worsen (Fidler, 1996, 1997; Heymann and Rodier, 2004; Bashford, 2006; Mack, 2006; Weir and Mykhalovskiy, 2006; Davies, 2008). China's failure to disclose the initial SARS cases on its soil is one example of how national sovereignty issues remain of primary importance in planning for effective global health policies. Indonesia has consistently refused to share samples of the H5N1 avian influenza virus. Since the country has been hit hard by avian influenza, its cooperation in tracking and studying the disease is critical. Citing the newfound concept of viral sovereignty, the Indonesian government has alleged collusion on the part of Western governments and pharmaceutical companies to steal such samples and create patentable vaccines from them that will be too costly for Indonesian citizens to buy (Fidler, 2008; Holbrooke and Garrett, 2008). Indonesian ministers have explicitly linked demands for the equitable provision of vaccines by private companies to compliance with international sample sharing protocols. Such tensions reveal the inherent weakness of the IHR. The WHO has no tools for enforcement and must rely on convention and peer pressure to encourage the compliance of member states.

New tools for new sources of information

New sources of information require new methods for processing that information, and such methods rely on norms and values that are different in official and unofficial contexts. One such new method is event-based surveillance systems. In contrast to classical surveillance, these systems include informal information or rumours gathered from a range of unfiltered sources. Such systems are becoming increasingly important. Some responses, such as the Global Public Health Information Network, the ProMed email distribution list and a more recently established HealthMap project designed to provide real-time information to a range of end users (Brownstein et al, 2008), use the power of the web and email to identify possible outbreaks. Second-generation IT tools include EpiSpider, which integrates information from ProMed and the Global Disaster Alert Coordinating System, to create enhanced 'situational awareness' of dynamic disease events (Keller et al, 2009). Another alternative to classical surveillance is syndromic reporting, based on clinical symptoms easily identified even by non-medical personnel. Some argue that such reporting tools can capture more relevant disease events in a surveillance system (Buehler et al, 2003; Reingold, 2003; Calain, 2007b). Such techniques may also be important when widespread epidemics threaten to swamp case-based reporting systems. During the summer of 2009, it quickly became apparent that swine flu cases were increasing so rapidly that sticking to a case-based system would place 'exponential' burdens on public health systems just when they are most strained. In such a circumstance, a mixed approach using proxy illness indicators (such as outpatient visits for flu-like illness, or hospital admissions for acute respiratory illness) for the majority of the population and laboratory testing for a subset of cases becomes a realistic alternative (Lipsitch et al, 2009). Such innovations in digital and mixed surveillance systems represent the future direction of health systems monitoring.

Commentators note that such 'infosurveillance' systems should not – and cannot – replace experienced public health practitioners with the skills and authority to make individual judgements about how and when best to act (Brownstein et al, 2009). Ironically, however, the turn to the informal and the unfiltered that such developments represent may elicit a greater formalization of decision-making elsewhere, lessening the role of individual decision-makers. For example, one response to the growth of information on outbreaks from unofficial sources has been a move towards a greater formalization of decision-making practices. In order to assist member countries in determining if an event counts as a PHEIC, the WHO has introduced a formal decision-making instrument based on risk-assessment techniques. In addition to these formal decision-making tools, a national IHR focal point in each country is intended to serve as a node in an international surveillance network. Thus the expansion of unofficial events included within surveillance has predicated a need for formal risk-assessment tools (Baker and Fidler, 2006). But the introduction of such formal risk regimes may mean that flexibility is sacrificed precisely when it is needed most, at the time when resilience and responsiveness are increasingly considered essential for responding to new dangers. Can resilience be programmed into formal risk assessment techniques? Or is it (just a little) oxymoronic to consider 'rules' for a flexible organization? Is it possible that open surveillance systems, of the kind promoted by the new IHR, may lead to less, rather than more, transparency?

Analysts of resilient or high reliability organizations have suggested that the organizations and individuals that most successfully respond to unexpected shocks are those that can determine when to discard inappropriate rules and hierarchies in the face of a dramatically altered reality (Weick, 1993; Hamel and Välikangas, 2003; Rayner, 2006). The ability to wrest sense from crisis depends to a certain extent on a balance between structure and chaos, between how much emphasis the organization places on training and hierarchy, and how much it gives to trust, communication and individual initiative. The structure of an organization determines the kind of story it can collectively construct about a fast-changing or unpredictable situation (Brown and Eisenhardt, 1997; Weick et al, 1999). Taking it further, the existence of multiple kinds of story-telling in an institution (which may take the form of simulations, vicarious experiences and other ways of imagining the diverse pathways leading to a catastrophic event) is itself a form of insurance against rigidity and narrow-mindedness: 'a system which values stories, storytellers, and storytelling will be more reliable than a system which derogates these substitutes for trial and error' (Weick, 1987). By the time an epidemic is upon us, it is too late to test the system. Story-telling, Weick suggests, is a good proxy.

A variety of alternatives to traditional expert-led governance of science and technology have been proposed that emphasize deliberation and reflexivity. Understanding how an issue is differently understood, or 'framed' by different knowledge-holders, thus becomes a part of the process of determining an acceptable solution (Smith and Stirling, 2006; Leach et al, 2010). By learning to see and accept that knowledge is necessarily and always imperfect, such approaches seek to build into decision-making an awareness of the inevitability of unintended consequences and, it is hoped, a corresponding humility that will make it easier to respond to such consequences when and if it becomes necessary. Complexity, ambiguity, contingency, plurality and ongoing re-evaluation are emphasized over simplicity, certainty, resolve, unity and finality (Stirling, 2006).

Can national health systems and global surveillance be compatible?

Developed countries with highly functioning health infrastructures stand to gain much from global surveillance efforts that may help them to protect themselves from the spread of infectious and communicable diseases. But if national health systems of developing countries are seen to be irrelevant to this global project, critics argue that there is a risk that funding and commitment to those systems will decline as the cart of surveillance gets put before the horse of robust national health infrastructures (Calain, 2007a; Wilson et al, 2008). Indeed, the increasing willingness of the WHO to incorporate informal data into surveillance systems has been taken by some as an indication of how global surveillance initiatives and health system strengthening are 'drifting apart' on the international agenda. The danger is that rather than funding much-needed national health infrastructure, funds from the WHO and other key public health organizations will be spent on surveillance that is of most benefit to countries with robust infrastructures, leaving poor nations out in the cold. 'If the main legacy of global surveillance policies consists merely of a summons to plug into a virtual "network of networks", and to welcome foreign investigators donning bio-protective equipment', writes Calain, for example, 'we will fail in our duty to protect the most vulnerable populations during a pandemic of some magnitude' (Calain, 2007b).

WHO has made few provisions for funding the official surveillance and reporting systems within resource-poor member countries. 'Core capacity requirements' establish minimum requirements for surveillance and reporting systems within all countries. Substantial resources are needed to meet the requirements, but while the WHO is required to 'assist' member countries in meeting their surveillance system obligations, there is no provision for WHO funding to enable member countries to comply with the regulations. Many developing countries simply do not have the capacity to comply with IHR 2005. Without a radical change in the way funds are distributed, some have argued, the WHO surveillance system will be little more than a faulty early warning system of benefit only to developed countries who invest their money in stockpiling vaccines rather than improving the health systems of developing countries (US Department of Health and Human Services, 2006; PLoS Medicine Editors, 2007).[2] Similarly, the real cost of global surveillance systems to developing countries may be considerable, with overlapping systems draining scarce human resources.

A key question raised by the changes in WHO IHR and by the critical literature is, therefore, whether surveillance systems and national healthcare infrastructures can be made compatible, if not actually mutually beneficial? One way of answering this question is to advocate surveillance systems that are 'holistic' or integrated and able to meet multiple kinds of information needs with one infrastructure (WHO, 2000a; Perry et al, 2007). With an eye towards the anticipated completion of the Global Polio Eradication Initiative (GPEI), the WHO has introduced an integrated surveillance programme that is meant to 'mainstream' the GPEI's extensive system of trained personnel, facilities and management structures (Heymann et al, 2004; WHO, 2004b). The impact of such top-down 'mainstreaming' on local communities is uncertain. Limited research on successful integrated regional surveillance systems emphasizes the importance of simplicity of reporting procedure, low costs, trust-building, communication and personal rapport between organizers and people in the network, and regular feedback of information (John et al, 1998, 2004; Calain, 2007b). Some investigators have suggested that strengthening regional surveillance systems to address outbreaks and epidemics can also improve local health systems (Kimball et al, 2008; Kruk, 2008). However, as already indicated, the language of integration, as presently used, may not go far enough in guaranteeing national or local self-determination in matters of health policy.

Looking to the future

As organizing narratives, globalization and surveillance cannot easily be separated. As the previous pages have demonstrated, the logic and assumptions of each contribute to a shared master narrative about infectious disease outbreaks that organizes much global health policy today. A series of dichotomies helps to distinguish and valorize interventions. Fast- versus slow-twitch models of disease, global versus local models of culture, and official versus unofficial models of knowledge provide categories according to which policies can be evaluated, designed and implemented. As a result, policy on the global scale has tended to be driven by narratives about sudden outbreaks that threaten to cross international boundaries rather than longer-term endemic problems the affect the most vulnerable people. Failure to heed narratives about such long-term changes (what might be called stresses to the system, rather than shocks) may make the whole global system itself more vulnerable over time. When they have been included, unofficial knowledge and local models of culture have often been so on terms that serve only to strengthen and justify a rigid, centralized protocol of risk assessment.

How best can resilience be fostered in relation to global health policy in a way that is sustainable for the communities most at risk? One answer is to provide ways in which these competing narratives can feed into each other: fast-twitch problems help signal slow-twitch transformations; local knowledge is seen to be a form of global knowledge; official knowledge systems feed unofficial ones. Such feedback loops are another way of introducing reflexivity into policy-making. Or, to use Weick's language again, this provides a wider set of stories that the collective global health community can tell itself about what might happen. The results are not simply discursive (although they are importantly that): they also include changes in what is seen to be the purpose and aim of global health policy. In other words, giving local people control over epidemiological information, or defining infectious disease events in terms of environmental change or migration patterns that occur over years (and decades), will change the overall contents of the box labelled 'global health policy'.

Making such changes will require us to take account of the complexity of the new global architecture of health policy without attempting to maintain rigid lines of control or allowing wasteful redundancy. Recognizing that organizational complexity does not necessarily entail conceptual complexity is essential. Just because there is a multiplicity of global health actors does not mean that there is a multiplicity of narratives about global health. A more nuanced description of the nature of the redundancy, chaos and/or lack of harmonization that characterizes this policy environment will require more comparative studies in the political economy of health policy in diverse contexts, such as those in this volume. Orienting this analysis to the end-users of health policy, rather than the designers, will help reveal a truer global map of health and disease

Notes

1   From 1 July 1997 to 1 July 1999, a total of 246 events of international public health importance were identified by the WHO outbreak verification team and disseminated on the outbreak verification list. Seventy-one per cent of those events were based on reports from informal or unofficial sources (including the web, listservs and NGOs – a varied lot), and only 29 per cent on the official WHO network or national health ministries of member countries.
2   In December 2005, the US Congress allocated US$3.8 billion to pandemic preparedness. US$3.3 billion of this went to the Department of Health and Human Services, of which three-quarters is devoted to stockpiling antiviral drugs and vaccines for use in the US, and only 3.8 per cent is committed to 'international activities'.

Chapter 3

Haemorrhagic Fevers: Narratives, Politics and Pathways

Melissa Leach and Barry S. Hewlett

Introduction

Haemorrhagic fevers have captured popular and media imagination as deadly diseases emerging 'out of Africa' to threaten the rest of the world. Associated with wildlife vectors in forested environments, viral haemorrhagic fevers such as Ebola, Marburg and Lassa fever figure high in current concern about so-called 'emerging infectious diseases', their hot spots of origin (Jones et al, 2008), and the threat of global spread. Outbreaks have been foci for rapid and sometimes draconian international policy responses and control measures. Ebola, in particular, has acquired iconic status as a disease-specific version of what Wald has called 'the outbreak narrative' (Wald, 2008, chapter 1).

Yet alongside and sometimes intersecting with this particular, scientifically shaped view of a deadly outbreak that requires rapid external response are a variety of other narratives about haemorrhagic fevers. These pose and respond to a range of questions: who is at risk, and how? How is the relevant system of interacting social–disease ecological processes to be framed and bounded, and at what scale? Should haemorrhagic fevers be understood in terms of short-term outbreaks – as epidemics – or as part of more structural, long-term social–disease–ecological interactions, with more endemic qualities? What of the perspectives of people living with the diseases in African settings? And what of uncertainties about disease dynamics, over longer as well as shorter timescales?

In this chapter we identify four particular narratives about haemorrhagic fevers that deal with these questions in contrasting ways. We begin with the iconic outbreak narrative that treats haemorrhagic fevers as an emerging global threat. We then consider a second narrative that casts the problem in terms of deadly local disease events requiring the mobilization of rapid containment and public health measures. A third narrative argues that local knowledge and socio-cultural practices are crucial to understanding and responding to haemorrhagic fevers. Finally, we address a fourth narrative that turns attention to longer-term interactions between social and environmental processes involved with disease patterns and vulnerabilities, as well as the areas of uncertainty, ambiguity and ignorance these generate.

As we explore, particular actors and institutions promote and adhere to these different narratives, drawing on different forms of knowledge and 'cultural models' (Hewlett and Hewlett, 2008) of disease to do so. Cultural model is here understood to mean a set of beliefs, assumptions and understandings about the nature and aetiology of a disease shared by members of a given population. Particular cultural models can inform and shape the content of narratives, but the latter are broader, incorporating dimensions of an epidemic storyline that go beyond the dynamics of the disease itself to encompass questions of how, why and for whom it is a problem; and more normative, in that narratives also contain exhortations as to what should be done about it. These narratives serve to justify contrasting institutional and policy pathways for responding to haemorrhagic fevers, with starkly differing implications for who gains and who loses. Nevertheless these different narratives also co-exist and overlap, as do the actors and networks associated with each. To some extent we can also identify a temporal sequence, with the dominance of the earlier narratives gradually receding and more recent ones coming into play. Yet there are also institutional, cognitive and political pressures that make certain narratives and associated pathways 'stickier' and more likely to dominate policy, while others receive less attention and fewer resources. In attempting to map a range of narratives that have emerged around haemorrhagic fevers in African settings, therefore, this chapter also reflects on the politics of disease control pathways. It considers the challenges of building responses that are sustainable in the face of ongoing social–disease dynamics, and which meet the priorities, needs and justice concerns of vulnerable groups – in this case, people living in haemorrhagic fever-prone African settings.

The chapter draws on literature and web-based sources together with interviews conducted by Leach with one major policy player, the WHO; Hewlett's extensive field experience with Ebola in Central Africa (Hewlett and Hewlett, 2008); and Leach's preliminary discussions of Lassa fever in West Africa in the context of long-term fieldwork on the region's social–ecological dynamics (Fairhead and Leach, 1996, 1998). Whilst far from fully comprehensive, the analysis is sufficient to suggest that in relation to other cases, haemorrhagic fevers may offer some positive lessons. A key thread running through this chapter tracks a shift from global scare stories to focused local responses in African settings, and then to responses that integrate local people's own system framings, goals and knowledge and become more effective and sustainable as a result. Yet we also argue that these responses do not sufficiently address longer-term ecological and social dynamics and more structural shifts that may be impinging on the nature and frequency of haemorrhagic fever outbreaks and regional vulnerability to them. What are the implications of this fourth narrative for institutions and strategies, and for further research?

Background

This chapter focuses on Ebola and Lassa fever, members of a larger group of viral haemorrhagic fevers. We restrict ourselves to these two because they are the two epidemiologically most significant haemorrhagic fevers in the African context, but also because they offer significant and interesting contrasts. As we shall see, Lassa more easily illustrates key issues concerning long-term dynamics that have been underplayed in the case of Ebola, which lends itself so easily to short-term outbreak narratives.

Biomedical cultural models represent Ebola haemorrhagic fever as a fierce and extremely 'rapid killing' viral disease that causes death in 50–90 per cent of clinically diagnosed cases. Passed via blood and other bodily fluids, it leads to rapid onset of symptoms (initially high temperature, shivering and aches, leading to gastric problems on approximately the third day, rashes and throat lesions by the eighth, often accompanied by spontaneous bleeding and renal failure, and then to extreme lethargy and hallucinations) and usually death within two weeks.

Ebola is one genus within the family of filoviruses that also includes Marburg. It is a zoonotic disease, whose natural reservoir is thought to lie in rats or bats in forest environments, although there is uncertainty and unresolved debate about this, as about precise viral transmission mechanisms. Transmission from primary vectors via apes touched or consumed as bushmeat is thought to be a major infection route. The first known outbreak occurred in 1976 in the Democratic Republic of Congo (DRC) (then Zaire), near the Ebola river from which the virus takes its name. There are five species of Ebola: Zaire (the most virulent, with an 80–90 per cent case mortality rate, and occurring in tropical forest areas), Sudan (40–50 per cent mortality rate, occurring in mixed savanna-forest environments), Bundibugyo (25 per cent mortality rate, occurring in mountain forest environments) and – less common and involving only a few individuals – Reston and Ivory Coast. There is no available antiviral or vaccine, and available treatment can address only symptoms. This high case fatality has led Ebola to be listed by the US government as a potential biological weapon in the highest-risk group (biosafety level 4).

Table 3.1 shows the locations of the primary African outbreaks of filovirus (Ebola-Zaire, Ebola-Sudan and Marburg), together with the number of cases.

Table 3.1 *African Ebola outbreaks*

Year	Location and number of cases					
	Gabon	Congo	DR Congo	Angola	Uganda	Sudan
1976			318			284
1979						34
1994	52					
1995			315			
1996	37, 61					
1999			73			
2000					425	
2001	65	57				
2002		13				
2003		143, 35				
2005		12		351		17
2007–2008			264		149	

Source: adapted from Hewlett and Hewlett, 2008, p5 and CDC (cdc.gov/ncidod/dvrd/spb/mnpages/dispages/ebola/ebolatable.htm)

Several points are of note. First, following the first three known outbreaks in 1976–1979 there was a gap until 1994. Since then, outbreaks have become more frequent. Second, while outbreaks are associated with very high case mortality rates (between 25 and 90 per cent, and over 75 per cent for all recent outbreaks involving the Ebola-Zaire virus) the overall number of deaths caused by these filoviruses has been relatively low – amounting to a maximum of a few hundred in years when major outbreaks have occurred.

Lassa haemorrhagic fever is caused by a single-stranded RNA virus (of the family Arenaviridae). It is endemic in Guinea-Conakry, Sierra Leone, Liberia and parts of Nigeria, and possibly also in other countries in the West African region. It is also a zoonotic disease, whose animal reservoir is a rat of the genus *Mastomys*. People become infected through direct exposure to the excreta of infected rats or – more rarely – by transmission from person to person via body fluids. Lassa infection is asymptomatic in about 80 per cent of cases, but causes acute illness in the rest. Fever and general weakness are followed by headache, chest pain, vomiting, diarrhoea, cough, fluid in the lung cavity, bleeding from orifices, and in the late stages sometimes disorientation and coma. Deafness occurs in 25 per cent of cases. In fatal cases, it kills rapidly, usually within 14 days. But compared with Ebola, the overall case fatality rate is much lower: around 1 per cent, rising to

15 per cent of hospitalized cases (http://www.who.int/mediacentre/factsheets/
fs179/en/). Nevertheless some studies estimate that 300,000–500,000 cases
of Lassa fever occur annually across West Africa. The overall number of
deaths is therefore much higher than Ebola, estimated at around 5,000 per
year (Birmingham and Kenyon, 2001).

These contrasts in mortality figures have led some to ask whether filovirus haemorrhagic fever outbreaks such as Ebola are 'much ado about
nothing' – locally devastating, but of marginal international importance
(Borchert et al, 2000). Others have hailed Lassa fever as 'an unheralded
problem' that demands more international attention (Birmingham and
Kenyon, 2001). Certainly, the numbers of people affected by each disease
are out of proportion to their international profile and the scale of Western
media attention. In the following sections, we reflect on reasons for and
consequences of this Ebola sensationalization and exceptionalism.

A global threat: tackling the plague emerging out of Africa

The first narrative that we consider – treating haemorrhagic fevers as an
emerging global threat – follows the contours of Wald's (2008) 'paradig-
matic story about newly emerging infections' rather closely. Popular, media
and fictional representations, as well as the biographical accounts of key
scientists, share a plot beginning with the discovery of an emerging infection, raising fears about its rapid spread through global networks to panic-
stricken publics in Euro-American settings, and documenting the work of
scientists to contain it.

Thus Laurie Garrett's *The Coming Plague* (1994) chronicles the 'discovery'
of both Lassa fever and Ebola in accounts replete with heroic European and
American doctors and self-sacrificing nurses and missionaries in remote
African settings. Lassa fever was named after the village in eastern Nigeria
where in 1969 an outbreak of the disease affected American nurses and
brought the disease to Western attention for the first time (Garrett, 1994,
p73). Tropical disease expert John Frame, nurse Pinneo and laboratory
scientist Jordi Casals in New York played central roles in the identification
of the 'mystery virus' as new, although a laboratory error meant that Casals
nearly died from it in the process. While Frame tracked outbreaks in Nigeria,
outbreaks in Zorzor, eastern Liberia brought WHO involvement and virol-
ogist Tom Monath onto the scene. Casals, Monath and Pinneo, together
with investigators from the US Centers for Disease Control (CDC) 'solved
the Lassa mystery' (Garrett, 1994, p90) in 1972 in the rural hospitals and
villages of eastern Sierra Leone, tracking the source of infection to *Mastomys*

natalensis rats. In 1976, Joe McCormick was sent by CDC to set up a 'one man research station' in Sierra Leone – which he did, following a period spent investigating Ebola outbreaks in Central Africa en route.

The Ebola discovery story begins in Yambuku, in the then Zaire, in 1976, with an outbreak of a mysterious disease amongst local people and then the nuns at Yambuku Mission Hospital. 'Soon the hospital was full of people suffering with the new symptoms. Panic spread as village elders spoke of an illness, unlike anything ever seen before, that 'made people bleed to death' (Garrett, 1994, p103). William Close, an American doctor based in Kinshasa, was called to help by the Zairean Minister of Health, and brought in a team from CDC Atlanta. Around the same time, an apparently similar outbreak occurred in the Maridi area of southern Sudan. A WHO team collected samples there and sent them to high security laboratories in Europe and the UK. By October 1976 the WHO had released a report stating that samples from Sudan and Zaire had revealed a new virus, based on confirmation from laboratories at CDC, Anvers and Porton Down, and had initiated a major international effort to try to stop the epidemics in Zaire and Sudan (Garrett, 1994, p116). 'Almost overnight, events would snowball into an effort necessitating over 500 skilled investigators, and mobilising the resources of numerous European and American institutions, all at an indirect cost of over $10 million' (Garrett, 1994, p116). Peter Piot, Karl Johnson, Joel Breman and David Heyman of CDC, and Pierre Sureau of the Pasteur Institute, were central hero figures in this work. But while several variants of the Ebola virus were identified and theories developed that it was a zoonosis, its animal vectors remained a mystery.

Garrett's journalism was not the only media work to popularize the haemorrhagic fever outbreak narrative in the mid-1990s. Ebola was the focus of Richard Preston's book *The Hot Zone* (1994), which became the box office hit film of 1995, *Outbreak*, and influenced much related popular writing and debate at the time.[1] Such works sensationalized not just the virus's heroic discovery and its deadly nature, but also constructed it as a threat to global populations, spread by globalized travel. Thus *The Hot Zone* portrayed Ebola as a 'predatorial virus' with global implications, and this rapidly became an 'urban legend' of global proportions (Weldon, 2001). In popular science writer Dorothy Crawford's account, this predatorial virus has agency of its own:

> the infamous Ebola virus which occasionally finds its way into the human population from an unknown animal host, causes epidemics of a highly lethal haemorrhagic fever. The virus punches holes in capillaries and blood teeming with viruses oozes into tissues and body fluids. So while the patient is prostrate with high fever, severe pain, generalized bleeding and catastrophic vomiting and diarrhoea, the

> *viruses in body fluids take the opportunity to pass to unsuspecting*
> *family members and hospital staff.* (Crawford, 2007, p17)

Along with a variety of other microbes, Ebola has 'gone global' thanks to the accelerating speed and scale of international travel:

> *We have seen infectious disease microbes exploiting international*
> *travel routes to infect naïve populations worldwide. Many, like the*
> *acute childhood infections, have established a global distribution, while*
> *others ... are hiding in the environment, waiting for their next oppor-*
> *tunity to strike.* (Crawford, 2007, p138)

In the haemorrhagic fever outbreak narrative, therefore, the system of concern is constructed at a global scale, with the virus seen to take advantage of new opportunities in a highly interconnected and mobile world. Concern about the potential use of Ebola and Lassa viruses in biological warfare and as agents of bioterrorism (Polesky and Bhatia, 2003) shifts the agency from the virus itself to humans who might deploy it, but dwells similarly on the devastating global implications of viral release.

This global threat outbreak narrative originates primarily from Euro-American sources – popular and sensationalized fiction and non-fiction newspaper reports, books and films about Ebola or Ebola-like outbreaks. Such books, films and other media are produced to sell, engage and entertain the public, but they also provide one of the most consistent sources of information about outbreaks to Euro-Americans. They draw on and contribute to a particular Euro-American cultural model of haemorrhagic fevers as a particular sort of disease requiring particular kinds of response (see Table 3.2).

Table 3.2 *Popular Euro-American haemorrhagic fever cultural model*

Common signs and symptoms	Flu-like, fever, vomiting, bleeding from orifices, skin rash or lesions, difficulty breathing, rapid death
Common causes – global threat	Mutant virus from foreign land (Africa, China), secret government labs, foreign terrorists
Common ways disease is transmitted	Airborne, touch
Treatment	None until high tech scientist discovers vaccine or other cure, otherwise everyone dies
Prevention and containment	Flee area of outbreak, isolate self and family, close schools and churches, wear masks
Prognosis	Not good until science discovers cure
Risk groups	Health workers and general public
Common human responses to outbreak	Panic, violence, competition

The media contribute to the Euro-American public's perceptions, knowledge and expectations about haemorrhagic fever outbreaks. Thus, for example, analysis of the approximately 60 newspaper articles about Ebola that appeared in 1995–1996 in Britain found that they all portrayed Ebola – in more or less sensationalized terms – as a horrifying disease emerging 'out of Africa' and threatening Europe and North America (Joffe and Haarhoff, 2002, pp10–11). For example:

> *A killer virus which turns body organs to liquid and makes AIDS look like a common cold could devastate Europe, health experts fear. The disease ... has been found in Germany, Italy and America and there has already been one case in Britain. (The Sun, 12 May 1995)*

> *Three suspected victims of the Doomsday Bug sneaked into Britain from Zaire without passports, it was revealed last night. The mother and two young children were allowed to roam London's streets for two days before immigration chiefs realised they were on the loose. (The Sun, 20 May 1995)*

> *Such infections could affect travellers and, in the era of air travel, an infected individual could import the disease into the United States. (The Guardian, 23 May 1995)*

However, Joffe and Haarhoff (2002) suggest that alongside these images of the disease invading European shores were images representing Ebola outbreaks as 'far-flung illnesses' associated with conditions in African settings. Thus certain media representations and people's readings of them interacted to construct Ebola as African, linking outbreaks with wild forests, poor African hospitals, 'bizarre' cultural practices such as eating monkey meat, and 'tribal rituals'. 'People who have contracted the disease, my impression is that they have done so in this, sort of, cave area, where the monkeys hang out' (broadsheet reader, cited in Joffe and Haarhoff, 2002, p9).

Such 'othering' by the media in the late 1990s, Joffe and Haarhoff suggest, served as a strategy for the containment of fear, presenting Ebola as posing little threat to Britain. Even as newspapers referred to the potential of Ebola to globalize, lay publics thus felt detached from these dimensions, tending to treat them as science fiction – perhaps encouraged in this by the science fiction works at the time which did indeed elaborate on the outbreak narrative theme.

The global outbreak narrative and the cultural model it is linked with have two major policy implications. First, the dramatic fear generated by a deadly disease has motivated national and international health and government officials to develop policy to prepare and respond to haemorrhagic fever and other outbreaks. Media popularization increases public interest and support for expenditures of government funds to prepare for and respond to outbreaks. Ebola in this sense is an 'exceptional' or 'master status' disease. It attracts more medical, public and media attention and resources than other diseases, such as Lassa fever, for example, that may in fact affect more people and cause more morbidity and mortality. The global threat narrative has contributed to the master status of Ebola and this in turn has stimulated the creation of policies and institutions at the national and local levels that have been shaped by the particular concerns raised by this vision of this disease. Thus the 1995 outbreak in Zaire, and the 'perception that the Kikwit outbreak was going to spread to the rest of the world' (interview, WHO, 8 July 2008) is reported as 'key to building political momentum' in the processes leading to the WHO's creation of a revised set of International Health Regulations (IHR) in 2005 (Heymann et al, 1999), regulations that are intended to guide the global response to all diseases with potential global impact (WHO, 2007c). The Kikwit outbreak, according to this view, helped crystallize a policy response within the WHO that resonated with a broader discourse of global health security that has been gaining rapid ground in recent years (e.g. WHO, 2007a).

The second policy implication of the global threat narrative is a lack of attention to the public and their knowledge in helping to contain outbreaks of haemorrhagic fevers. Popular fiction and non-fiction films and books alike emphasize the roles of medical doctors, nurses, scientists and government officials. In the end, dreadful outbreaks are contained by incredible and often last minute discoveries and efforts by scientists. Publics are rarely shown or discussed in these narratives and when they are, they are often represented either as ignorant and backward (especially in African settings) or as panicked and ineducable (especially in European and American ones). Media-based representations of the public in outbreak narratives contribute to the lack of serious attention to the knowledge and perspectives of the public in policy, and negative images of the public in international and national policies that aim to contain outbreaks.

Deadly local disease events: the building of universal rapid response

A concern with haemorrhagic fevers in their African settings – rather than as global disease threats – is central to a second narrative. This takes a more local focus, constructing haemorrhagic fevers as devastating disease events that require containment because of their impact on local populations.

This narrative has a long history in medicine and public health, and is adhered to and promoted by many international and national health institutions. In many respects it is the most powerful narrative of the four described in this chapter, providing key representations on which the global threat narrative draws, and providing a frame of reference for the third narrative that we consider below.

A biomedical cultural model of disease, described in the background section of this chapter, is used to explain the signs, symptoms, transmission, prevention and prognosis of Ebola and Lassa. This narrative is transmitted in medical schools and schools of public health around the world, contributing to relatively uniform and global views of correct ways to respond to local outbreaks. These emphasize disease containment at source through a universal kind of rapid response by external agencies. The system and its dynamics are framed in local terms and over the short term, whether in responding to 'outbreaks' (Ebola) or to cases as they arise in an endemic situation (Lassa). This narrative and the biomedical cultural model on which it is based directly shape dominant pathways of policy and intervention to contain Ebola and Lassa. Attempts to influence policy thus require, above all, influencing this narrative.

Thus the outbreak alert and response programmes to Ebola of the WHO and CDC from the 1990s established a standardized set of medical and public health strategies to contain the disease. Programmes of rapid response to notified outbreaks had to be triggered by national government request, and denial has sometimes been a cause of delay. Once on site, externally led teams would institute responses centred on establishing isolation units for the infected and implementing barrier nursing techniques; tracking and controlling those who had had contact with infected individuals; mobilizing the community to respond and providing health education to inform the public of symptoms and modes of transmission. Responses also involve identifying individuals who have had contact with infected individuals (contact cases) in order to watch and control their activities for 21 days (the viral incubation period), and limiting 'dangerous' local behaviours such as the washing and burial of corpses without recommended precautions (Hewlett and Hewlett, 2008, p5).

Such outbreak responses are linked to surveillance and early detection strategies. Thus after the large-scale outbreak of Ebola in Bandundu region, DRC, CDC Atlanta developed a surveillance and prevention programme to help detect and prevent future outbreaks in the region (Lloyd et al, 1999). This was based on early recognition by trained doctors, and the use of a laboratory diagnostic test on skin specimens from patients suspected to have died from the disease. While this programme was set up at the regional scale, its focus was nevertheless resolutely on local outbreaks, constructing the system of concern as one which coincides spatially and temporally with the outbreak itself.

In some contrast with Ebola, in this 'deadly local disease event' narrative Lassa fever tends to be framed as an endemic disease that throws up particular cases, clustered relatively regularly in particular seasons and centring on a spatial 'hot spot' – the so-called 'hyperendemic' centre of the disease in Sierra Leone extending to other locales in Liberia and Guinea. Ebola, on the other hand, is presented as a disease prone to sporadic outbreaks, or epidemics. The more endemic character of Lassa fever shapes the standardized strategies that have emerged to deal with it. These include rapid transport of suspected cases from their village homes to centralized isolation and laboratory facilities; surveillance to identify all close contacts of a patient for three weeks after the start of their illness; and the initiation of searches for undiagnosed or unreported cases, as well as treating identified cases with the antiviral drug ribavarin (Merlin, 2002). However, a core challenge is in getting cases identified in order to proceed with treatment. This is difficult given that the initial clinical symptoms are non-specific and in these resource-poor settings, funds for polymerase chain reaction equipment that could rapidly confirm the presence of the virus are lacking (Birmingham and Kenyon, 2001). Thus although around 16 per cent of people admitted to hospitals in Sierra Leone and Liberia are estimated to have Lassa fever, doctors must often rely on diagnosis by elimination, excluding other conditions such as TB and malaria before presuming Lassa. Despite public education campaigns illustrating biomedical symptoms on posters in community health centres, a large proportion of Lassa fever cases in Sierra Leone's rural areas are presumed to go unreported to medical staff (interview, director, Mano River Lassa fever research network, Kenema, April 2009).

In this narrative, then, the goal is quite narrowly defined around early intervention and limiting disease mortality, with the focus on vulnerable local African populations. At least in the case of Ebola, the focus is relatively short term – dealing with haemorrhagic fever disease events as shocks (outbreaks) as they arise. Lassa fever presents a contrast, requiring more sustained engagement of health teams and measures to deal with its more endemic character.

This narrative, like the first, is co-constructed with notions of scientific authority. Epidemiology, virology and clinical medicine are the dominant forms of knowledge considered to be central to disease response and control. For haemorrhagic fevers, as emphasized at the WHO (interview, Geneva, 8 July 2008), 'epidemic control is not rocket science; it involves the simple principle of breaking the cycle of transmission'. Key roles in this are also acknowledged for 'frontline' health workers in implementing public health and control measures. In contrast, local populations have often been presented within this narrative as ignorant, and mired in negative cultural practices – although as we shall see in the next section, the early field experience of outbreak response practitioners encouraged many to revise their views.

Thus elaborating on the details of themes sketched in the 'global threat' narrative, this local response narrative encompasses consideration of 'cultural factors' that are seen to contribute to the emergence and spread of haemorrhagic fever events. In the case of Lassa, for example, 'traditional burial ceremonies' for infected corpses are identified with risks of disease spread (Richmond and Baglole, 2003). Beliefs in traditional remedies, and misunderstandings of miscarriage (a scientifically identifiable symptom of Lassa) as attributable to witchcraft, are associated with delays to timely presentation of cases for treatment (Merlin, 2002). Medical staff in Sierra Leone lament community traditions that encourage the eating of rats, and identify dry season festivals where this happens at scale as a major cause of Lassa outbreaks (interview, Kenema, April 2009). In the case of Ebola, research in Gabon into three outbreaks between 1994 and 1997 identified a range of problematic practices, including family members remaining close to the patient to nurse him/her; hugging and touching the dead at funerals, and traditional healers' treatments such as cutting a patient's skin with unsterilized knives and applying blood to the skin (Kunii et al, 2001). The researchers presented as evidence of local ignorance the fact that only two-thirds of the population of a village suffering from an Ebola outbreak knew the name of the disease and only half could explain what kind of disease it was in scientific terms (the rest attributed it to sorcery and evil spirits) (Kunii et al, 2001).

According to this narrative, local communities and their 'culture' are granted agency and responsibility for spreading disease. And culture itself is seen as a problem to overcome. The beliefs and practices at stake are seen as requiring reform through education, as part of externally implemented control measures.

Such top-down responses and control measures have often proved unsustainable, however, facing resistance from local populations. In the case of Lassa, for example, Richmond and Baglole report people's mistrust of medical facilities and rumoured Lassa treatments there: 'People don't go to medical facilities … [they fear that] Especially when they say they have Lassa fever, they will be given injections to kill them' (Richmond and Baglole, 2003, p1274). In the case of Ebola in Gabon in 1995–1996, for example, American and French control measures were perceived as so inappropriate and offensive by villagers that they aroused deep suspicion. International responses to a further outbreak there in 2001 met with fierce local armed resistance (Milleliri et al, 2004; see also Bausch et al, 2007). Hewlett and Hewlett (2008) document in detail which, and how, particular aspects of the response strategies caused local anxiety. Particularly significant were the prevention of people's ability to carry out customary burial practices, and the hiding of sick and dead relatives in tarpaulined isolation units, which led people to suspect that their body parts were being stolen. These particular instances which incited worry and resentment interplayed with a broader distrust of international teams 'parachuted' in from outside.

Yet despite such instances, the late 1990s to early 2000s witnessed a greater entrenchment of this biomedically grounded, local disease event narrative, along with arguments for its wider application across the world. As the WHO argued, the Ebola outbreak in Kikwit, DRC

> *signalled a need for stronger infectious disease surveillance and control worldwide, for improved international preparedness to provide support when similar outbreaks occur ... there are new and more diverse partners able to rapidly respond to international outbreaks.* (Heymann et al, 1999, p283)

Thus was institutionalized in the WHO Global Outbreak and Response Network (GOARN), bringing together multiple agencies in a process sometimes likened to 'herding international cats' – ranging from scientific to humanitarian agencies. Ebola is described as 'peppering the history' of GOARN's creation and indeed several of its orchestrators spent earlier parts of their career at the frontline of Ebola outbreak control in the 1990s (interviews, Geneva, 8 July 2008). In the narratives of those at WHO involved in GOARN's creation and implementation, the responsive, network style of GOARN's operation enables 'each agency to play to its own strengths' (interview, 8 July 2008) in adapting to specific outbreak conditions. Nevertheless the key elements of response are generic, consisting of preparedness and early containment. In these respects the GOARN network is framed as suited to dealing with uncertainty in the sense that outbreaks will arise, but their risk, timing and location cannot be predicted (Heymann, interview 8 July 2008). A flexible response network that can be mobilized as and when needed can, in this context, be seen as a strategy for resilience.

While it is recognized as 'easy to get the boy scouts in' to the drama of dealing with an outbreak, getting them to stay on is more difficult (interview, Geneva, 8 July 2008). Thus the key challenge within this narrative is now seen to be around building national capacity for epidemic preparedness and response. Some countries (e.g. Uganda) are applauded as exemplars in this respect, making efforts build up effective links between local health centres and the national capital. Others are decried for their lack of effort (e.g. DRC). Where infrastructure and resources are lacking, effective use has been made of the surveillance infrastructure established for the global polio eradication campaign. New technologies are also expected to enhance outbreak response, with mobile diagnostic kits, in particular, predicted by some to bring about 'a revolution as great as that brought by mobile phones' in the disease context (interview, Geneva, July 8 2008).

While the international community was expanding its ability to parachute in external teams to deal with Ebola, however, Lassa fever – initially high profile – has increasingly tended to receive less attention from the WHO and other international agencies. This is despite its higher prevalence and mortality effects. With its less rapid killing and less outbreak-like nature, it had always fitted this increasingly established outbreak-event model less well. As one senior WHO officer put it, 'we have not really dealt with Lassa – we prefer to deal with these outbreak-like haemorrhagic fevers, like Ebola' (interview, Geneva, July 2008). Moreover, from 1991 Lassa fever's hot spots in the forests of Sierra Leone and the border regions of Liberia and Guinea became engulfed in the regional conflict associated with Sierra Leone's decade-long civil war and its overspill and refugee crises in neighbouring states. The regional Lassa research centre in Kenema, Sierra Leone was closed – to be re-established slowly only from 2003 – and the disease lost the limelight in the face of more immediate concerns facing both local populations and international agencies.

Local knowledge and culture matter: Integration for acceptability

In a third narrative, haemorrhagic fevers are seen as long present amongst local populations who have developed culturally embedded ways to live and deal with them. Local knowledge and cultural logics and models can, so the argument goes, inform and be integrated into response strategies, helping to make these more context-specific, locally appropriate and acceptable. To the extent that these arguments have been taken on board within local outbreak response strategies such as through GOARN, so overlaps between this and the previous narrative are evident.

In the accounts of several scientists involved in the early Ebola responses in the mid-1990s, the realization that 'culture matters' emerged through direct field experience 'on the ground'. Thus one recalled evocatively the encounters that helped him and his colleagues to realize that Ebola responses were fundamentally 'not just about a virus', and that Western-style responses were often culturally inappropriate, provoking local fear and anxiety. For example in Gabon in 1996, he recalls: 'the eerie silence in a village with all its house doors boarded up. Entering a house where an old woman lay dying, her profound terror was matched by my own terror; in my white isolation suit I was either God or the devil' (interview, Geneva, July 2008).

In this field-experience view, a set of realizations emerged through the direct experience of outbreak response teams. These included appreciation that haemorrhagic fevers are 'weird', with the power to evoke the most profound fear amongst suffering communities; that top-down Western responses were often denying people basic human rights, such as burial of their dead; and that if the key to breaking the cycle of transmission is creating social distance between people, then this could be done more effectively by building on ways that people were also doing this themselves; 'you cannot deal with an outbreak without getting people on side' (interview, Geneva, 8 July 2008). WHO scientists involved in Ebola outbreak responses recount many stories where appreciating local cultural logics, and seeing that local practices that initially appeared bizarre were actually rational to their performers, proved important to their work.

In elaborating these realizations and in responding to them, however, this narrative also constructs the inputs of anthropologists and anthropological knowledge and tools as vital to response strategies. Thus in what is described by WHO staff as an organic, ad hoc process, anthropologists began to be involved in response teams. One was Barry Hewlett, whose pioneering 'outbreak anthropology' (Hewlett and Hewlett, 2008) has been pivotal in developing this narrative, and in its uptake by the WHO which from 2001 came to include anthropologists in integrated Ebola response teams. When his coincidental presence during the 1996 Gabon outbreak proved enlightening and helpful, Barry Hewlett subsequently persuaded WHO through personal contacts to invite him onto the teams responding to the outbreaks in Uganda in 2000–2001 and DRC in 2003, initiating an inclusion of anthropological perspectives in outbreak situations that several other anthropologists have continued.

Central to this narrative – and a key contribution of anthropology – is a focus on elucidating and re-valuing local cultural models of disease and framings of system dynamics, and on identifying valuable, health-enhancing local knowledge and cultural categories which can be blended productively with scientific knowledge. Thus, for instance, explanations of Ebola origins in terms of sorcery, dismissed as evidence of local ignorance in narratives one and two, are shown to make sense in their specific socio-political contexts. During the 2003 Ebola outbreak in DRC, four teachers were killed – and anthropological perspectives helped elucidate the local political–cultural dynamics through which this epidemic was being used as an excuse and context to settle old political–economic scores. This is a well-recognized phenomenon (interview, Geneva, 8 July 2008), but anthropological perspectives prove helpful in illuminating the nuances of particular cases, and the ways in which particular aspects of technological, medical and bodily practices intersect with people's views and experiences of wider politics (see Leach and Fairhead, 2007).

Table 3.3 *Local cultural model for epidemic illness (gemo) amongst Acholi people, Uganda*

Description	Bad spirit that comes suddenly like the wind and rapidly affects many people
Signs and symptoms	Mental confusion, high fever, rapid death
Cause	Lack of respect for *jok* (spirit), sometimes no reason
Transmission	Physical proximity, wind
Treatment	Talk to spirits via traditional healer

Amongst Acholi people in Uganda, for example, local framings of disease dynamics include the concepts of both endemic and epidemic (*gemo*) disease. Local perspectives on Ebola draw on both biomedical and sorcery explanations, and epidemic and endemic models (Hewlett and Hewlett, 2008). In the 1999–2000 Ebola outbreak, the international teams initially did not realize that the local people had an existing cultural model to explain the nature, transmission and prevention of epidemic illness. However, assisted by Hewlett's work, this model and the elaborate social protocols which it triggered were successfully integrated into response strategies.

Table 3.3 summarizes the Acholi's cultural model for epidemics that was utilized in the 1999–2000 Ebola outbreak.

Once the Acholi identified an illness as *gemo*, they would implement a protocol for its prevention and control. Elements of their protocol include isolating the patient in a house at least 100m from all other houses; having a survivor of the epidemic feed and care for the patient; identifying houses with ill patients with two long poles of elephant grass, one on each side of the door; limiting general movement and advising people to stay in their household and not move between villages; and, finally, keeping patients who no longer have symptoms in isolation for one full lunar cycle before moving about freely in the village. From a biomedical perspective, the protocol constitutes a broad-spectrum approach to epidemic control which also makes sense in relation to the biomedical cultural model employed by international teams responding to the outbreak. This complementarity was able to be exploited in pathways of response that blended local and scientific knowledge.

Despite evidence of such complementarities, it is also worth pointing out that local cultural models are transmitted and acquired in very different ways from the cultural models associated with the first two narratives. Local cultural models are based upon lived experiences with haemorrhagic fevers and other outbreaks, and transmitted within and between extended families. In contrast, biomedical and Euro-American cultural models are transmitted and acquired one-to-many via teachers, professional training, books, films and so on.

This 'local knowledge and culture matter' narrative carries a range of implications for pathways of response to haemorrhagic fevers. It emphasizes understanding and building on local knowledge and practices, identifying their health effects and guiding responses to harness those aspects that are health enhancing, while educating to avoid those that are health reducing. This narrative also suggests that community engagement must be central to policy approaches to containing outbreaks. In this respect, anthropological involvement has led to significant policy shifts. For instance, establishing isolation units was previously one of the first tasks of the outbreak response team while health education and community mobilization followed. Once anthropologists participated in control efforts, however, the priorities were reversed, as community engagement and understanding was seen as essential if people were to support and utilize isolation units. Further, this narrative bolsters an argument for communication and education approaches that take account of and work with local perspectives. For example, NGOs addressing Lassa fever in Sierra Leone in the late 1980s used participatory theatre and role plays to understand people's views of the links between rats and disease, and to build from these a set of mutually acceptable strategies for limiting people's contact with the disease vector (Leach, field notes, 1988).

This narrative also offers ways to understand local resistance and adapt accordingly. For instance, in DRC in 2001, the high screens used to hide victims' bodies were found to contradict funeral norms, and were modi-fied. The narrative also emphasizes humility and respect for local practices as an essential dimension of outbreak control, whether by international or national team members. In this view, empathy and emotional support have to be added to an epidemic control team's goals. Defence of the human rights of those suffering from haemorrhagic fever has to be balanced along-side disease control aims (see also Jeppsson, 2002; Bausch et al, 2007; and Edstrom and MacGregor, this volume). Local rights and ethical concerns must be given due regard in outbreak responses and associated research and public health investigations (Calain et al, 2009). In this respect, there is a strong emphasis on social justice as a goal in pathways of disease response. Overall, this narrative highlights the need for responses to be locally context-ualized and adapted to local circumstances. Context matters: technologies and practices suited to one place might be rejected in another.

In contrast with Ebola, in the case of Lassa fever there appears to have been virtually no anthropological study. Equally, with the exception of the participatory theatre example above, there is no evidence of responses incorp-orating local knowledge. But the disease nevertheless throws up many ques-tions which anthropological knowledge and attention to local cultural logics could help inform. Staff of the Mano River Union Lassa Fever research network recognize that addressing these could complement the public health-oriented 'knowledge, attitudes, practices and beliefs' studies that they have already carried out, going beyond the biomedical model on which these have been premised (interview, Kenema, April 2009). Are there, for instance, local categories and ways of distinguishing Lassa that might be helpful in the diagnostic challenge? How are symptoms that arise in Lassa understood and assigned causes, and what are the moments at which something that might correspond to Lassa is suspected? What aspects of hospitals are feared? Within the terms of the 'culture matters' narrative, addressing questions such as these could help facilitate effective, sustainable and socially just responses.

By 2008 the incorporation of anthropologists into integrated outbreak response teams had become institutionalized, at least within the WHO. The Director of Outbreak Alert and Response Operations (interview, Geneva, 8 July 2008) claimed that 'we have anthropologists at the frontline of our teams now'; that 'we would be fearful to go to the field without an anthropologist', and that 'anthropological integration is now a key pillar of our response strategy – as important as isolation'. He notes that 'this was not the case ten years ago'.

However, discussions at the WHO also revealed an intriguing 'Ebola exceptionalism' in this respect. For no other disease under the purview of GOARN, it seems, is anthropological knowledge regarded as important. This appears to reflect both the 'exotic' nature of haemorrhagic fevers: 'they are all about burial practices'; and the apparently exotic locations and 'traditional cultures' in which many outbreaks have occurred – isolated forest communities with unfamiliar, and to Western eyes bizarre, beliefs and practices. This constructs anthropology in a very particular – and old-style – way, as dealing with 'the primitive' and 'the other' in ways that echo, again, the othering of African practices in the first, global outbreak narrative. The African 'other' and haemorrhagic fevers are again equated, this time with anthropology as both broker and characterizer.

In this vein, anthropology is constructed as less appropriate or necessary for dealing with epidemics such as avian influenza, SARS and swine (H1N1) flu which have taken place in more globalized settings, where 'tradition' has broken down and 'cultures' have become homogenized (interview, Geneva 8 July 2008). For such epidemics and settings, instead, it is argued, 'social mobilization' is sufficient. In a related vein, most technical guidelines for responding to outbreaks state 'special attention must be given to the actual perception of the outbreak by the community... In particular, specific cultural elements and local beliefs must be taken into account to ensure proper messages, confidence and close cooperation of the community' (WHO, 1997). Thus, for whatever reason, the perspectives of international agencies perpetuate a particular notion of 'culture' as confined to local settings; the impression is that rural Africans have culture, while people and institutions in more globally linked settings do not. Yet as we have discussed, particular cultural models are associated with all three of the narratives discussed thus far (Euro-American, biomedical and Acholi).

WHO staff within GOARN also note the pervasive problems of bringing natural sciences and behavioural sciences together – 'WHO is weak in this'. In this sense, the incorporation of anthropologists in response teams appears as a 'blip' in the institutional business-as-usual of dominance by epidemiologists and medical scientists – a blip made necessary by the peculiarly difficult, 'other' character of haemorrhagic fevers, rather than a frontrunner in a broader process of institutionalized interdisciplinarity in epidemic framing and response.

Mysteries and mobility: Taking long-term ecological and social dynamics seriously

For all their contrasts, these narratives share a focus on short-term responses to haemorrhagic fevers, conceiving of these as short-term shocks, be they outbreaks or cases to be dealt with as they arise. Different again is a fourth narrative that turns attention to longer-term ecological and social dynamics and more structural shifts that may be impinging on the nature and frequency of outbreaks, and on local and regional vulnerability to them. However effective the integrated teams of narrative three may be in dealing with particular outbreaks, they leave begging a number of questions about dynamics of response if the system is framed over larger temporal and spatial scales.

The relevance of such longer-term and broader-scale perspectives is underlined by evidence of an increase in frequency and severity of Ebola outbreaks, and of the highly uneven patterning of severity in Lassa fever's endemism across West Africa and over time. Some virologists now argue that identifying and addressing the underlying causes of the emergence and spread of infectious diseases is vital to interrupt potentially dangerous cycles of viral–animal–human co-evolution. As the WHO Director of Outbreak Alert and Response Operations put it (interview, 8 July 2008), with haemorrhagic fevers large socio-ecological changes mean 'there is a constant ecological frontline, with the virus exploiting new niches'. One response to such a situation is simply to deploy the outbreak-focused pathways of disease response suggested by the three narratives above, addressing each outbreak as it occurs, at source. This is the dominant perspective in WHO and other major policy agencies. It emphasizes strategies of control aimed at stability, and established responses aimed at resilience, in the face of 'known' short-term shocks. But what if viral–ecological–social dynamics, perhaps over longer timescales, throw up new kinds of viral mutation and dynamics? Questions also need to be raised about the sustainability and appropriateness of 'rapid response' mobilization for ever-shifting, more frequent outbreaks, including the strain this may put on institutions and resources. Virologists Kuiken et al (2003) argue that while to date research efforts have concentrated on improved surveillance and diagnostic capabilities to pick up and respond to outbreaks, 'more attention needs to be given to the identification of the underlying causes for the emergence of infectious diseases, which are often related to anthropogenic social and environmental changes. Addressing these factors might help decrease the rate of emergence of infectious diseases and allow the transition to a more sustainable society' (p641).

From a range of origins and perspectives, a nascent – and as yet fragmented – narrative is therefore emerging. This highlights the social and environmental dynamics of haemorrhagic fevers and vulnerability to them, and the longer term stresses in play, as well as pathways of research and response required to understand and address these.

One line of argument, forwarded particularly by those social scientists, international agencies and NGOs interested in health systems, focuses on the poverty, inequality and 'structural violence' (Farmer, 1999a) in regions where haemorrhagic fevers are rife. Declining health systems and overcrowded hospitals in which viruses multiply are one manifestation of this. Indeed the notion that 'poor hospitals are key amplifiers' (interview, Geneva, 8 July 2008) has long been a central tenet of understanding of the dynamics of Ebola. Overcrowded and poorly constructed settlements associated with impoverished and conflict-affected communities also provide ideal conditions for viral spread, and in the case of Lassa fever, for exposure to vectors. *Mastomys natalensis* rats congregate in domestic rice stores and people are particularly vulnerable where these are poorly built or inside their dwellings. Temporary mining camps are a particular hot spot (interview, Kenema, April 2009). Processes of migration and urbanization pose particular challenges for addressing haemorrhagic fevers given their capacity to spread very rapidly amongst crowded urban and peri-urban populations. Yet to date, there appears to be rather little analysis either of the dynamics involved, or of possible responses that address them – beyond the application of narrative two-like outbreak control measures. This is an area where further research and thinking are needed, towards effective disease responses amidst inevitable mobility.

Whatever the precise dynamics, this line of argument suggests that tackling haemorrhagic fevers cannot be separated from tackling poverty and its causes, and building accessible and equitable health systems. Pathways of disease response thus involve moving from 'reactive to sustainable control' in which the training and funding of frontline health workers, and integration of strategies with the broader building of health systems, is key (interview, Geneva, 8 July 2008).

This narrative can also focus on long-term environmental and socio-ecological dynamics. Thus deforestation through agriculture and logging, and its political, economic and poverty-related causes has been assumed to contribute to haemorrhagic fevers, by bringing populations closer to their forest animal viral reservoirs and secondary vectors. Haemorrhagic fevers in this respect exemplify broader narratives, put forward by certain epidemiologists and environmental scientists, that relate zoonotic infectious diseases to long-term environmental dynamics. Thus Jones et al (2008) show that emerging infectious diseases (EIDs) are increasing, that the majority (60 per cent) are zoonoses, and that of these, 72 per cent originate in wildlife. They find that 'wildlife host species richness' is a significant predictor for the emergence of zoonotic EIDs with a wildlife origin. In the identification of EID hot spots, the forest fringes of West and Central Africa appear prominent.

Such research focuses attention on factors that bring people into contact with wildlife. In particular, deforestation on the 'forest frontier' is given attention – people's encroachment into forests, and their greater contact with forest wildlife (bats, rodents and so on) that are animal reservoirs for disease, or vectors (e.g. apes). In such narratives, forest ecosystems frequently appear in one of two popular guises, each of which figures large in the work of disturbance ecologists and conservationists. The forest is either 'virgin', a pristine ecosystem in need of protection, or 'viral', a place within which lurk dangerous pathogens in need of containment (see Hardin and Froment, forthcoming). In policy terms, these dual images combine in prescriptions that focus on reducing contact between people and wildlife – separating people from the virgin/viral forest through protected areas or resettlement. For instance Jones et al (2008) suggest that 'efforts to conserve areas rich in wildlife diversity by reducing anthropic activity may have added value in reducing the likelihood of future zoonotic disease emergence'. In this respect, arguments about forest ecosystems and emerging infectious disease resemble 'fortress' conservation measures, which have been widely recognized as having negative effects on the rights and livelihoods of people living in forest areas (see for example Fairhead and Leach, 1998).

The 'bushmeat crisis' is also prominent in long-term socio-environmental narratives about haemorrhagic fevers (Hardin, forthcoming). Poverty, unemployment, conflict, hunting technologies, the opening of access through logging and extractive industries (e.g. gold and diamonds), and the growth of urban markets for bushmeat are recognized as contributory factors to the expansion of practices which bring hunters and bushmeat traders into closer contact with disease-carrying animals. Here again, it is conservation-oriented responses that have found easiest alliance with disease control concerns, emphasizing the expansion and increased securitization of protected areas, the criminalization of hunting and trade, and restrictions on wildlife and human movement. As Hardin (forthcoming) notes, alternative narratives about the bushmeat trade – focusing on its contribution to livelihoods and food security (e.g. Brown, 2003) – have received far less attention in relation to disease issues. Yet these would suggest alternative response strategies, for instance aiming to reduce people's dependence on bushmeat whether through alternative sources of livelihood for traders or alternative sources of protein (such as fish and dried fish).

Climate change is a further factor to have been drawn into the forest–haemorrhagic fever calculus. The linkages between climate change and health have recently become a major topic of donor, research and policy concern. Infectious diseases are discussed in this context, with climatic variations and extreme weather events expected to have profound impacts both in accelerating deforestation, and on the distribution, reproduction and survival rates of pathogens and vectors (see Patz et al, 2005). While much of the current climate change/infectious disease debate is characterized by general statements and hype – given the political profile of climate change issues – others call for evidence of recent, specific climate change–disease interactions to inform policy responses. For instance, the WHO message in this area is described as 'very clear' (interview, Geneva, 8 July 2008): there are weather events that affect health, leading to a requirement for better vector control, for educating populations on the risks and for surveillance systems that can give a review of likely events.

Across these various versions of the long-term socio-environmental dynamics narrative, at least as manifest in mainstream, policy debates, three related features are striking. First, they often contain a somewhat linear view of the relationship between climate change, deforestation and encroachment on the forest frontier, wildlife contact and disease. Second, the envisaged policy responses tend to focus on control – of people–ecosystem interactions, trade and livelihood activities – frequently in ways that re-enact top-down conservation and disease control measures. Third, socio-ecological dynamics are presented as known, or at least as knowable; able to be represented and managed as risks. In these respects, this long-term environmental narrative has a great deal in common with the first, global outbreak narrative discussed in this chapter.

Yet other strands of work contest and complicate this top-down disease–environment framing, suggesting the possibility of alternative narratives that might support pathways of response oriented towards an ecosystem–disease focus. Thus research in historical ecology (e.g. Balee, 2002) questions a linear framing of forest dynamics, along with dominant views of the impacts of climate change on forest ecosystems. West and Central African forests are not 'virgin' ecosystems undergoing new disturbance, but have been shaped by interacting and non-linear anthropogenic and climatic influences over centuries and millennia (Fairhead and Leach, 1996, 1998; Hardin, forthcoming). Research in environmental and climate history suggests far more dramatic responses to past climate changes than have been appreciated, implying possibly more dramatic future shifts (Maley, 2002; Fairhead, 2008); yet the implications of this for haemorrhagic fever dynamics have yet to be spelt out.

Ecological research raises unanswered questions about the relationship between forest ecosystem change and animal habitats and behaviour, and thus reservoir and vector prevalence. In the case of Ebola, the natural reservoirs and transmission cycle remain ambiguous, with competing theories – centred on bats and rodents – in play. Ebola's natural transmission cycle, the nature of its reservoirs and means of transmission remain 'an enigma' (Morvan et al, 2000). Disease dynamics may also respond to ecosystem dynamics in non-linear ways. Thus researchers at the Max-Planck Institute suggest that outbreaks of the Zaire strain of the Ebola virus are epidemiologically and ancestrally linked, and that the virus has recently spread across the region in waves rather than being persistent for long periods of time at each outbreak locality (Walsh et al, 2005). Pinzon et al (2004), using satellite data, have shown that the majority of Ebola outbreak events are associated with sharply drier conditions at the end of the rainy season, which they suggest may act as trigger events to enhance transmission of the virus from its cryptic reservoir to humans. They suggest that this link might help unravel the enviro-climatic coupling of Ebola outbreaks, which might in turn help lead to the development of early warning systems.

Detailed research informed by perspectives in cultural and political ecology highlights how links between ecosystem change, vector dynamics and disease are mediated by patterns of land use that shape people's contact with animals (see Lambin, 2008). Here, too, many questions remain unresolved, and causative patterns are uncertain. As research in landscape history and oral testimony has shown, forest–population–land-use dynamics in West and Central Africa are not all one-way. The interactions of settlement, soil use, farming, fire, animals and local institutional arrangements have led to processes of forest advance and biodiversity enrichment as well as decline, over overlapping temporal and spatial scales (see Fairhead and Leach, 1996, 1998). These land-use dynamics, often overlooked and obscured within scientific and policy convictions that one-way deforestation is under way, raise new and as yet little-researched questions about interactions with disease and vector ecology.

For instance, both Ebola and Lassa are most common in the forest-savanna ecotone. Denys et al (2005) in Guinea find that the rat species causing Lassa (*Mastomys natalensis*) is found only in houses in the southern part of the forest-savanna ecotone, but in all habitats in the northern part. The south is associated with higher Lassa incidence. They relate this to the fact that *natalensis* cannot survive in forest so in forest villages there is more intense circulation of viral loads. In contrast in the north *natalensis* is more dispersed across savanna landscapes and also competes with a second, non-Lassa carrying species, *Mastomys erythroleucus*. If, as landscape history studies would suggest, population growth and increased intensity of farming in the forest-savanna ecotone lead to extension of woody vegetation in savanna and the expansion of forest 'islands' around villages (Fairhead and Leach, 1996), then this could over time lead to reduced competition and an increase in *Mastomys natalensis* and Lassa viral load in villages further north.

Identifying such ecosystem–disease interactions more precisely could, in turn, inform ecosystem-based interventions to address disease. This research has the possibility to dissolve the separation between a disease, such as Ebola, that has been predominantly viewed as intermittently epidemic, and one such as Lassa, that has come to be seen as endemic, by providing tools for assessing both the short- and long-term drivers of disease within the same social-ecological frame. Notions of 'integrated vector management' and of habitat ecology interventions to address malaria are of this kind, and form part of a growing body of work on ecohealth (Lebel, 2003). However, to date the research has not been done to inform how such interventions might be constructed for haemorrhagic fevers.

Investigating these social–land-use–ecosystem interactions requires multi-disciplinary approaches that draw on forms of knowledge and understanding not included in any of the three narratives we considered earlier. The relevant conceptual terrain thus comes to combine environmental science (ecology, natural history, climate science) with social science (anthropology, history) in new transdisciplinary approaches.

There are also key roles for local and popular knowledge in elucidating long-term dynamics, not just of the body and of disease as in narrative three, but of local ecology and history. Rather than rely on expert-led assessments of socio-environmental dynamics, one might ask, for instance, how people living in haemorrhagic fever-prone areas themselves frame processes of ecological and land-use change, and their interactions with human health; how they conceptualize vectors and their interactions, and what metaphors they use in understanding these. Going further than the 'community participation' urged in many ecohealth approaches (e.g. Lebel, 2003), such work could take inspiration both from studies of local environmental knowledge and its challenging of dominant scientific narratives of landscape change (e.g. Fairhead and Leach, 1996; Leach and Mearns, 1996), and from the 'local culture matters' narrative of disease outbreaks outlined earlier. Combining these could yield alternative, locally relevant ecology–disease narratives that could in turn support response pathways geared to local sustainability goals.

To the extent that scientific research and international discussion focus on long-term socio-environmental dynamics, most work attempts to pin them down: to bring long-term shifts into a realm where they can be understood and controlled. Thus as a medical scientist in the WHO put it, 'there is value in putting a risk index on this shifting situation; science is needed, and scenarios' (interview, Geneva, July 2008). The assumption is that ignorance can be transformed into more calculable and manageable forms of uncertainty and risk, and with this, greater control achieved.

But in some areas, at least, ongoing ignorance may be the reality. Full predictability and control of non-linear ecosystem shifts and people's interactions may be an illusory goal, with the possibility of surprise ever present. Strategies may therefore need to focus on robustness – designing flexible adaptive response to long-term shifts as a complement to the resilience to short-term shocks already provided by narratives two and three's strategies. Devising such strategies for robustness around ecosystem–health dynamics currently represents a frontier area. Possible elements might include what Kilbourne (1996) terms 'holistic epidemiology' – widened to include historical ecology, cultural economy and local knowledge – and institutional arrangements to link it with strategies that enable communities to adapt and adjust land use. They include conceiving of policy and response over a larger temporal and spatial scale than 'the outbreak', to track and be positioned to respond to processes that increase threat and vulnerability. It also requires a broader set of actors and networks, linking those with a focus on epidemics alone to those involved with broader environment, development and health systems processes. What is envisaged, then, may not be a major new, enlarged global infrastructure aimed at 'controlling' long-term dynamics, but a network of actors who can address these in a more flexible, inclusive and participatory way.

Conclusions

Each of these narratives – of global outbreak, of local disease event requiring external response, of local knowledge and cultural logics, and of long-term socio-environmental dynamics – thus constructs haemorrhagic fevers in different ways. They pick out different temporal and spatial scales; they use and validate different kinds of knowledge, and they assign cause, blame and vulnerability differently. Each suggests somewhat different pathways of response, involving different combinations of actors.

Elements of each of the narratives outlined in this chapter must undoubtedly contribute to the vital task of addressing haemorrhagic fevers in the decades to come, underlining the need for further elaboration of the kind of understanding and strategy implied by each. Yet this chapter has also highlighted problematic conflicts between them, shaped by institutional and political pressures, and by the operation of power. The differences in the framing of Ebola and Lassa fevers, as respectively epidemic and endemic, highlight the effects of a bias at the global institutional level towards identifying and responding to short-term shocks as opposed to long-term drivers. Thus global and rapid response outbreak narratives, and their central biomedical and epidemiological precepts, have dominated the powerful international apparatus that orchestrates haemorrhagic fever responses. These have often conflicted with the narratives of people living with the disease, resulting in perceived abuses of rights and local resistance that has undermined responses. Yet field experience also shows the potential for narratives recognizing that local knowledge and perspectives matter to be drawn into responses, shaping approaches, goals and technology use so as to render them more effective, sustainable and socially just. A key challenge for the future is to ensure that these complementarities and forms of integration are sustained, even as institutional pressures favour top-down, globally and security-framed outbreak responses.

We have also seen the disjuncture between outbreak narratives that focus on short-term disease risks, aimed at building stable and resilient responses to them, and the kind of long-term environmental and social dynamics highlighted by the fourth narrative. Taking the latter seriously has implications for programme appraisal and design, suggesting the need to move beyond a reliance on risk assessment and rapid response to a more strategic adaptive learning approach. It has implications for response mechanisms and their entry points – suggesting alternatives grounded in broader health system-building, or via ecosystems and land management. It has implications for monitoring and indicators of success, suggesting the need to understand long-term drivers of change in context and to link development interventions more broadly to improving the resilience/robustness of people and places to both existing and potential vulnerabilities to haemorrhagic fevers. And there are implications for surveillance – especially towards rethinking approaches to be more inclusive, adaptive and responsive in the increasingly likely conditions of disease persistence, multiplying 'hot spots' and increased frequency of outbreaks.

Finally, a key challenge involves connecting the insights and implications of the 'local knowledge and culture matters' narrative, with narratives focused on long-term socio-ecological dynamics. Thus far, the latter have, as we have seen, tended to be top-down – with current discourses around climate change and infectious disease featuring in new forms of globally driven intervention that threaten to ride roughshod over local concerns. When locally grounded, understandings and interventions tend to be dominated by the formal science disciplines of epidemiology and ecology. Including insights from long-standing work on cultural ecology and ethno-ecology, and placing a concern with local framings more firmly within the emerging field of ecohealth, may help generate more inclusive, acceptable and robust approaches to dealing with haemorrhagic fevers in fast-changing social and ecological systems.

Notes

1   This in turn can be seen as part of a much longer-established tradition of 'plague writing' in English literature, extending back at least as far as Defoe's 1665 journal of the plague in London (Healy 2003).

Chapter 4

SARS, China and Global Health Governance

Gerald Bloom[1]

Introduction

For a number of months early in the 21st century an atypical viral pneumonia dominated the world's headlines. Severe Acute Respiratory Syndrome (SARS) emerged in southern China in late 2002. By August 2003 it had caused 8422 cases and 916 deaths in 32 countries (WHO, 2003). After a short delay, the governments of affected countries and the international community mobilized a major response, which successfully contained the outbreak (Abraham, 2005). Despite the modest number of deaths and its short duration, the outbreak generated a lot of media attention and a great deal of concern that it might be the killer pandemic which so many scientific articles, future scenarios, novels and films had anticipated.

Once the epidemic was controlled it largely disappeared from public consciousness, but its influence lived on in the form of competing narratives and their influence on the direction of development of national and international health systems. These narratives were constructed by different actors to explain the course of the outbreak. They reflected a combination of different types of knowledge, including biomedical and scientific, and the understandings and interests of the stakeholders who created them. This paper explores these competing narratives as a way to gain insights into how health development pathways of response are understood and constructed. It focuses in particular on the impact of the outbreak in China, where it originated, and where responses to the epidemic had a profound effect on the shaping of that nation's domestic and foreign health policy.

The SARS outbreak has achieved iconic status in the public health community as an outbreak that was controlled by an effective public health response. The overarching story of 'a big epidemic which might have been' played an important role in convincing China's policy-makers to take national health reform seriously and in motivating key actors in the global health community to invest resources and political capital in building international capacity to respond to potential epidemics. The SARS outbreak illustrates the high political cost to a national government of the possibility of being seen to respond inadequately to the emergence of a new disease – and what a government will do to avoid it. It also provides an example of an effective multilateral response to a global challenge, at a time when powerful forces in the US favoured unilateralism. This chapter outlines how this narrative was strongly influenced by the understandings and interests of the key actors at national and global levels and how, in turn, the narrative influenced both the reform of China's health system and the global response to potential epidemics. The case of SARS demonstrates that the response to epidemics must be understood not simply in the context of pre-existing institutional and governance landscapes, but that outbreaks and the responses to them often re-shape those very terrains, introducing new relations, new institutions and new expectations.

There are three versions of the 'epidemic which might have been' narrative. One reflects the perspectives of international experts, the international English language media, officials of the WHO and a community of experts on global health governance. It focuses on potential clashes between, on the one hand, scientists and those seen to be acting on behalf of a scientific understanding of the public good and, on the other hand, national political leaders and bureaucrats who are portrayed as influenced by short-term benefits. It is a story about the identification by experts of a potential epidemic threat, their efforts to overcome the tendency of politicians and bureaucrats to cover up or respond slowly to threats, and actions by the WHO and the international media to ensure there was a rapid response.

Another version reflects the perspectives of a policy network of Chinese Ministry of Health officials and health system researchers, who were seeking greater support by the political leadership for health system change and of reformist government officials and analysts of China's development experience, whose focus was on the need to establish rules-based systems to influence the performance of weak local administrations. It is a story about the successful containment of the epidemic through an effective response by the Chinese government, after a relatively short delay.

The sub-text of both versions is the attempt by a major organization (the WHO or the Chinese state) to adapt to a rapidly changing context and win political legitimacy. The WHO is seeking to create a niche for itself amongst a number of health-related organizations by building a reputation for scientific expertise and leadership in responding to global health challenges. China's party state is constructing the institutions of a modern, science-based economy in the most populous country in the world. The powerful shaping story of an organization identifying and responding effectively to the major threat that SARS represented played an important role in building the legitimacy of both.

A third version of this narrative tells of a growing partnership between these organizations in confronting national and global challenges.

Other narratives have much less prominence. One is that the epidemic might have been controlled without the major economic disruption which did, in fact, occur. Another is the unstated fear of what might have happened if SARS had spread to localities and countries with poorly organized health systems and where people had impaired immunity due to malnutrition and infection with other organisms, thereby amplifying the pandemic. The following sections trace the development of the different narratives and link them to the actors who played an important role in constructing them. They draw on existing accounts of the outbreak in the social science and political science literatures, as well as the author's long personal experience of research into health systems and governance in China.

Context

The SARS outbreak occurred at a time of great change and contention in global economics and politics and of growing engagement by the international community in health-related issues. A number of scientific publications raised the possibility of the emergence of a new pathogen that could trigger a major pandemic (McMichael, 2001; Weiss, 2001). Several contextual factors were particularly important influences on the response to SARS.

The first factor was the growing recognition that international boundaries are porous and national well-being is linked to that of other countries. The threat of epidemic disease is one of a number of potential threats. The interest in security was greatly amplified in the aftermath of the attacks on the World Trade Centre in New York in 2001 and the associated fear of bioterrorism. Abraham (2005) recognizes this context in labelling SARS as the first epidemic of the post 9/11 world and points out that it took place during the initial phase of the war in Iraq. The intensity of the media interest may have reflected the heightened concern about security.

The second factor was the vision of a unipolar world then favoured by the US government. That country was leading a war in Iraq with only minimal support from global governance arrangements and it would not engage with several global initiatives, including the response to the threat of climate change. Newspapers were reporting significant tension between the Secretary General of the United Nations and the US government (*LA Times*, 2002; UN Wire, 2002). At the same time, a variety of views about new forms of global governance were emerging.

The third factor was the growing international awareness of the challenges of ill-health and the efforts by the WHO to redefine its role. Since the

LIVERPOOL JOHN MOORES UNIVERSITY
LEARNING SERVICES

publication of the Alma-Ata Declaration in the late 1970s (WHO, 1978), the WHO had faced growing challenges to its pre-eminent position. The World Bank built its expertise in health systems development and by the late 1990s was managing a substantial portfolio of health projects and playing a leadership role in multi-agency support to a number of Ministries of Health. A number of bilateral government agencies, large international NGOs and new charitable foundations had established important global roles. Meanwhile the WHO was in the midst of initiatives to recover its leadership position. In 2000 its Director General commissioned a high profile body to produce a report on Macroeconomics and Health (WHO, 2001), which was followed by national reports aimed at influencing policy. The organization was also returning to one of its original mandates of overseeing surveillance of infectious disease and coordinating international responses. This was stimulated by perceived failings of the global response to the spread of HIV and by new scientific understandings of the role of zoonoses as a source of human infection. Fidler (2004) argues that SARS occurred at a critical time in the creation of an international capacity to respond to potential epidemic outbreaks and illustrated the importance of global governance in addressing this kind of problem.

The fourth factor was the changes taking place in China, the epicentre of the outbreak. Since the early 1980s China had been managing a successful transition to a market economy associated with rapid economic growth. By the late 1990s, policy-makers were becoming increasingly aware of the need for action to address growing social inequality and perceived failures of the social sector, including health. The SARS outbreak coincided with the coming to power of a new leadership committed to addressing these problems. As we shall see, the SARS outbreak would have a marked impact on the attitudes to public health of these policy-makers.

Finally, the fifth factor was China's changing role in the global economy and changing image in the international media. In 1997 the ending of British colonial rule in Hong Kong was a major story in the English language media. The spread of SARS to Hong Kong and other communities of the Chinese diaspora highlighted the existence of a network of communities with links to China. In 2001 China joined the World Trade Organization, a symbolic statement of China's growing links to the global economy. The enormity of the changes taking place entered the consciousness of the American and British media in 2005 with the purchase of two iconic companies, IBM and Rover, by Chinese companies. The reporting of the SARS outbreak by the English language media reflected this growing awareness of China as important, mysterious and somewhat threatening.

Science, global public goods and health governance

This section outlines the dominant international narrative, which emphasized the role of scientists as objective advisers on global public health and
of the WHO as a potential source of political legitimacy for action. It draws
on a recent book by Fidler (2004), which recounts the story of SARS as
a conflict between the global public interest and the narrow national and
political interest of the Chinese government, which withheld information on
the outbreak. Fidler presents this episode as a major turning point in global
health governance, suggesting that global responses to epidemics have been
hampered by the 'Westphalian' approach, which gives priority to national
sovereignty at the expense of the global public. He then characterizes
SARS as the 'first post-Westphalian' epidemic in which the WHO played
an important role in ensuring that all countries provided accurate reports
on the outbreak and mobilizing a rapid response. This narrative presents the
shared understanding that a group of global health policy-makers, relying
on expert scientific advice, gained about the SARS outbreak, and their
subsequent response to the epidemic. It places the WHO at the centre of
the effort, granting it a major coordinating role amongst a largely tractable
group of member nations motivated to cooperate in the interests of both
national and, importantly, global health and security (Fidler, 2004).

The first case of SARS is believed to have occurred in Foshan City,
Guangdong Province, in November 2002. This was soon followed by a
number of cases of atypical pneumonia and the provincial health authorities issued a confidential report on them in January 2003. According to
Chinese law at that time, the provincial authorities were not obliged to report
the outbreak to higher levels. Despite efforts to control information flow and
avoid the negative consequences of a health scare, the news spread through
the internet and mobile telephones; the following telephone text message was
forwarded 126 million times between 8 and 10 February: 'There is a fatal flu
in Guangzhou.' Stories began to appear in the local media and there was a
rise in public concern. The WHO made its first official request to the Chinese
government for information on this outbreak on 10 February. The next day
the government reported that the outbreak was under control (Fidler, 2004).

But the virus spread quickly to other countries. A professor of neph-
rology from Guangdong visited Hong Kong in February and transmitted
the infection to several people staying at his hotel. They subsequently
travelled to Hong Kong, Hanoi, Singapore and Toronto, where outbreaks
followed. In Hanoi, the illness was identified as a new disease by Dr Carlo
Urbani, a WHO epidemiologist who subsequently died of the disease. On
12 March, the WHO issued a global alert about cases of a new atypical
pneumonia which was followed three days later by a statement from the

Director General that SARS had become a worldwide health threat. Within a week the WHO had launched a global scientific effort to identify the SARS pathogen, involving 11 laboratories in ten countries. Epidemiological evidence collected from the outbreaks in Canada, Hong Kong and Vietnam soon suggested a common origin in Guangdong Province. The WHO sent a team to China to help the Chinese authorities investigate the Guangdong outbreak, but their visit was delayed. By late March, the WHO reported that a coronavirus had been identified as the causative pathogen. The epidemics continued to spread in Canada and Hong Kong (Fidler, 2004).

The situation in China remained unclear. The government provided information on the spread of SARS to other provinces, but by the end of March, it had still not agreed to a visit by the WHO team to Guangdong. In early April, the WHO issued an advisory recommending that people planning to go to Hong Kong or Guangdong Province consider postponing non-essential travel. Shortly thereafter a Chinese doctor publicly accused the Chinese government of covering up a major SARS outbreak in Beijing and the story received intensive coverage by the international media. With unease amongst both the Chinese population and the international community growing, the WHO became increasingly insistent that the government provide full disclosure about the size of the problem. For a few days the WHO itself became the major source of reliable information on the Chinese outbreak. Eventually, the Minister of Health was dismissed and the Deputy Prime Minister took charge of the response to SARS. China then implemented a highly organized campaign, which included the identification and isolation of suspected cases and controls on travel. Chinese television began to provide daily information on the state of the epidemic. By the end of June, China's epidemic had subsided (Fidler, 2004).

The English language media played a significant role in framing international understanding of the epidemic. Their stories expressed the fear that the epidemic could have a major impact on populations in Europe and North America. SARS had become a major political issue in Canada, which was experiencing an outbreak, and other countries were also concerned. A number of stories presented the outbreak as a major global threat and focused on heroes, who acted bravely in the face of danger from a virus or from political and bureaucratic forces. Some reports drew parallels between the Chernobyl accident and the SARS outbreak, linking the latter to the drama of the ending of the Soviet Union (Goldgeir, 2003; *Time Magazine*, 2003). This, in turn, was part of a wider narrative of the emergence of a unipolar world dominated by the US. Some even spoke of an empire, which would act, to some extent, in the global public good. The underlying framing of these stories was of a major challenge thrown up by nature to which an agreed scientific response was needed to protect all humanity, with a particular focus on the residents of the advanced market economies (for an analysis of the 'global outbreak narrative', see Wald, 2008; and narrative one in Leach and Hewlett, this volume). Advocates of global public health governance used such concerns about shared global threats – and the potential for shared public goods – raised by the SARS outbreak to illustrate the need for a multilateral approach.

This narrative must be understood within the wider context of growing efforts to reform global governance of infectious disease (Fidler, 2004). Framed by the interests and understandings of a large group of policy-makers, epidemiologists, health ministers and officers of NGOs and charities, this narrative draws on the concept of global public goods to lend legitimacy to comprehensive, multilateral and top-down approaches to managing epidemics that are seen to threaten the global community. Efforts by such actors to reform the architecture of global health governance based on the concept of public good date to the 1990s (Kaul et al, 1999). During the same period, the international community became involved in co-funding health services in low income countries. One form this took was so-called 'sector-wide approaches', in which several donor agencies reached a multi-year agreement with the host government to implement a health system development plan. Another was the creation of the Global Fund to Fight AIDS, Tuberculosis and Malaria to finance disease-specific interventions. At the same time non-state actors, advocacy groups, large charitable foundations and large non-government service delivery organizations took on new and more important roles than they had previously held (Lee, 2003b). Meanwhile, the health problems of low-income countries were given much greater publicity in the advanced market economies. Political leaders of the latter countries made public commitments to support efforts to address these problems including the highly public agreement of the G8 in July 2005, which included major commitments to address health problems in Africa. They also faced pressure to protect their population from the spread of disease to their own country. The combination of empathy and generosity with guilt and fear had an important influence on the response by governments of these countries to a perceived threat of an epidemic.

Meanwhile, there was growing scientific concern about the possible emergence of new infectious diseases. The WHO had established the Global Outbreak Alert and Response Network (GOARN) in 1997 to collect and analyse information from both government and non-government sources. Amongst other things, it used search engines to mine information sources for indications of a new outbreak. By 2003, the American Institute of Medicine issued a report calling attention to emerging infectious diseases as possible global security threats and advocating strengthening the capacity for a coordinated global response (Institute of Medicine, 2003). According to David Heyman, former Executive Director of Communicable Diseases at the WHO, the SARS outbreak provided GOARN with its first major success story, showing it to be a coordinating centre appropriate to the new mixed institutional landscape and capable of responding to major threats to global health (Fidler, 2004).

The core of this narrative is the confrontation between the WHO and the Chinese state. Under existing international law China was under no obligation to report the outbreak. But the Chinese government eventually engaged with the international community and retreated from a stance based on national sovereignty, because of the new institutional developments in global health governance of which GOARN is an exemplar. According to this telling of the story, the outcome of the confrontation between the WHO and the government of China was the recognition that aspects of the response to outbreaks must transcend the principle of national sovereignty. For example, a precedent was set establishing the de facto right of the WHO to issue travel advisories based on the best scientific advice, despite the economic harm this could cause to states. According to Fidler, this represented a shift of power from nation states to global governance structures – a sharp move towards new post-Westphalian governance arrangements (Fidler, 2004).

At one level the story is a reminder of the biological reality that dense transport networks, which speed the spread of new pathogens across national boundaries, make rapid global responses necessary. A World Health Report on public health security uses the example of SARS to illustrate the impact of an effective response and the potential consequences of a failed one (WHO, 2007a). However, this narrative relies on accepting some implicit assumptions that may be contested. First, it implies the prior existence of an international legal order, the so-called Westphalian system, that fully respected national sovereignty. But such a supposed system is contradicted by the reality of frequent cross-border military interventions, the use of a variety of mechanisms to influence economic policies (including so-called 'conditionalities' in many World Bank loan agreements with low-income countries), and support for action to change 'rogue' regimes. Once the Westphalian ideal has been called into question, any narrative based on a so-called post-Westphalian model loses some traction.

Second, its concept of global governance suggests an uncontested understanding of the public good. In this view, the WHO represents a public good in its function as a repository of expert knowledge to be used in the fight against a deadly pathogen that threatens us all. The example of the emergence, rapid spread and eventual isolation of a new pathogen provides a strong case for this view of global governance. However, the situation is rarely so clear and there are many legitimate differences in understandings about the potential costs and benefits of alternative actions. For example,

Smith (2006) draws attention to the high economic cost of the response to SARS and of the important influence on this response of public perceptions of risk. This points to an inevitable trade-off between the biological estimates of risk and the cost of response (overall and for different groups of people). This is essentially a political judgement. In practice, the legitimacy of the WHO rests, to a large extent, on the representative nature of the World Health Assembly. In the case of SARS, it would appear that the Chinese government viewed the WHO as a source of objective scientific information. However, we have limited information on the degree to which the WHO is viewed, more generally, by opinion leaders in different countries as a source of international legitimacy for public health governance.

Third, it implies that the big story concerned the initial acknowledgement of the significance of the outbreak and the rapid identification of the new organism, and it says much less about the capacity of countries to organize an effective public health response. The following section shifts the focus from the WHO to one in which the Chinese state is the central player.

Building China's regulatory state

At the height of the SARS crisis, several articles in the international media drew an analogy between the outbreak in China and Chernobyl, in the former Soviet Union, where a nuclear accident contributed to a crisis of legitimacy, which eventually led to a change in regime. Some analysts have questioned this analogy, suggesting instead that the SARS crisis most probably strengthened the state and, in particular, the legitimacy of the leaders who had come to power shortly before the outbreak (Saich, 2006). Several explanations can account for China's delayed response to SARS. For one thing, the outbreak occurred during a major leadership transition, when senior political leaders were focusing on consolidating their position. Political priority was given to social stability and economic growth at this time and discouraged local officials from disclosing information that could create a panic. Finally, the Chinese Ministry of Health did not previously have the authority to require local government leaders to disclose potentially deleterious information. Furthermore, an initial belief by local government officials that this was an outbreak of avian influenza, which would lead to large culls of domestic flocks with major local economic consequences, may also have led them to conceal information (Kaufman, 2006). Once it recognized that SARS was in fact a new disease, combined with action by whistle blowers and the international media, a growing public unease, and the pressure of the WHO, the Chinese government eventually altered its stance (Saich, 2006). Having recognized the seriousness of the

situation, political leaders then mobilized an effective response, which led
to a rapid result.

SARS can accordingly be understood as a chapter in the history of efforts
by the Chinese leadership to manage a transition to a market economy and
construct appropriate institutional arrangements in a context of very rapid
change (Saich, 2006). These changes include urbanization, large population movements, rapid industrialization, demographic transition and an
explosive growth in the density of transportation and information linkages. Organizations formed during the era of the command economy faced
major challenges in adapting to this new reality (North, 2005). It is possible
to draw a parallel between China in the early 21st century and the US a
century earlier, when a series of scandals and government responses led to
the gradual construction of a regulatory state, based on rules-based institutional arrangements to support an advanced market economy (Yang, 2004;
Tsai, 2007). This story of gradual transformation and institution-building
is becoming an important narrative for understanding the current phase of
China's transition from a command to a market economy. It is also a nationalist story of the emergence of China as a modern and increasingly powerful
international actor.

The SARS outbreak occurred at a turning point in China's development. The political leadership had been managing a transition to a market
economy for over 20 years, through a combination of radical devolution of
economic decision-making to local governments, individual enterprises and
households, and retention of strong political control. This was associated
with rapid economic growth, but was accompanied by growing inequalities
between successful and less successful localities. Also, the creation of institutional arrangements to regulate complex relationships between organizations lagged behind the development of those organizations (see Tsai,
2007; also Yang, 2004 for the gradual creation of rules-based systems in the
financial sector and Meessen and Bloom, 2007 and Bloom et al, 2008a for a
description of a similar process in the health sector). One expression of the
problems in the health sector was a series of scandals concerning the safety
of medical products and the cost and quality of medical care. Prior to the
late 1990s the government often tried to cover them up, but this became less
and less possible as channels of information proliferated.

One important aspect of China's management of economic transition
has been its substantial devolution of government functions. In the health
sector, this meant that each level of government was responsible for its
'own' health facilities. Higher levels of government had limited means to
influence the performance of local health facilities other than through the
power of higher-level Communist Party members to control the appointment of local government leaders. Local government leaders had strong

incentives to suppress information that they felt might damage the reputation of their county or themselves. By the late 1990s, the central government was making a substantial effort to alter the balance and make local governments more accountable for their performance. This included an opening-up of opportunities for researchers and journalists to identify and publicize problems (Zhang et al, forthcoming).

Health rose up the political agenda through the 1990s (Wang, 2008). The initial source of pressure for change came from health facilities, which were struggling to meet the rising expectations of their employees without commensurate increases in their government budgets. A series of research studies documented the growing problems of the health sector (Meng et al, 2004; Eggleston et al, 2006). Public concern about the rapidly rising cost of medical care and its quality and safety grew over time. In late 1996 the Ministry of Health convened a national conference which identified a number of problems and agreed a broad reform agenda. The next year the central government issued a policy document, which supported major reforms (State Council, 1997). Implementation was constrained because the political leadership continued to prioritize economic growth. The central government was also concerned that some local governments would not use any additional funds to improve their health services.

A general perception had taken hold that health facilities were overstaffed, charged unfair informal fees and encouraged excessive use of pharmaceuticals. This was associated with a more general concern about ethics and the need to make public services more accountable. The Communist Party and local representative bodies made anti-corruption a major political priority. In the late 1990s they began to focus on so-called 'unprofessional behaviour', such as the demands for under-the-counter payments from patients and kickbacks from pharmaceutical suppliers (Fang, 2008). Health facilities were asked to sign agreements to uphold ethical standards and their performance was monitored through periodic visits, public opinion surveys and offices to which people could report complaints. The most dramatic illustration of this growing concern to regulate the quality and safety of the health system took place in 2007, several years after the SARS outbreak, with the conviction and sentencing to death of the head of the Food and Drug Administration on charges of corruption. These anti-corruption measures set the stage for more systematic efforts to establish rules-based institutional arrangements in health and other sectors.

By the beginning of the 21st century, the Chinese media regularly reported the problems of poor rural residents and policy-makers were drawing attention to these problems (Wang, 2008). They published stories on education, medical care and housing for poor people, which they characterized as 'the three burdens on the shoulders of the people'. This was occurring in the lead-up to the Sixteenth Congress of the Communist Party at which a major change in government leadership was anticipated. In November 2002, Hu Jintao took over as President and said he would lead a reorientation of government priorities.

The focus of political leaders during late 2002 was on the Sixteenth Congress of the Communist Party and the change in leadership. This transition was completed in March 2003 at the two-week meeting of the National People's Congress. The new government announced a major policy shift in favour of the construction of a 'Harmonious Society' which gave greater priority to spreading the benefits of development and strengthening the social sector, including health. In late 2002 the government launched two new health financing schemes: the new cooperative medical system (NCMS) established county-level health insurance to be financed jointly by household contributions and budgetary allocations by both central and local governments, and medical financial assistance allocated public funds to subsidize medical care for very poor people. The government decision to earmark funds for rural health services represented a major policy change. Implementation began in a small number of pilot counties and spread rapidly and NCMS became a visible sign of the government's commitment to take the concerns of rural people seriously (Zhang et al, forthcoming).

SARS emerged in the midst of these changes. The delay in responding to the outbreak and the perceived cover-up led to an erosion of trust and threatened to lead to panic. This was particularly threatening at a time of leadership change. However, the rapidity and effectiveness of the response quickly restored calm. The government used well-established management systems for setting targets, organizing a top-down response, mobilizing the population to both identify and isolate people who might be infected, and restricting travel (Kaufman, 2006). The Deputy Prime Minister took charge of the response, giving it a very high political profile. Public statements by the political leaders described the response to SARS with metaphors harking back to the period of the mass mobilization, command economy (Saich, 2006). This reinforced the narrative of a party state drawing on a long-established capacity to respond to major challenges. When the crisis was over, the government implemented two initiatives to strengthen its capacity to mount similar responses in the future. It renamed the existing chain of outbreak response stations Centres for Disease Control, strengthened the national disease surveillance system and funded the construction of many new buildings for the county centres for disease control. These initiatives reflected the perspectives of a top-down organization, which wanted accurate information and facilities to house a greatly expanded public health bureaucracy. They also responded to successful lobbying by the programme for epidemic disease control to take on this new role and secure additional funding.

This narrative views SARS as a shock, which empowered a new political leadership to consolidate its authority and accelerate its reform agenda. The government had already indicated a shift in policy in favour of health system development and reform and had launched new rural health financing programmes. However, it faced great difficulties in translating these programmes into substantial improvements in poor rural areas. Some senior Chinese health policy analysts told the author that the location of the outbreak in Beijing had an important influence (personal communication). Government officials and leaders themselves had to live for several weeks with the fear of a major epidemic, facing serious travel restrictions, frequent body temperature monitoring and the possibility of compulsory quarantine. Then the powerful Deputy Prime Minister took over the response and raised the political profile of health, sending a powerful message to both the general population and these government officials. The government soon called for a rapid expansion of the rural health insurance schemes and by 2008, almost all counties had established a scheme and the central government had very substantially increased its financial contribution to them. The government allocated a significant amount of money for an existing disease prevention bureaucracy to construct a surveillance system and network of buildings (Wang et al, 2008). The government also made it clear to local politicians that they would face serious consequences if they failed to report an outbreak. This underlined the political priority now given to health and reinforced the role of the Ministry of Health.

Chinese government ministers were eager to promulgate a narrative about SARS that conveyed a vision of a highly organized bureaucratic response, well controlled by a centralized government. In reality, the management of institutional change and development in a complex and highly devolved sector represented a major challenge for the government. If the SARS outbreak had unfolded somewhat differently – and the Chinese government not been so successful in controlling the outbreak – the government would have faced serious problems. For example, if SARS had spread, it would have found it difficult to enforce compulsory hospitalization, unless it had also agreed to finance all treatment. Also, several years after the new county centres for disease control were completed, county governments had not substantially increased the budgets of their public health programmes and the government had not defined how counties would establish priorities and design programmes. Despite the strong rhetoric of health system reform which the government narrative around SARS put forward, the effective impact on public health services of investments made in response to the narrative of the 'epidemic which might have been' was disappointing.

An alternative narrative to the view of reform as a combination of large public investments and the top-down implementation of new organizational arrangements focuses on public attitudes to health service providers and the need to build trust. It emphasizes incentives, motivations, understandings and ethics, and the role of government and other agencies in establishing and enforcing rules and ethical standards. It reflects the views of senior politicians, Communist Party officials focusing on combating corruption, the media and a growing advertising industry. In 2005, the Development Research Centre of the State Council, a source of policy advice to the highest political level, published a report (DRC, 2005), which highlighted these problems and called for a radical change in policy. It pointed out that perverse financial incentives were contributing to rapid rises in health-care costs and that sickness had become a major cause of the descent of households into poverty. This report led to much greater coverage in the mass media of problems and abuses in local health services. It also led to high profile attacks on doctors by political leaders. In 2009 the government made a further commitment to allocate a fixed amount of money per person to public health services. It now faces the challenge of defining the health problems to be addressed and ensuring that local governments provide effective services.

The SARS episode illustrated the growth of information sources in China, which now include the mass media, mobile telephones, a variety of websites (which became an important source of SARS jokes) and the international media. These information flows contributed to national conversations about the kind of risk that SARS posed and the efficacy of government action – influencing both personal responses and attitudes to government. In response to the increasing importance of consumer choice and the influence of a facility's reputation on government decisions, health facilities have been showing a growing interest in strategies to win the trust of the community and build their reputation through posting pictures of staff, establishing telephone complaint lines, commercial advertising and so forth. These measures illustrate the growing importance of public attitudes and opinions to the performance of China's health system and the ongoing work of building new social contracts within which to embed health systems (Bloom et al, 2008b).

One can anticipate continuing tension between efforts by the central government to control information flow, lead health system reform and establish an effective regulatory framework and the ongoing efforts to strengthen mechanisms of local accountability for the use of public funds and the expansion of communication channels. On the one hand, scandals and the exposure of problems threaten the legitimacy of the regime, but on the other hand, effective responses and the gradual creation of effective regulation and accountability mechanisms reinforce its legitimacy. New institutions will be constructed out of this tension. Top-down management and regulatory systems, market-like mechanisms for building and maintaining reputations and the active participation of local account-ability mechanisms and the media are likely to co-exist in the institutional arrangements that emerge. The dominant narrative which emphasizes the creation of highly organized bureaucratic organizations tends to obscure an alternative narrative that emphasizes the need to build institutions that make providers of health services more accountable for their performance and build trust in health facilities and the government officials who oversee them (Bloom et al, 2008c).

China engages in global governance

This chapter began with a story about the WHO and global govern-ance in epidemic outbreaks and then explored China's efforts to build its response capacity. The first narrative suggested the emergence of a 'post-Westphalian' international order, which seemed to imply the prior existence of an order based on national sovereignty. It emphasized the need to set limits on national sovereignty without addressing how power relations have influenced decision-making at the international level. The second narrative focused on the emergence of a strong regulatory state in China. This section outlined a narrative in which the response to SARS is seen to presage new international governance relationships, in which a strong Chinese state will play an increasingly important role.

One of the most dramatic outcomes of the crisis was the appointment of Margaret Chan, who led Hong Kong's response to SARS, as Director General of the World Health Organization, and her subsequent decision to make global public health security the topic of her first World Health Report (WHO, 2007a). She is the first Chinese citizen to lead a major inter-national organization.

In April 2003, immediately after China acknowledged the magnitude of the SARS outbreak, Wen Jiabao, the newly appointed Premier, attended a special ASEAN Summit to discuss SARS. He affirmed that the Chinese government gave high priority to its response to SARS, making health the subject of his first major diplomatic mission. According to Lee et al (2009), Wen's quick engagement with the international community on health-related issues was part of a concerted effort by the government to adjust its traditionally defensive stance towards the outside world. Modifying a long-standing concern to protect China's national sovereignty from outside interference at all costs, this new approach was calculated to encourage cooperation with the international community for access to finance and expertise to help strengthen the Chinese health system. It also reflected a growing awareness that some problems were in their very nature trans-national, requiring international cooperation for a successful resolution. And finally, China's leaders hoped to build the country's image as a respon-sible state, countering the economic and political impact of scandals that might damage China's reputation.[2]

China has been building its relationships with international organiza-tions for many years. Jacobson and Oksenberg (1990) document how the government used these relationships to support its management of transi-tion and reposition itself in the international community. Bloom et al (2009) describe a strategic partnership between the Ministry of Health, the World Bank and the UK Department for International Development, to imple-ment a ten-year rural health development and reform project, which began in 1997. The government used the project to test new ideas from abroad and the project implementers used their partnership with international agencies to strengthen their hand in negotiating with county governments about their implementation of the project and of health system reforms. The World Bank, on the other hand, highly valued its role as an international repository of expertise on health system development and provider of tech-nical advice to the government of China. China is now an important actor in the World Bank, whose chief economist is Chinese. Its changing rela-tionship with the World Bank illustrates the symbiotic relationship that has emerged between the Chinese government and the leadership of a number of international organizations.

According to this third narrative, the SARS crisis provided a forum in which the Chinese state and the WHO began to forge a new kind of relationship. Schnur (2006) describes the delicacy of this process in his discussion of the interaction between the Beijing Office of the WHO and the Chinese Ministry of Health, at a time when the former was pushing the government to accept the seriousness of the challenge and accept assist-ance in mounting an effective response. Within this narrative, China is seen to struggle to balance the need for national autonomy with a desire for a greater role on the world stage, while the WHO is beginning to learn how the changing balance of power between countries might affect its relation-ships with national governments. The discussion of the SARS outbreak in the 2007 World Health Report (WHO, 2007a) implicitly acknowledged the key role that China played in managing the response to SARS, speculating about what might have happened if there had been an outbreak in a country that could not act in such a coherent fashion:

> *Had SARS been allowed to establish a foothold in a resource-poor setting, it is doubtful whether the demanding measures, facilities and technologies needed to interrupt chains of transmission could have*

> *been fully deployed. If SARS had become permanently established as yet another indigenous epidemic threat, it is not difficult to imagine the consequences for global public health security in a world still struggling to cope with HIV/AIDS.* (WHO, 2007a, p40)

Within this third narrative, then, the construction of effective responses to new outbreaks must involve strengthening the capacity of both nation states and international organizations in new kinds of partnership. The Chinese approach to development and its response to emerging health challenges are anticipated to become increasingly influential in international policy discussions. The SARS outbreak and the appointment of Dr Chan to lead the WHO may mark an important turning point in the role of China in global health governance.

Hidden narratives

Other narratives about the SARS outbreak and its aftermath have been given much less prominence. Some policy-makers and social scientists have questioned the assumption that if the response had been inadequate, the world would have experienced a global SARS pandemic with disastrous health and economic consequences. Although this is a possible outcome, it is impossible to assess its likelihood. The response to the H5N1 avian influenza virus was based on a similar assumption that it was essential to eradicate the virus. So far, there have been a number of minor outbreaks of human disease, but no major pandemic. In several countries attempts to eradicate the virus have been unsuccessful and it looks like it is becoming endemic in some localities, with hard-to-predict consequences (Scoones and Forster, 2008). This points to the need for a more nuanced understanding of the uncertainty surrounding the risk of pandemics and of the need to acknowledge ignorance when devising strategies for response. How both uncertainty and risks are perceived can have significant impacts on the types of responses that are considered. Indeed, perceptions of relative risks can powerfully determine pathways of response. It can be argued, in retrospect, that one driver of the response to SARS was a highly emotional reaction to a perceived threat amplified by the media. This reaction may have been amplified, in some cases, by public distrust in the accuracy of government statements. One result was very high costs in lost production and trade. It will be difficult to convince the international community to respond the same way to every new threat; more reflective ways of agreeing responses and building trust in the judgements of political and scientific authorities in situations of incomplete knowledge are needed.

Another narrative concerns the much larger epidemic which might have happened if the virus had reached a population with increased vulnerability to infection (due to the co-existence of malnutrition and infection with HIV and other pathogens) and where the government had limited capacity to respond to a health challenge (Foresight, 2006; Bloom et al, 2007; see Nightingale, Edstrom and MacGregor, this volume). The response to SARS by countries with relatively well-organized government administrations provides little guidance for action in this context. One can imagine highly organized measures by national and international agencies, which might isolate an outbreak and prevent a catastrophic pandemic. However, the success of such measures would depend on both their effectiveness and the willingness of local people to accept them. There are strong political barriers to an explicit discussion of this kind of international action and the factors which might justify it and there is only limited international capacity to mount this kind of intervention. Outbreak narratives have diverted attention from the development of practical measures to improve resilience to health challenges in countries where the population has a heightened vulnerability to infection and the health system has a limited capacity to respond. Other chapters in this book address this issue.

The growing divergence between a vision of global health governance, based on the predominance of nation states coordinated by a single international agency, and an increasingly complex reality with a variety of organizations influencing national and international decision-making, most clearly applies to the poorest countries with populations most susceptible to infection. Many are ex-colonies, which were not recognized as autonomous nation states until the second half of the 20th century. The global health system reflects the legacy of colonialism in the disproportionate influence of rich donor countries over global health policy, the actions of the World Health Organization and the health policies of many low-income countries.

Many actors are now involved in decisions about the finance and organization of health services in low-income countries. There is plenty of evidence that the incoherence of international support has had a deleterious impact on health system performance. However, this is a continuation of a long-standing situation in which low-income countries have been influenced by a variety of different international actors. In this context it is difficult to identify where the old 'post-colonial' relationships end and a new 'post-Westphalian' public health regime begins. It is also difficult to predict the impact on these relationships of the emergence of China and other 'developing' countries as important global actors.

Conclusions

The SARS outbreak provided a sharp reminder of the dangers the world faces from new and unexpected diseases. The successful response provided an important counter-argument to Malthusian fatalism and despair about the capacity of international organizations to act effectively. A recent World Health Report (WHO, 2007a) has placed the need to build national and global capacities to respond to potential health emergencies on the policy agenda. The challenge is to translate a general concern into effective ways of identifying major threats, assessing their significance and mounting an effective response. This will involve, amongst other things, a clear understanding of the roles of all actors and the creation of global governance arrangements that provide a voice to all stakeholders.

The SARS outbreak and the immediate and longer-term response marked a major change in the involvement of China in global initiatives. The WHO is the first big international organization to be led by a Chinese citizen and it is conceivable that the process that began with SARS could lead to strengthening of rules-based international law concerning surveillance, reporting and responding to outbreaks of potential epidemic diseases. This would require new ways of building international agreement on rules that transcend national borders.

The SARS outbreak presages both the renewed engagement of nation states and international organizations in building effective global responses to public health challenges and the growing importance of non-state actors. It drew attention to the many actors who influence the understanding of an outbreak of a new illness and of the alternative responses. The drama was played out in a complex environment in which it was impossible to separate scientific understandings from stakeholder interests and political and geopolitical considerations. The media played an important role in raising the pressure on governments to respond to the challenge of SARS and there are indications that governments responded to this pressure. The main message from the story of SARS is the need to integrate concerns about the problems of disease into political discourse and create mechanisms the population can trust to lead a response. It also underlines the increasingly important influence of a variety of non-government organizations and information channels on every aspect of the response to new health-related challenges.

Notes

1   The author would like to acknowledge very helpful comments and suggestions by Joan Kaufman, Pei Xiaomei, Fang Jing, the editors of this volume and the participants at the workshop on epidemics organized by the STEPS Centre.
2   For example, scandals about the quality of pharmaceuticals, toys and milk products have had wide international coverage and may have influenced the global public perception of the quality and safety of Chinese goods.

Chapter 5

Constructing AIDS: Contesting Perspectives on an Evolving Epidemic

Jerker Edström

Introduction

A mysterious new disease first named 'gay-related immune deficiency' (GRID) surfaced in the US in 1981. GRID was soon renamed the Acquired Immune Deficiency Syndrome (AIDS), and a viral pathogen, the human immunodeficiency virus (HIV), was identified as its causative agent in 1983. This new illness initially affected mainly marginal groups, such as gay men and injecting drug users in San Francisco and New York or sex workers in Kinshasa. Today, HIV/AIDS is one of the main health and development challenges in large parts of sub-Saharan Africa, affecting men, women and children. Over the past 30 years, HIV/AIDS has gradually revealed itself to be much more than a health issue, with far-reaching social, political and economic implications for individuals, communities and institutions throughout the globe. At the same time, scientists and health professionals have had difficulty identifying the detailed pathways by which the virus is transmitted and designing effective ways to break the cycle of transmission, particularly in areas of high prevalence. Due to these challenging social and biomedical aspects of the disease, HIV/AIDS has been more hotly contested than perhaps any new disease in recent times.

In this chapter I reflect on how the HIV pandemic and local epidemics (sometimes settling into endemics) have been constructed and contested over the past 25 years. This is not an authoritative review of evidence or the academic literature, but rather subjective reflections garnered over many years of engagement with multiple kinds of stakeholders. As someone with a long-standing interest in both development and HIV since the mid-1980s, I eventually elbowed my own way into the melee during the mid-1990s, with a focus on 'supporting community action on AIDS in developing countries' – the strap line to the name of the International HIV/AIDS Alliance (or 'the Alliance'), which I took part in building up for just over a decade. I have thus had the relative privilege of attending and partaking in some of these debates. In this chapter, I give my impressions of how different sets of actors have tended to approach the issue. Drawing on different forms of knowledge and exhibiting differing attitudes towards uncertainty and ignorance, these actors formulate four main narratives about the HIV/AIDS epidemic, which are characterized by a respective focus on risks, vulnerabilities, threats and rights.

Framing the core problem

Fundamentally, the risk of any problem or crisis can be expressed as a function of its source, a threat (or hazard) and the vulnerability of the subject of concern, such that:

$$\text{Risk (of A)} = \text{Threat (by B)} \times \text{Vulnerability (of C)}$$

This may apply at an individual level or at more aggregate community and national levels, but the identification and description of the various elements is a matter of contention and often comes down to political choices and positions, which evolve in historical trajectories of contested narratives. The terms may at times themselves appear value laden and the analysis tends to suggest implications for rights and responsibilities within the equation – particularly when B and C are conceived of as human beings. From a health perspective HIV was initially approached in terms of 'outbreak' narratives, focused on transmission risk and safeguarding public health; from a security perspective, HIV is typically viewed as an external (societal) 'threat' of some kind, even if brought by deviant foreign bodies; from the perspective of affected citizen groups, the issue of injustice and 'rights' is often the main concern; whereas, from a development actor view, the epidemic has typically been linked to 'poverty' and – more centrally – 'vulnerability', as described in Figure 5.1.

Considering the 'angles' from which the topic is being approached can be useful in inter-relating different debates. On this 'map' the vertical Y axis would take us from a hegemonic 'North', concerned with control, status quo and order (often with conservative and top-down tendencies) to a contesting 'South', where inequality, aspiration and change are driving concerns (often with reformist, dissident, plural bottom-up perspectives). The horizontal X axis takes us from an individualist 'West', primarily concerned with freedoms and choice, towards an 'Eastern' orientation of more collective thinking and concerned with community, sustainability and balance. In this chapter, I will explore each of these four narratives in turn, as I see them having unfolded over time.

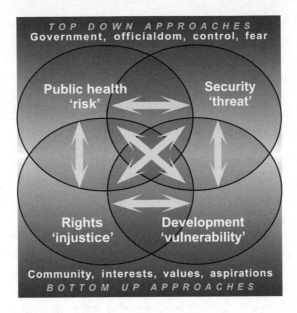

Source: Edström et al, 2006

Figure 5.1 *Four approaches to HIV*

The risk narrative: individuals and their behaviour

The first narrative that I would like to examine understands HIV in terms of individuals engaging in risky behaviour. Risky individuals, in this narrative, are social deviants whose sexual and drug-taking activities endanger themselves and those in their community. This narrative was initially driven primarily by members of the biomedical community drawing on epidemiological models of disease prevention and transmission, often riding on conservative fears over societal threats expressed in outbreak narratives of popular media in the mid-1980s. By 1987 the WHO had launched the Special Programme on AIDS (later named the Global Programme on AIDS, or GPA) and in the following year a global summit of health ministers was held in London, which focused on HIV prevention and control.

In these early years scientists and health officials commonly used the language of health risk to identify those factors, or 'disease precursors,' most likely to contribute to infection. These precursors associated with an unusually high morbidity or mortality rate, included demographic variables, individual behaviours, family and individual histories, and various physiologic changes. In the context of HIV, 'risk' has been defined as:

> *the statistical probability of becoming HIV infected through specific*
> *behaviours (e.g. sex without a condom), patterns of behaviour (e.g. sex*
> *with multiple partners) or specific situations (e.g. one sexual partner*
> *has multiple partners, but does not tell his or her regular partner)...*
> *Yet ... the methods of epidemiology have predetermined that our*
> *understanding of "risk" will be focused on individual behaviours.*
> (Mann and Tarantola, 1996, pp430–431)

The 'precursors' indeed quickly focused in on individual risk behaviours, but the specific behaviours in question had certain further consequences. The early and powerful outbreak narratives fuelled by media panic (in a receptive and morally conservative Reagan–Thatcher era of a 'return to family values') elicited initial widespread fear. In the process, emerging understandings of risk factors linked to particular sexual and drug-taking behaviours – which were broadly seen as 'marginal' – had an 'othering' effect and rapidly created stigma and discrimination against those essentially labelled as health risks. Practically, this led to individuals being categorized as threats and to subsequent attempts to reduce the supply of threats by removing them or limiting their mobility. Examples included panic over Haitian 'boat people' arriving in the US, forced quarantine for HIV-positive people in Cuba, slightly later the incarceration and intermittent executions of HIV-positive sex workers in Burma, and brothel evictions and closures in Bangladesh and Cambodia. The early construction of 'risk groups' in the US was based on the 'the four Hs' – homosexuals, hookers, heroin addicts and Haitians. In other words, we were being warned that we were dealing with 'social deviants', bad blood and immoral or dangerous people of African descent. Tellingly, the fifth H – haemophiliacs – was not generally considered a 'risk group', as they were not seen as particularly likely to pass on the virus and were instead described as 'innocent victims', or as having contracted the virus through 'no fault of their own'. This 'exemption clause' for haemophiliacs suggested that implicit in this popularized construction of risk groups was not so much the fact that they themselves faced serious health or infection risks: rather, they were seen as 'vectors of transmission' (like mosquitoes or rats in other epidemics) or some kind of health risk *incarnate* – embodied 'precursors' to potential disease in other people.

The predicable controversies over where to locate the risks shifted the debate more squarely onto specific behaviours, with several interesting results. One outcome was essentially a consensus between progressive public health experts and sexual rights activists (and others concerned with human rights) that 'supply reduction' – by criminalizing people at risk, locking them up, or restricting their mobility – was not likely to be effective.

There were many reasons, including instrumental ones such as the long window period between infection and symptomatic disease, the low uptake of HIV testing and the marginalization of those most centrally involved, that would make it more difficult to address transmission by driving risky individuals further underground. However, the earlier draconian public health reactions never fully disappeared and 'criminalization' has recently returned to AIDS responses.

Another outcome of the shift towards a focus on risk behaviours was that of 're-labelling', sometimes by defining putative 'population groups' on the basis of behaviour, such as 'men who have sex with men' (MSM), or on the basis of new names for existing occupational groups, like 'sex workers' (SW) for people selling sex – usually assumed to be women. In some cases this re-labelling was about broadening group definitions, rather than focusing specifically on risky behaviours. Sex worker, for example, was actually a term that emerged in the 1980s from the sex workers' rights movement in the US and was intended to refer to – and unite – a broad range of people in the sex industry (Quan, 2006).[1]

'Injecting drug users' (IDU), on the other hand, was a label that narrowed the focus amongst drug users and did indeed get closer to the key risk behaviour in that area, namely sharing the injection equipment. In the case of MSM, however, it certainly broadened the category, but missed its target for at least three complications:

- It did so to a point where many men who have sex with men are invisible or not programmatically included, since the behaviour itself is not necessarily associated with any identification of being a man who has sex with other men.
- It was feared to potentially undermine the political project of claiming rights for sexual minorities (Young and Meyer, 2005).
- It did not actually name the risk behaviour in question.

If we were able to be truly explicit about the key behaviour of concern here, we should have termed it something like 'people who have unprotected anal sex with different partners', which – importantly – includes many women.[2] All this has set off many intricate and in several ways important debates about identity, behaviour, citizenship and stigmatization versus empowerment. At a practical level, we have finally ended up with new, less controversial names for groups of individuals thought to be most at risk or likely to pass on the virus. The term 'harm reduction' has been particularly effective at allowing us to acknowledge certain kinds of behaviour without judgement, whilst helping to reduce the harms associated, such as through exchanging clean needles and syringes, or using condoms in commercial sex.

A different outcome of the shift to a risky behaviour narrative was a move towards broader-based health promotion with information, education and communications strategies aimed at raising the awareness of the public, thereby changing behaviours towards safer ones, essentially reducing the *demand* for unsafe practices. This includes, on the one hand, simple promotional messages such as, in the words of Nancy Reagan, 'Just say no', to providing people with a broad range of accurate facts and education, on the other. At the time, an array of organizations from the reproductive health movement entered the more liberal end of this spectrum, such as Family Health International, John Snow International and universities like Johns Hopkins University. Underlying these approaches were a number of essentially similar 'behaviour change models', all predicated on a rational choice theory of individuals' behaviour (AIDSCAP, 1996). Many campaigns failed to change behaviour, however, and 'new and improved' iterations, such as behaviour change communication interventions were developed. These were still predicated on a view that risky behaviours result from calculated choices, that choosing to take major risks is not (truly) rational and therefore that you can re-educate people to make the 'right' decisions. Based on the existing evidence mostly coming out of studies in the US, consistently providing young people with access to a broad range of information has been somewhat successful, while abstinence programmes have not (Lloyd, 2007; Kirby, 2008). Education for behaviour change also overlaps with harm reduction. Targeted interventions based on peer education (such as amongst gay men, sex workers or injecting drug users) aim at introducing behavioural adaptations that reduce relative infection risks rather than attempting to eliminate the basic behaviour. Such programmes have often been shown to be far more effective than less closely targeted interventions (Plummer et al, 2001).

A positive trajectory in these developments was that of taking real infection risks seriously and finding more effective ways of engaging those individuals most crucial to transmission, which included outreach and peer education. This required a coming together of public health approaches with activist groups amongst those affected. Some of these targeted interventions with sex workers, gay and bisexual men or injecting drug users were highly effective in reducing HIV transmission when human rights-based and when they engaged and involved the communities affected.

There was also a less positive pathway of response that emerged from the shift towards broader generic health promotion based on educating the general public about health risks. Specific individuals' situations tended to be neglected, with abstract models of individual behaviour and choice lacking social and economic context. It is these models that have continued to sustain largely ineffective campaign and prevention efforts over the decades.

The initial 'outbreak' narrative around HIV/AIDS based on risky individuals displays some similarities to those by which other epidemics, such as SARS or Mexican swine flu, have been understood. However, there are also major differences, resulting from a combination of the virus's slow progress (in terms of the development of visible symptoms in the host), its transmission through stigmatized behaviours and its initial apparently universal fatality rate (in the absence of a cure or vaccine). Another major difference with the early response to HIV was the fact that groups of affected individuals themselves began to mount challenges to a risk framing of the disease, and in turn formulated their own alternative narratives of the epidemic. These alternative narratives resonated with a view emerging amongst public health practitioners that individual human rights were essential to good public health. Such a narrative, based on rights, would eventually emerge as an important way of framing responses to the disease. But first, a narrative based on vulnerability to disease came to the fore.

The vulnerability narrative: Sensitive to context

During the late 1980s to the early 1990s, development actors and institutions began tentatively to consider the potential long-term implications of AIDS. From the early 1990s the United Nations Development Programme's (UNDP) HIV and Development Programme led a growing challenge to what was increasingly seen as the WHO's excessively vertical and health-dominated approach to the AIDS epidemic. Arguably this narrative reached its peak by the mid-1990s, when the WHO's role had diminished and its Global Programme on AIDS was dismantled. In its place a joint United Nations' Programme on AIDS (UNAIDS) was created in 1996 with a mandate to advocate for a multi-sectoral approach as well as to coordinate the contributions of the various development agencies of the UN system. Following the establishment of UNAIDS, the World Bank scaled up its own Global AIDS Programme in 1998. In the years preceding the demise of GPA, international development NGOs, such as CARE, Save the Children Fund or ActionAID, were also setting up new AIDS programmes and donors were busy trying out new community support structures, including NGO 'umbrella mechanisms', such as the Southern Africa Training Programme and the International HIV/AIDS Alliance.

With the involvement of this tapestry of actors and institutions, a new narrative began to take shape based on the concept of vulnerability. Unlike the epidemiologists who had mainly driven the first narrative with a focus on individuals and risky behaviours, members of the development community involved in running both NGOs and new government programmes conceived of the AIDS epidemic within a much broader framework of poverty, education, welfare and migration. They used the concept of vulnerability to refer to interlinking contextual features that placed population groups in precarious situations, making them vulnerable to a range of threats, including disease, and their potential impacts. The broader focus of this narrative matches up with a corresponding shift in the development field itself, which had expanded beyond a narrow focus on poverty and economic growth towards a more multi-disciplinary approach to vulnerability and livelihoods. This was partly in reaction and response to the conservative social and economic policies of the 1980s, including the neoliberal economic policies of the World Bank and the IMF. The UNDP Programme on HIV and Development published a report that depicted the epidemic as a series of unfolding waves, starting with the initial epidemic burst, which leads to increased burdens for care, broader social and economic impacts and, finally, the potential erosion of governance, social order and security (Cohen, 1993; Reid, 1993). According to this vulnerability narrative, AIDS was a 'shock' to political, social and health systems with the potential for large and increasingly aggregate effects. Poverty was granted a big role in this framing of the disease, helping to render certain people vulnerable to the disease, while at the same time disease was understood to render people vulnerable to poverty, setting up a vicious cycle.

Within this group of diverse actors, the term vulnerability came to be both influential but later also contested, with varying emphasis placed on the degree of resilience or agency granted to the vulnerable individual or population, and the relative importance of prevention and impact mitigation. The concept of vulnerability is complex, as it can and is used in the senses of vulnerability 'to exposure' as well as 'to impacts' (Chambers, 1989). Whilst this is also true in the case of HIV (Bloom et al, 2007; Edström, 2007), development writers tended to define it exclusively with reference to impacts (Barnett and Blaikie, 1992; Devereux, 2001; Gillespie and Loevinsohn, 2003; Morton, 2006) whilst writers on preventive health have focused on vulnerability to exposure or infection (e.g. Bates et al, 2004). The fact that this key word is used in different senses has obscured debates and encouraged the conflation of issues on poverty, gender and AIDS as well as leading to proposing ill-founded vicious cycles.

The concept of a vicious cycle of poverty and AIDS has been, and continues to be, influential despite evidence that the relationship between poverty and HIV is not symmetrical: the fact that HIV makes people vulnerable to poverty does not mean poverty necessarily makes people more vulnerable to HIV. Development academics and other actors closely engaged with HIV and sensitive to this evidence have sought to complicate the old cliché that 'poverty drives the epidemic', introducing an alternative version of this narrative that emphasizes the importance of inequality rather than poverty in determining vulnerability to disease. They point out that at the aggregate level, HIV prevalence does not correlate with gross national income per head, nor does it seem to be associated with the percentage of population under a poverty line of US$1 a day (Barnett and Whiteside, 2002; Gillespie and Greener, 2006). A greater proportion of absolutely poor people in a population does not go with a greater level of HIV prevalence, generally. In sub-Saharan Africa, HIV prevalence does, however, show a highly significant correlation with inequality in income distribution, which in turn tends to correlate with higher rates of growth, mobility and export-led market driven development strategies, as recommended by the World Bank. That is, African countries with more pronounced wealth gaps and more rapid growth tend to display significantly higher HIV prevalence rates.[3] Rather than simple poverty driving the epidemic, proponents of this alternative narrative suggest that inequality in contexts of rapid development, mobility and societal transition appears to drive the epidemic.

The idea that vulnerability is context dependent is not controversial and appears obvious. It is not always easy, however, to describe the importance of environment without losing sight of the role of individual actions. While the risk narrative perhaps over-emphasizes the individual and neglects social context, the vulnerability narrative suffers from the opposite weakness, often neglecting the agency of vulnerable individuals who take action based on their own decisions. By appealing to multiple factors of inequality and disadvantage, powerful accounts of 'structural violence' as accounting for health crises (e.g. Farmer, 1996) were integrated into narratives that particularly viewed combinations of poverty and women's disempowerment, rather than the risky behaviour of individuals, as the root causes of AIDS.

A common feature of vulnerability narratives is that of framing gender in strongly general and binary terms, which can lead to an almost essentialist view of women as uniquely vulnerable. Conversely, men are often constructed as the counterposing problem, or threat. Such binary constructions of gender are deeply embedded and persist despite evidence of a far more nuanced reality. For example, even the most common generalizations about extra-marital sex – as an overwhelmingly male behaviour – often do not stand up in the face of evidence. In an analysis of Demographic and Health Surveys (DHS) data on HIV sero-discordant couples (where one partner remains HIV negative) from a broad range of African countries, Mascolini (2007) finds that in 4 of 11 countries studied, women were the infected partner in a majority of cases. Confirming the robustness of the results he also found that a significant proportion of women's infections occurred ten or more years into the marriage. This is at odds with the common perception that unfaithful men are by far the main link between high risk groups and the general population.

It appears hard for this vulnerability narrative to reconcile the notion of the vulnerable female victim with the idea of resilient African women willingly deploying sexuality through selling sex as part of a livelihood strategy. Development narratives often construct such women quite differently from the idea of 'sex workers' used to describe women who sell sex in other settings, such as Asia. Of course, traditions of polygamy and diffuse family structures create grey areas around what can be called commercial or transactional in the way of sexual relations. However, in parts of South Africa shifting demographics, mobility patterns and declining marriage rates, along with Christianization, seem to be accompanied by increased bartering of sex for income (Hunter, 2007). This is familiar from histories of rapid development in Southeast Asia. Both in terms of transactional sex and especially for recognized sex work, the vulnerability narrative tends to justify calls to prevent women from entering sex work, or assisting in their exit, dismissing women's autonomous choices in favour of a vision of rescuing vulnerable women. Sex workers themselves tend to protest against this characterization, calling for greater rights and representation.

Whilst inequality, age and gendered power relations do matter to the epidemic, the dominant version of the vulnerability narrative has not always captured the complex ways that they intersect and play out in local contexts. A vulnerability-based analysis has been inadequate to capture such additional factors as the density and mobility of sexual and drug-taking networks, not to mention the prevalence and behaviour of the virus itself in local groups. Despite its reference to issues of poverty and structural drivers, the vulnerability narrative tends to lend itself to quite an abstracted and generalized view from above. An alternative narrative that is consonant with these concerns but more context-specific suggests that the issues around gender or social and economic injustice that matter most to the epidemic are not 'general' but those 'at the margin' and 'at the intersections' – that is, those of sex workers (under any description), men who have sex with men, drug users and others marginalized in society. This alternative narrative suggests that these women and men still remain woefully marginalized in our responses in higher-prevalence settings. This marginalization extends to the global level, where, for example, female sex workers remain unrepresented in predominant feminist agendas.

According to this alternative narrative of vulnerability, participatory methods, skilfully employed, have the potential to reach critical members of a given vulnerable population. In order to be most effective, these methods should be tailored not simply to 'vulnerable groups' but specifically to so-called 'key populations', that is, to those who are most vulnerable to contracting and passing on the virus and also, critically, most key to the response, that is, with a potential to mobilize and build up social capital. This approach to 'empowerment for prevention' has been developed in a major multi-country project, the Frontiers' Prevention Project (FPP), which has shown some significant shifts towards safer behaviours in target groups involved in India, Ecuador and Cambodia. However, it also represents a departure from the more common development approach by integrating public health and human rights perspectives.

Both the dominant and alternative strains of the vulnerability narrative emphasize the structural determinants of poverty and inequality. The dominant narratives of mainstream development actors tend to conceive of interventions as externally supported to ameliorate vulnerabilities of large sections of populations but often lack the input of, or attention to, truly marginalized populations crucial in the transmission, or control, of the virus. The alternative narrative, of those engaged in development as well as HIV prevention with marginalized groups, has tended to allow for responses that are more closely tailored to the specific settings in which they are applied as well as to the structural obstacles to empowerment and agency for these specific groups, which speaks to issues of justice and equal rights. This alternative narrative has been more sensitive to issues of voice and agency in formulating responses, viewing key populations as central actors in advocating for their own protection and for impacting on HIV in low or high prevalence settings alike.

The rights narrative: Contesting the stigma of HIV

Many of the preceding narratives emerged in an era when treatment for HIV was not yet available or was considered by policy-makers to be out of reach for people in the global South. Meanwhile, in the global North, with development of antiretroviral (ARV) treatment and increasing pressure by activist groups such as ACT UP, the language of responses to HIV began to shift from primarily prevention and control of a fatal disease to one of chronic disease management. As part of this shift, a narrative of the disease gradually emerged that considered access to treatment as a right, on a par with treatment of other manageable diseases. Aside from its origins in Northern treatment activism and links with sexual rights (and other human rights) movements, this rights-based narrative drew on a broader rights-based approach to development which was gaining currency more generally, based on the principles of 'equality and equity, accountability, empowerment and participation'.[4] Both the risk and vulnerability narratives outlined above were consonant with a respect for human rights and the constellations of actors who formulated this rights narrative built strategically and opportunistically on elements of the preceding framings, and in many cases the same people were actors and sometimes in new positions of relative influence. However, both the risk and vulnerability narratives, with their respective focus on protecting the uninfected majority from infection or protecting broader communities of women and children from the impacts of disease and deaths on families, had neglected those people most directly affected by the epidemic – those who were themselves infected or labelled as a risk. The rights narrative, more than the proceeding two narratives, gave special attention to those most directly affected by the disease in the present, and particularly to those living with the virus whilst negotiating multiple levels of stigma (e.g. being a sex worker as well as HIV positive).

The rights narrative grew out of a history of tireless efforts and mobilization amongst HIV affected groups and supporters of those infected, such as ACT UP in New York or the AIDS Support Organization (TASO) in Uganda, both established in the same year as WHO's GPA (1987). The rights narrative emerged more squarely in the 1990s when the perceived importance of human rights and care and support for those infected had greatly increased. The first patient activist health conference in Africa took place in Cape Town in 1995. Throughout the decade civil society networks – such as the Global Network of People living with HIV, the International Community of Women living with HIV/AIDS, the International Centre for AIDS Service Organizations, and the International Network of Sex Work Projects – increasingly mobilized those living with or affected by HIV to become active in this project. To different degrees these were supported by regional and national network structures, but most were driven by highly committed and inspiring individuals.

Other highly successful national level coalitions and networks developed: the Treatment Action Campaign (TAC) in South Africa focused on policy activism; and the Alliance National Contre le Sida à Sénegal (ANCS) sought to increase civil society mobilization and support. Such national groupings tended to connect with other local movements, government officials, politicians, global development institutions (such as UNAIDS or the Global Fund) but also international actors and private agencies, including international NGOs (such as Médecins Sans Frontières (MSF), Oxfam or the Alliance).

Along with lobbying particular policy-makers in government health services and international agencies, coalitions were formed to put pressure on pharmaceutical companies and the international community. This included demands for changes that helped bring down the price of ARV drugs and consolidated commitments to massively expanding and rolling out treatment in the South.

Proponents of the rights-based narrative argued that infected people needed support even before treatment came within reach. NGOs, governments and faith-based organizations (FBOs) developed models for home and community-based care and peer support in places such as Burkina Faso, Cambodia, India and Zambia. This was part of a broader global mobilization for care and treatment. The sense of solidarity and peer support it developed was key in shaping new identities and a sense of purpose. An influential and defining account of 'therapeutic citizenship' in relation to HIV described this process as a shift from 'bio-sociality' to 'bio-politics' (Nguyen, 2005). Along with the calls for rights-based responses, NGOs such as MSF have urged responsibility along with rights, in particular pushing for adherence to ART in order to avoid, or slow down, the evolution of drug-resistant strains of HIV (Robins, 2004; MacGregor, this volume). With these developments, and increasingly close links between HIV-positive groups and health services along with a 'normalization' of HIV as a manageable chronic illness, some analysts have suggested that a rights-based narrative has ultimately domesticated, tamed or dampened activism (Robins, 2005).

Within a rights-based narrative, defining who counts as an HIV citizen can be controversial. In the dominant version of this narrative, people living with HIV and AIDS have taken centre stage, and are increasingly privileged by development actors. However, alternative versions of this narrative have continuously sought to widen the focus beyond those living with HIV, as sexual rights movements and sex workers rights groups in different countries have engaged with the response to HIV from the outset. Whilst categories such as MSM or sex workers have been seen as problematic, stigmatizing or 'othering' diverse exotic sexualities in the South under blanket terms, they have also been seen to be liberating (offering legitimacy and resources) and as offering new avenues of empowerment and unity for groups, such as men identifying as MSM in India (Boyce, 2007; Khanna, 2007). Crucially, definitions of key groups in HIV often overlap for individuals (e.g. you can be MSM, a sex worker, injecting drug user and HIV positive at the same time and have different peers and allies in each sense), so alliances between networks can provide a broader base for activism and organizing. Amongst those who have engaged with groups in different countries, it is also clear that PLHA movements have benefited from collaboration with other civil society networks, with engaged NGOs and AIDS service organizations. It is essential to recognize, in this, that overlapping HIV-related subject positions have been co-constructed in interaction with the global AIDS response, through alliances between individuals and groups of differently identified and self-identified categories. Rather than seeing the framing of rights and citizenship in HIV as purely related to ARV therapy, we need to see it in more diverse actor-oriented terms of engagement and emergent solidarities contesting access to scientific evidence and resources.

If international development institutions were relatively dominant in generating a vulnerability narrative around AIDS policy in the early to the late 1990s, a much more diffuse and diverse constellation of civil society actors (many of whom were also in government and international institutions) came into prominence and influenced the emergence of a rights-based narrative for understanding and organizing responses to AIDS in the mid-1990s to early 2000s. Coming together around a human rights framing, these coalitions' diffuse tentacles and flexible strategies for influence arguably primed demand for a major scale-up in the global response to AIDS and opened up doors for major and previously unlikely players to enter the fray to ensure 'supply' in the new era of 'universal access'. In this process there was also often a perceived need to simplify messages, which – although not uncontested – paved the way for scaling up more standardized packages of services, leading to less politicized and more medicalized and corporate responses.

The security narrative: A 21st century perspective

The fourth narrative, which was officially heralded at the turn of the millennium and emerged more strongly in the years following 9/11, views HIV as a threat to security. This narrative, like the preceding three, has existed in some form throughout the history of the epidemic. Indeed, a version of this narrative framed the initial reaction to the new virus with alarmist language of 'outbreaks' or a 'new plague,' similarly to how Ebola was first received (Leach and Hewlett, this volume). The idea of HIV as an outside threat has taken many forms. In the early days, AIDS was often constructed as an outside threat – from Haitians in New York or from peace keepers in Cambodia, etc. In more recent times, however, a renewed and clearer security framing has gained prominence, driven largely by US government foreign policy since the millennium (especially post 9/11) and becoming institutionalized in large programmes such as the President's Emergency Plan for AIDS Relief (PEPFAR) and the Global Fund to Fight AIDS, Tuberculosis and Malaria (GFATM).

This security narrative can be traced back to the idea of 'national security' defined in the wake of the Second World War 'as the integrity of the national territory and its institutions' (Morgenthau, 1948). Based on the construct of the nation state and the concept of political realism, a national security narrative played a key role in the US justifying its exercise of global power in the Cold War period. Many in the international community believe that such a national security-driven approach has outlived its usefulness, particularly since many sources of insecurity in today's globalized world are beyond the reach of unilateral state action: e.g. global warming, financial crises, terrorism or pandemics. One response has been to argue for the adoption of a people-centred model for security instead. The 'human security' paradigm, which emerged in the 1990s, is often framed as more useful for understanding global vulnerabilities and argues that the focus of security should be for the individual rather than the state (UNDP, 1994).

According to a security narrative, one potential outcome of HIV is the threat of conflict. UNDP's waves of the epidemic model predicted a fifth wave of impact resulting in social disintegration, the weakening of armies and national defence, leading to the eventual collapse of governance after some 25 years, unless transmission was brought under control at an earlier stage (Reid, 1993). However, despite significant increases in HIV prevalence in several countries of sub-Saharan Africa for more than 25 years, we have yet not seen any government fall to AIDS. On the contrary, some suggest that the resources and infrastructure mobilized under governments in the response to AIDS may have strengthened the hand of several governments (De Waal, 2006).

While AIDS is often described as a global threat in this narrative, it is in fact the perceived national threat to the US that has motivated much of this framing. Projections about a spread of generalized epidemics to significant large countries like Nigeria, India, Russia and China from the CIA's National Intelligence Council allowed US President Clinton to declare AIDS an issue of national (not human) security for the US in April 2000, when the UN Security Council first discussed the effects of AIDS on peace and security. These US intelligence projections (National Intelligence Council, 2002) were used to boost momentum for the establishment of GFATM in 2002. It also facilitated President George W. Bush's mobilizing multiple billions of $US for PEPFAR, announced in 2003. Whether these projections were well founded is disputed (Chin, 2008). A broad security framing also influenced the redesign of the US institutional architecture for AIDS funding that accompanied PEPFAR. Here, the United States Agency for International Development, traditionally a bastion of liberal politics, lost its prime responsibility for international HIV support and was clearly subordinated under the Office of the Global AIDS Coordinator, the AIDS Tsar, and alongside the Centers for Disease Control in Atlanta, the National Institute for Health and the Department of Defense.

Around the turn of the millennium, several complementary as well as contradictory appeals to the threat of HIV and AIDS fed into the broader momentum for establishing the GFATM (also known as the Global Fund and sometimes nicknamed the 'Global ATM'). The fact that several diseases were included was not merely a compromise or a rational agreement on relative priorities: it reflected a far deeper fear of infectious pathogens operating together to refuel smouldering endemics or to create new epidemics. The emergence of extensively drug-resistant tuberculosis (XDR-TB), particularly affecting people living with HIV in South Africa, illustrates the potential risk of viral interactions in immune-suppressed population groups generating new 'millennium bugs' with dangerous implications for drug resistance and drugs development, not to mention for balancing rights and responsibilities between governments, NGOs and affected groups (see MacGregor and Nightingale, this volume). In such contexts, the rights-based narrative described above is seen by some as inadequate to address broader health threats from HIV infection. If the marginalized and vulnerable become potential vectors for new and more transmissible pathogens, security narratives are likely to gain currency, reintroducing an old dilemma: whilst a human rights discourse has proved essential to engaging affected groups in responding to HIV, security narratives have typically driven them underground.

These developments must be seen in the broader context of post-9/11 global politics, where security narratives have continued to flourish in a range of fields. It seems plausible that concerns about HIV/AIDS have contributed to a broader shift towards security within the field of international health, as reflected in the WHO's 2007 report *Global Public Health Security in the 21st Century* (WHO, 2007a).[5] It is hard to disentangle the precise way that the broader 'human security' discourse had already rendered security narratives more sensitive to progressive or medicalized framings (Elbe, 2006, 2009) but it seems plausible that HIV and associated developments such as 'health security' have added to this trend. Of course, medicalized framings are often not seen as progressive by actors with vulnerability or right-based narratives. Whether this represents a new and less draconian orientation in security approaches, or some 'fusion' of perspectives into a more managerial corporate approach, is difficult to determine. In fact, this same period has also seen major corporate and private philanthropic institutions enter the field with major resources to scale up responses (for example, the Bill and Melinda Gates Foundation and the Clinton Foundation from 2003). What is clearer, however, is that the attention to rights and the structural vulnerabilities of the most marginalized groups have taken second place, as an increasingly dominant security narrative privileges expediency and scaleability. Large institutions (state or private) now clearly take precedence over individuals. Earlier lessons about focusing on priority marginalized groups or the structure of their disempowerment have faded into the background.

Furthermore, the earlier heated debates about prevention, sexuality and gender have been marginalized and replaced with faith-based policies for abstinence and strict monogamy, or medical interventions in the form of surgical circumcision. Whilst AIDS activists and civil society groups have earlier been accused of exporting Western liberal values on gender and sexuality – something which some of us are unapologetic about (e.g. Altman,

2001) – those closely engaged in community responses to HIV view the proliferation of faith-based organizations and PEPFAR's earmarking of funds for 'abstinence and faithfulness' programmes as part of a calculated export of a different set of Western (more conservative and Christian) values in a broader game plan of global geopolitics following the collapse of communism and the rise in the West of a perceived 'Islamic threat' from the East.

This brief sketch illustrates that while actual 'security threats' of AIDS may be overblown, they can have a powerful impact on rapidly mobilizing significant resources. In turn, they influence other chains of events where issues of governance, sovereignty and 'voice' become fundamentally altered. Securitization has increased resources and built up imbalances in some areas, with resulting arguments over verticalization and exceptionalism versus health systems strengthening and mainstreaming on the other. At the same time, broader security perspectives have themselves become more medicalized and less obviously draconian. As a result, new approaches for incentives and routine testing are presented as 'normalizing', whilst their implementation continues to be contested by affected groups and strong tensions with human rights remain.

Conclusions

Narratives about AIDS and the corresponding pathways of responses they have helped to justify have evolved tremendously in the 25 years since the disease emerged. At the outset, old fashioned public health-driven narratives based on notions of individual risk led to responses that proved largely inappropriate and ineffective, except when adapted in the face of contestation from affected groups, which taught us the importance of attending to human rights in developing responses. With time, vulnerability narratives taught us positively to use more imagination (sometimes too much) and consider complex contexts as shaping vulnerabilities and risk, as well as the epidemic itself impacting on complex contexts, but it often took our gaze off the all-important virus. When drawing on the lessons from engagement with affected groups, vulnerability narratives were sometimes effective in engaging and empowering those at the heart of the epidemic but at the margins of local communities and society.

Rights-based narratives were helpful in learning how to improve risk or vulnerability focused analyses, particularly by giving voice to the people at the heart of the epidemic's very dynamics. At the centre of this lies HIV-positive living which, along with making treatment a reality in the South, has changed the entire syntax and logic of effective comprehensive AIDS responses. Rights-based narratives, actors and their interests are, however, diffuse, which holds both important potentials for alliances and constant risks of disintegration (sometimes due to avoidance of multiple levels of HIV-linked stigma).

It is clear that appeals to collective security threats may mobilize the resources and political incentives required to mount a response to HIV on the scale required to have any impact. But, whilst resourcing, 'normalizing' and medicalizing the response may improve how health systems can manage HIV treatment and disease interactions, continued failures to address prevention will make the response increasingly unsustainable. This could potentially also threaten improved health and care in relation to other diseases over the long term in highly affected countries, which underlines a justification for a high-level concern for broader health security. The challenge lies in the recognition that most effective responses have been focused, context sensitive and rights based, whilst a security narrative can undermine such responses. There is evidence to suggest that HIV epidemics can be brought down to lower levels and if utilized selectively and in tandem, certain elements of each narrative have the potential to contribute to a more effective response to the epidemic.

HIV and other epidemics can be usefully compared in terms of the different characteristics of the pathogens that cause them. HIV's long latency periods and its transmission via highly stigmatized behaviours account for some of its particular traits. This may in fact explain why the AIDS epidemic is one of the most contested epidemics: people infected with the virus can live lengthy and active lives during which they can become active participants in a disease narrative and response, yet the stigma attached to HIV combined with the virus's serious health implications ensure that this participation will be from a position of discrimination. Unlike many other past epidemics, HIV affected groups and civil society have mobilized both locally and globally to create change on an unprecedented scale (which may be harder in epidemics of more transmissible pathogens).

The broader structural issues that matter to HIV transmission are population mixing, mobility, inequality and change (departures from traditions and established livelihoods, changing family and social structures, values etc.), but also specific features of individual lives, relationships and bodies that affect transmission. Attempting to stop a virus at national borders has rarely been effective, if ever. We have no evidence that investing in rural development, combating widespread hunger through food assistance or efforts to boost traditional family values would have any significant impacts on curbing the epidemic at scale, although often very important for other reasons and possibly helpful to slowing the pace of spread at the margin.

HIV challenges us to square the circle by relating individuals (who are hard to categorize and control) to structural contexts and forces (which are hard to measure and often even harder to control). We know enough now to see that complex dynamics in multiple domains influence the pathways of the epidemic. We also know that affected individuals respond to, and thus alter, the epidemic and that the virus's own evolution influences its course. Individuals have agency, resilience and their own wills, which play a central role in their ability to respond. At the same time, their actions take place in a social context, so citizenship, networks, social capital and political action are key to any successful response.

To date, the biggest failure in HIV is the response to prevention in high prevalence settings. Certain tools and techniques marshalled by all four narratives can be meaningfully applied here and calls for combination prevention are increasingly sounded. This includes a basic role for accessible large-scale measures such as those justified by traditional public health promotion narratives, which include better and earlier sex education, condom availability and access to effective HIV and STI treatments (both of which can lower individual infectiousness and susceptibility) or safely conducted male circumcisions (which can lower men's individual susceptibility and potentially population level vulnerability). However, a top priority is now a stronger focus on the 'core dynamics of the epidemic', we need new and better socio-epidemiological science, building on lessons from the risk and vulnerability narratives, to define and adjust hierarchies of priority groups (as well as their inter-linkages), whilst also learning better from evidence and experience in lower prevalence settings. We need highly intensive, holistic and empowering approaches for key populations that draw on both the vulnerability and rights-based approaches in all epidemiological contexts. These include, for example, addressing the needs and rights of sexual minorities and sex workers in relation to sexual health, substance abuse, legal discrimination at work, law enforcement practices and child care.

Notes

1   The popularity and adoption of the term 'sex worker' into modern language is traceable to the GPA, where Priscilla Alexander worked and several sex workers were advisers. GPA's then Director, the late Jonathan Mann, made the brave decision to include it in documents instead of 'prostitute'. Cheryl Overs – a sex workers' rights activist from Australia – was one adviser to the GPA who, along with Paulo Longo from Brazil, went on to establish the Global Network of Sex Work Project (NSWP) and both of whom were to influence my thinking about AIDS significantly over many years and continue to do so (although Paulo sadly died in 2004).

2   As a more general reflection, sensitivity to explicit descriptions of sexual behaviour, self-censorship and vague innuendo may be some of the more important causes of watering down analyses and losing sight of the virus.

3   Whilst HIV prevalence is highly imperfect as a marker of epidemic dynamics and although incidence of new infections would be far better as a marker, data on incidence are very difficult to come by or generate. The significance of the correlation means that it is no doubt related with the actual link to transmission.

4   www.unhchr.ch/development/approaches-04.html.

5   WHO also offers a working definition of health security as 'health issues with potential security implications', that is, generally those health emergencies of an acute, rather than a chronic, nature that have serious public health consequences and potential cross-border implications. www.euro.who.int/globalchange/Topics/20070227_4.

Chapter 6

Local Practice versus Exceptionalist Rhetoric: Case Studies of HIV/AIDS Programming in South Africa

Hayley MacGregor

Introduction

This chapter addresses debates about the future direction of global HIV/AIDS policy processes. It employs a case study approach to examine how particular narratives have come to define policy at national and local levels in one severely affected country in a 'hyperendemic region', namely South Africa. Specifically, it examines the thesis advanced by De Waal (2006) that a shift is currently occurring in the framing of the nature of the epidemic, with corresponding implications for both the kinds of interventions adopted at the national level and their efficacy.

The scholar Alex De Waal has been a vocal proponent of a revision of the priorities and underlying ideological tenets of HIV/AIDS programming. De Waal (2006) argues that from the outset 'AIDS exceptionalism' has been the defining feature of the global response to HIV/AIDS, both in the framing of the nature of the disease and the responses to it. Exceptionalism, he contends, is predicated on the assumption that HIV/AIDS is an extraordinary disease that necessitates its own unique set of responses, which are distinct from the conventional public health approaches to potentially fatal infectious diseases. The exceptionalism that De Waal draws attention to has been a feature of the dominant narrative by which the HIV/AIDS epidemic has been understood, and addressed, to date. This exceptionalist account places emphasis on the global scale of infection, the severity and incurable nature of the illness, the long latent period which facilitates spread, the ability of the virus to sustain high prevalence in 'hyperendemic' areas, and the predictions of massive social and economic upheaval that could cause a humanitarian disaster in heavily affected countries. De Waal suggests that it is such an exceptionalist narrative that has led in the past to the framing of HIV/AIDS as an 'emergency' by governments (see for example Abuja

Declaration, 2001)[1] and agencies such as PEPFAR and UNAIDS, a 'global threat' that has been compared by some to nuclear proliferation and climate change (see for example Piot and Seck, 2001; Piot, 2005). The epidemic has been discussed in US security reports in the context that humanitarian crises might cause political upheaval and threaten fragile states, especially in sub-Saharan Africa.[2] To this analysis one might add that the 'health security' perspective (see for example WHO, 2007a) includes the implicit fear that areas of now endemic HIV infection provide an immuno-compromised population pool that might disastrously accelerate the cross-border spread of potential new pandemics such as avian flu.

In terms of the responses to the epidemic, De Waal (2006) maintains that the historical origins of this exceptionalist narrative can be traced back to the significant involvement of the gay activist lobby in the US at the outset of the epidemic. The prevailing neoliberal ideology further strengthened an emphasis on the individual privacy and dignity of those affected, and encouraged the enshrining of exceptionalism in the sense of HIV-positive people requiring unique treatment. This is evident in the provision that the respect of individual rights should be paramount. Associated assumptions were based on the idea that the education of individuals will lead to behavioural change. In other words, prevention efforts incorporated the notion that people can be persuaded to behave in 'epidemiologically responsible' ways if they know their HIV status, and are given biomedical knowledge of the forms of transmission.

The crux of De Waal's critique of the exceptionalist narrative is that the 'global threat' rhetoric has not been matched by an equivalent level of action. The dominant responses[3] that have grown out of this narrative are largely informed by human rights discourse. Based on the importance of individual rights, responses issuing from the exceptionalist narrative are a far cry from the more coercive public health approaches mobilized in response to a perceived global 'emergency', such as the mandatory testing and treatment, and disease notification procedures that were implemented during both the SARS and avian influenza outbreaks (see Bloom and Scoones, this volume). African governments, even if they might have harboured other inclinations, have been in a position where they have needed to access the newly mobilized global resources to respond to the epidemic. The conditions associated with funding have been set in an exceptionalist framework, thus ensuring that policy blueprints privileging individual human rights above the need to act aggressively or intrusively in the face of a perceived global threat have dominated. An important example would be the very widely instituted directive that HIV testing must be preceded by consent and counselling, and the resultant insistence in many countries on the need for lay or professional health workers to have completed training in order to counsel, at not inconsiderable expense and resultant delay in the opening of testing services. Thus, whilst the exceptionalist emphasis might have strengthened civil society and activism in sub-Saharan Africa, De Waal argues that the associated responses have not been particularly effective in combating what is indeed an epidemiologically complex epidemic (associated as it is with shifting viral dynamics, the phenomenon now of endemic levels of prevalence in certain areas, and the associated spread of lethal drug-resistant forms of other infectious diseases such as TB).

Several factors have contributed then to a growing call, from De Waal and others, for a revision of exceptionalist responses. These calls are based partly on adjustments to the global statistical estimates of the projected scale of HIV infection. The UNAIDS *Report on the Global AIDS Epidemic* (2008), for instance, indicates that the global percentage of people living with HIV has stabilized since 2000 (although the authors point out that, with 33 million people living with HIV in 2007, the level is still unacceptably high, with declines not universal). In addition, concern has been expressed regarding the strain on health systems of the burden of the disease and its special response measures. Resource limitations also call into question the feasibility of calls for 'universal access' to ARVs that are a cornerstone of human rights activism.[4] Furthermore, there is much dispute about the strengthening versus undermining effects on health systems[5] of the influx of vertically channelled funds for HIV/AIDS following the increase in large global health initiatives.[6] Others, like England (2007),[7] even contend that there has been a disproportionate emphasis on HIV/AIDS in health and funding budgets. Piot et al (2009, p4), however, contest the 'myth' that too much money is being spent on HIV/AIDS, claiming that the gains suggested by the more recent global statistics are patchy and should not be a reason for complacency. The increasing medicalization of responses associated with the concerted focus on access to drug treatment, to the detriment of prevention initiatives, has caused alarm in some quarters, and intensified disputes as to the efficacy of the latter measures. Barnett and Whiteside (2002) have pointed to the neglect of structural factors driving the epidemic. Pisani et al (2003) argue for closer attention to variable modes of transmission (who is becoming infected and by which means) to enable targeted interventions suited to the setting, a context-sensitive strategy echoed in a recent paper by Piot et al (2009). Whiteside (2009) has recently suggested that AIDS remains exceptional for certain parts of the world (where overall prevalence is unacceptably high) because of the cumulative impact on the entire social fabric, whilst in other countries, by this criterion, there is exceptionality only for groups of individuals, such as men who have sex with men.

The shift in the framing of HIV infection from a terminal to a chronic condition as a result of the gradual expansion of large ARV treatment programmes is a significant factor in prompting thinking towards AIDS revisionism. Fears about drug resistance foreground the dangers of non-compliance to drug regimes. With respect to the goal of treatment adherence as well as the concern to achieve effective behavioural change, there is a growing interest in the use of psychological techniques. As the dominant narrative regarding HIV/AIDS has gradually shifted from considering the disease to be acute and 'epidemic' to considering it to be endemic and chronic (with hyperendemic encapsulating a place somewhere in between), an additional question is raised about the similarities now between chronic HIV/AIDS and chronic non-communicable diseases. The suggestion that aspects of policy and clinical management might be similar adds another dimension to the discussion about the merits of vertical disease initiatives versus more 'integrated' horizontal programmes.

It is thus evident that the debates surrounding the exceptionalist narrative are multifaceted and as yet unresolved. The intention of this chapter is not to argue for any one position, but to explore further the issue of exceptionalism in *responses* to HIV/AIDS, and De Waal's observations specifically regarding the effects of a rights-based framing. Even if the epidemic remains exceptional in its impact in certain high prevalence countries, the very realities now of the scale of infection and the resource limitations in precisely such hyperendemic settings, might in fact make an argument for unique measures for those who are HIV positive untenable in a practical sense. If this is indeed an important time for considering alternative narratives with which to understand and frame responses to HIV/AIDS, then it seems a worthwhile moment to examine the current situation in local contexts where certain policies, predicated upon the protection of individual human rights and associated assumptions about individual 'epidemiological' responsibility, have been applied. This is the intention in examining the case studies in order to prompt further thought regarding different understandings of rights and responsibilities, given complex realities, resource limitations and a range of actors. Such an approach takes cognisance of anthropological analyses of the social processes whereby rights discourses come to be locally interpreted (see Cowen et al, 2001), and also ethnographic evidence that the application of 'rights talk' can in practice have unintended effects and mask very different realities (see Englund, 2006). Have there been unintended consequences of policies based on exceptionalist narratives? What local strategies have emerged to accommodate different perspectives and tensions and can these be relevant in the development of alternative narratives about the disease that would promote different public health measures?

In order to unpack these perspectives and the assumptions underpinning them, the chapter draws upon the concept of 'framings', 'the different ways of understanding or representing a social, technological or natural system and its relevant environment' (Leach et al, 2007, p19). In other words, different narratives about the causes and response to a particular problem differ partly because of the way they frame the system in which the problem is seen to arise. Of particular relevance here are the ways in which narratives and their associated framings come to be enshrined in rhetoric by particular actors, whilst the politics and pragmatics behind the scenes might with time enable a seemingly paradoxical set of practices. In such instances it is relevant to examine the extent to which the words that encompass the narratives constitute an intended or even unconscious politics of representation. Similarly, it might be possible to identify the pivotal issues that have enabled some broad or even global framings to be transformed, and to map this process of reinterpretation as they find footholds in local contexts.

The case studies examine this theme by exploring specifically the gap between the principle of AIDS exceptionalism enshrined in the dominant AIDS narrative and what has developed in practice. To what extent have exceptionalist narratives translated into pathways of response with meaningful impacts? Which developments have prompted modifications and which groups have been most affected by the resultant gains and losses? The case studies illustrate two key policy areas that pertain to people with HIV/AIDS but that also reveal dimensions of broader debates about rights and responsibilities. The different framings of the issues in these case studies reveal how the principle of AIDS exceptionalism has been influential in civil society rhetoric and at national government level. At the same time, however, pragmatic factors have encouraged revealing shifts in practice that facilitate implicit compromise behind an enduring surface discourse of rights. The exceptionalist narrative, and its associated pathways of response based on a rights-based sensitivity to individuals, seem dominant at the level of rhetoric. On closer inspection, however, it becomes apparent that there is a greater diversity of response in practice. These responses represent the 'answers' produced by alternative narratives of the disease which remain implicit or much less forcefully expressed.

The first case study examines the ongoing discussion in South Africa regarding appropriate social assistance for people with HIV/AIDS. This story intersects with a protracted debate in the post-apartheid era about the definition of 'disability' and thus eligibility for the state disability grant. Opinions diverge as to the appropriate side of the inclusion/exclusion line to be assigned to the range of manifestations of HIV/AIDS: the healthy HIV positive; those who are 'merely' chronically ill but remain variably functional (especially considering the option of ARVs); and the AIDS sick, incapacitated by full-blown illness. The difficulty in distinguishing between these groups increases the ambiguity as to whether to treat someone living with the virus as having a disability, or requiring management of a chronic (albeit 'hyperendemic') illness, or having the potential to spread an incurable infectious disease of epidemic proportions. The exceptionalist narrative has kept the lens of responses focused on the rights of the individual, even in the face of the risks to others. With respect to the grant debate, the activist lobby has in fact fixed upon the 'chronic' label to argue for a special cash benefit for anyone diagnosed HIV positive. With the seriousness of TB-HIV co-infection alarmingly evident, this status as a unique chronic illness has also been extended by activist groups to TB, for the purposes of advocating for inclusion in the suggested chronic illness benefit. However, the appraisal in general of TB, and in particular drug-resistant TB, has consistently placed this disease much more firmly in a category of 'public health threat'. This has had the effect of sanctioning as appropriate a response involving far more coercive interventions, in keeping with a framing of a dangerous and potentially epidemic disease. In the final analysis then, this case study raises the possibility that the dynamics of co-infection might have the potential to shift, even just implicitly, the discourse around HIV from one based on individual rights to a greater emphasis on population-wide control, even if couched in the language of 'responsibility'.

The second case study unpacks the dynamics behind the changing role being assigned to lay counsellors in the testing and management of HIV infection. Here particularly it is the appraisal of HIV/AIDS as a chronic disease that has added impetus to a shift in approaches. In this example it becomes revealing to examine in greater detail the distinction between narrative and response, or between rhetoric and practice. The counselling that has been seen internationally as the hallmark of best practice in rights-based testing methods is in danger of becoming rudimentary. In the face of concern to keep in check the associated epidemics of TB and HIV, as well as fears of drug resistance on both counts, it has been relegated to second place behind strategies to achieve adherence, also placed under the rubric of 'counselling'. In chasing adherence targets, individual responsibility is emphasized at the clinic level, as knowledge of the disease is imparted as the key to behaviour change. Yet this focus easily translates into pressure for a kind of individual moral compliance that can be seen as ultimately complementary to an aim of epidemiological control at a population level. The seeming dichotomy between the rhetoric of rights and the practices harnessed in the attempt to enforce adherence becomes less apparent when the gap between the framing and the implementation of the policy is considered more closely.

The analysis presented in this chapter is based upon past experience of working in South Africa on disability grant restructuring whilst employed by the Human Sciences Research Council in 2003. It also draws upon interviews conducted in Cape Town and Pretoria in October 2008. Before presenting the case studies and analysis in detail, it is necessary first to contextualize the discussion by explaining the significance of the post-apartheid context for HIV/AIDS and disability policy, and to provide some necessary background to the South African healthcare system.

The context of South Africa

South Africa provides a relevant national context in which to pick case studies: the arrival of democratic-style freedoms for the majority of the population coincided with a frightening increase in HIV infections.[8] Southern Africa is now characterized as a 'hyperendemic area'.[9] The end of apartheid, an era of human rights abuses, was also marked by the enormous emphasis given to rights in the new constitution. It has been argued that the rights discourse has been a prominent 'social glue' in the endeavour of nation building since independence (Wilson, 2000). It is of obvious relevance that the 1994 constitution guarantees health as a right of citizenship. It is this significant provision which assisted the HIV/AIDS activists of the Treatment Action Campaign (TAC) to successfully challenge the state to provide universal access to ARVs in 2003. Such action became necessary in the light of President Mbeki's persistent denial of the viral aetiology of AIDS, and the concomitant inaction of the Department of Health in responding to an epidemic that had become a major national cause of mortality. Fassin and Schneider (2003) have argued that the struggle that ensued over understandings of AIDS and appropriate responses should be analysed as a bodily legacy of a history of oppression and as a space where other contentious political issues were contested by proxy. Given the political moment characterized by an enormous recognition of the significance of individual political freedoms, it is not surprising that the HIV/AIDS activist sector so readily adopted a rights-based agenda that was already a feature of global policy initiatives. Schneider (2002) contends that the principles built around protection of rights were in fact already enshrined in the AIDS Plan developed in a participatory process from 1992 to 1994, prior to the ANC government even being elected. However, it is worth pointing out that alternative perspectives exist: Leclerc-Madlala (2005) argues that in general in the country universal principles of human rights have not always characterized popular responses to HIV/AIDS, and in other contexts a rights-centred approach has at times conflicted with local notions of social justice or customary law (see Jensen, 2001); Posel (2004) comments on situations where certain sectors of the population have perceived the new rights dispensation to be a 'burden'.

The constitution also guarantees the right to social security which has become increasingly relevant in discussions of disability and chronic illness.

In practice such basic needs-based rights are compromised by resource limitations and the state has had to resort to promises for the 'progressive realization' of rights. Disability grants nonetheless constitute an extremely important form of income for those with chronic conditions such as mental illness (MacGregor, 2006) and for people with HIV/AIDS (Collins and Leibbrandt, 2007). The disability rights approach of international disability activists has taken root locally and provisions such as free primary health care for those experiencing disability have been introduced.

The change in government in 1994 enabled far-ranging reforms in the health sector, with the introduction, for example, of a district health system and the extension of provisions for free primary health care. The introduction of 'integrated' primary health care[10] has relevance for current discussions about coordinating TB and HIV care. A further striking state intervention (in a middle-income country with an established health service), has been the deliberate increase in the use of lay people in service provision. Schneider (2009) describes how this started in the mid-1990s, the state working with NGOs. Disease-specific interventions were developed, largely for TB and HIV and to fulfil needs for home-based care and counselling specifically. According to her calculation, there are now 40,000 'community care givers' funded by provincial governments, not including those in the non-profit sector. In her opinion, the practice whereby government has outsourced services to NGOs as intermediaries[11] ('labour brokers') has been suggestive of a tendency to keep lay workers out of the civil service in more informal and flexible arrangements. Mobilization on the behalf of lay workers might, however, be encouraging government to move towards a more formalized policy, recognizing their place as workers in the health system with rights under employment law.

In terms of healthcare financing, plans to institute a national health insurance scheme finally seem to be concretizing into policy. At present South Africa has a large private health sector that services wealthier patients. In his June 2009 budget speech, the new Minister of Health declared it unacceptable that more than half of the percentage of total gross domestic product (GDP) spent on health caters for just 14 per cent of the population. He has pledged to remove out of pocket health expenditure by introducing a system of universal healthcare coverage as a matter of urgency. The South African treasury claims that South Africa's annual health budget is funded exclusively through government resources, including the ART programmes (Hanefeld, 2009). The country does, however, receive significant sums from global health initiatives (GHIs), in particular the Global Fund (Round 3 US$66 million; Round 6 US$55 million) and PEPFAR (US$590.9 million in financial year 2008), and these have had a significant impact on the roll-out of ARV therapy in the public sector. Hanefeld describes how, on account of the state's denialist stance, GHIs (as well as other civil society initiatives) were important in assisting the development of ART programmes prior to 2003.

In terms of the state response to HIV/AIDS, the National Strategic Plan (2007) has targets for increasing access to ART.[12] However, cracks have already appeared in the programme infrastructure, with one province experiencing a budget shortfall in the 2008–2009 financial year and temporarily suspending the ARV programme. At the South African AIDS conference in Durban in early 2009, sustaining a supply of drugs in the national ARV programme was a large point for concern. Mark Heywood, the director of the AIDS Law Project (ALP), warned that whilst South Africa has the most extensive ART programme in the world, the existing structures are under strain. Based upon recent calculations, he predicted that the budget for ARVs in the 2009–2010 financial year (through the government's conditional grant allocations to the provinces) is going to experience a R1 billion[13] deficit (Healthlink Bulletin, 2009). More concerted government efforts and planning are urgently needed to achieve several of the targets outlined in the strategic plan, as the case studies will illustrate.

Case Study 1: Defining disability in the age of HIV/AIDS

Since the introduction of a new constitution and bill of rights following the democratic transition in 1994, the system of social security provision in South Africa has undergone restructuring and so-called 'rationalization'. This includes the attempted standardization of how disability grants (a monthly payment equivalent to roughly two-thirds the value of the minimum wage) are disbursed, an important and contentious feature of welfare provision in a country where nearly 20 per cent of the adult population is HIV positive.[14] This restructuring has led to charged debates over how to define who counts as disabled.

In particular, the HIV/AIDS epidemic has raised serious public health questions related to the purpose of social security in the context of chronic illness (such as, for example, the cost and value of such monetary provision versus other interventions, and the relationship between treatment adherence and the receipt of cash payments). Debates continue as to whether an HIV-positive status constitutes a 'disability' and whether a disability grant is the most appropriate support for people with serious chronic illness. These issues have generated considerable attention in media and policy circles on account of widespread professional and popular concern regarding the introduction of 'perverse incentives', not only to be classified as and remain 'disabled', but also to purposefully contract diseases such as TB or become

LIVERPOOL JOHN MOORES UNIVERSITY
LEARNING SERVICES

HIV positive. Discussion has come to centre upon narrowing the definition of 'disability' for the purposes of the grant, and creating a separate form of chronic illness benefit.

It became evident during fieldwork that an exceptionalist, rights-driven narrative of HIV/AIDS remains prominent in activist and legal circles in South Africa. In interviews with key players in these domains, there was no evidence of explicit questioning of the applicability of this paradigm. When I questioned directly about alternatives to a rights-based approach, this was usually met with some surprise and lack of enthusiasm. Several informants went further to give a standard explanation for this: the history of human rights abuses under apartheid meant that any compromise on this front was not possible or even desirable. More than once comparison was made with other countries in the region, for example Botswana, where routine HIV testing has been tried. Such a measure might be possible there, but not in South Africa, was the standard response. The position of activists has been to advocate for a chronic illness benefit with the needs of those with HIV at the forefront. In some instances the rights of those living with HIV to receive state support (even if they are healthy) are implicitly placed ahead of those who are merely poor or unemployed.

Official government discourse is also concerned to stress the rights of those who are HIV positive, although more evidence exists in the arena of social security of a shift in terms of actual planning, particularly on account of concerns to assist a broader constituency of people with chronic illness on equity grounds. A policy emphasizing the importance of equity argu-ably has equivalent moral high ground in the post-apartheid context to one advocating for specifically addressing the human rights of people with HIV. The idea within the Directorate of Social Security to address all chronic illness as a whole and situate it alongside 'disability' also makes adminis-trative sense in terms of a comprehensive social security provision. The constituencies that were more open to explicitly discussing alternatives to the exceptionalist-driven narrative and had clearly been grappling with the challenges for some time were academics in health economics and public health. The former were uncomfortable on account of equity issues, and the latter had both equity and population level public health concerns.

While concerns over how best to assess disability have been present in some form since 1994, they intensified with the state's commitment to roll out universal ARV provision in late 2003. From the perspective of public health professionals, discussion centred around the relationship of grant receipt to ARV provision. There were fears that more stringent criteria for grants for those with HIV and the allocation of a temporary grant only during periods of significant illness would have negative consequences for ARV provision. For example, those who entered programmes early might be less likely to get a grant than those who delayed until the illness became severe enough to meet eligibility criteria. Pertinent questions included: should the grant be linked to stages of illness and, if so, how? Should the grant be temporary or permanent?

In 2004 the government announced that all disabled people would be entitled to free health care, with the result that the Department of Health was faced with the same challenge of defining and assessing disability. Consequently, a decision was made to develop a 'harmonized assessment tool' (HAT) that could be used by departments of both Health and Social Development.

It has become self-evident and accepted within the Directorate of Social Security that the application of the HAT and the narrowing of the definition of disability will result in many people with chronic illness, and in particular those who are HIV positive and in receipt of grants, no longer being eligible for disability grants once the new HAT system is introduced. Margie Schneider, a consultant from the Human Sciences Research Council, has proposed that a chronic illness grant be developed to take the strain off the disability grant by distinguishing between those who are unemployed and those who are chronically ill (Schneider and Goudge, 2007). Under the proposed chronic illness grant, recipients would not be evaluated on the severity of their illness but would instead be eligible for funds intended to provide prophylactic benefits. The aim is to reduce the progression of the illness and to forestall the development of 'activity limitation' and thus 'disability'. In the case of HIV, this would involve purchasing food to ensure adequate nutrition to strengthen the immune system, and to ensure that individuals could attend clinics regularly to receive ARVs and participate in treatment support programmes, thus boosting adherence also.

It remains to be seen what impact the political upheavals of late 2008, which resulted in the fall from power of the controversial Health Minister Mantu Shabalala-Msimang, will have on both the proposals for a chronic illness benefit and the implementation of the new harmonized assessment tool. More concerted action on HIV/AIDS-related initiatives has already been evident, and provisions for a more specific and dedicated form of income benefit for this constituency is one proposal that many activists hope will be actualized.

The perspective from HIV/AIDS-related civil society organizations

Civil society organizations and actors have been vocal in arguing that there is a need for a specific form of social security that would cover people infected by HIV. ALP, TAC and the AIDS and Rights Alliance for Southern Africa (ARASA) have called for better social assistance for people with chronic illness, maintaining that the disability grant is not meeting their needs. The focus in particular is on grants cancelled in the case of those infected by HIV and those institutionalized with TB (TAC, 2008). The ALP collaborated with the TAC to produce a briefing document on the issue (Booth and Silber, 2008) for the South Africa National AIDS Council's (SANAC) Treatment, Care and Support technical task team.

Significantly, the emphasis in the SANAC document suggests that the rationale for a grant has been strongly influenced by drug resistance concerns. There is a clearly stated aim for the grant to improve adherence to ARVs and also to address the increase in MDR and XDR-TB. TB as a disease is second in the list of relevant conditions (UNAIDS, 2008), and the concern here is to aid treatment compliance by providing people with the financial means to attend clinic appointments regularly. Booth[15] even suggests linking receipt of the money conditionally to drug compliance.[16] Importantly, the ALP position in this respect is to insist that the grant would be permanent. However, Booth rejects as stigmatizing and lacking in evidence the popular claim that grants constitute a significant 'perverse incentive' to remain ill or that people would become infected with HIV in order to receive monthly cash. On balance the available research supports his assertion.[17]

In terms of civil society advocacy, the current position of the National Association of People with AIDS (NAPWA) is undoubtedly the most indicative of a stance of AIDS exceptionalism, advocating special measures for those with HIV/AIDS. In the week of 20 October 2008, NAPWA held protests regarding the issue of grants for HIV/AIDS. Staff in the Department of Social Development spoke of the unreasonable nature of their demands, and expressed the desire that they would cooperate with the SANAC civil society initiatives and demonstrate a willingness to negotiate.

Civil society groups have had to respond to concerns about the equity issues associated with providing social security to those who are HIV positive but remaining well. Nattrass (2006) suggests that ongoing poverty and high unemployment remain a key concern for many people in South Africa, regardless of their HIV status. Zackie Achmat, stalwart of the TAC, has acknowledged the difficult question of social justice, and the TAC has partly dealt with this concern by being proponents of a general basic income grant.[18] Paul Booth[19] of the ALP responds to Nattrass' argument by putting forward the position that people who are HIV positive require a grant to enable them to be healthy so that they can gain equal access to participate fully in society. Nattrass has also made forceful arguments for the institution of a basic income grant, as have others when considering the problem of the disability grant in the case of HIV/AIDS (see for example Hardy and Richter, 2006).

Lack of standardization remains a key concern. There are still no central directives to address the lack of standardized HIV grant allocation procedures across provinces. The TAC became aware that some provinces were even advocating that doctors should stop grants when CD4 counts rise above 200 with ARV treatment. Additional research in the Western Cape by the AIDS and Society Research Unit (ASRU) at the University of Cape Town supports the contention that the criteria for the allocation of grants are often obscure in the case of HIV/AIDS and decisions are largely dependent on the stance of the individual doctor, whose recommendation still carries great weight in the existing system. The comment of an HIV-positive woman interviewed as part of the ASRU research illustrates painfully the arbitrary nature of the process: 'It depends of the heart of the doctor sometimes... [talking about extension of the original disability grant time period]. If the doctor has got your sympathy then he can do that' (De Paoli et al, 2008). The comment of a doctor illustrates the other perspective and the difficulty of practising in a context of significant generalized poverty and unemployment, where grants and old age pensions support many households: 'The most difficult thing about being a doctor is that you have to write disability grants. It is like you are God; you just have to look at the person's face and decide about whether they qualify or not' (De Paoli et al, 2008).

HIV/TB: Accommodating co-infection in the narrative

Public health practitioners in particular give significance to co-infection with TB and the increase in drug-resistant TB when arguing for particular measures to address the HIV/AIDS epidemic. The grant/benefit debates indicate how prominent this issue has become, prompting the supposition that the need to control the public health threat of TB is starting to provide a proxy way of talking about and implementing limitations to the rights of people with HIV/AIDS.[20] It appears that the relationship between these two conditions has become key to providing spaces where exceptionalist measures can be bypassed whilst the explicit discourse about HIV/AIDS continues to be uncompromising in its upholding of individual human rights. When I questioned activists from the TAC and ALP about their stance regarding the limitation of the rights of people with MDR and XDR-TB through the forced institutionalization that has been implemented by the Department of Health, no one was resisting the policy itself. The point was made rather that they would advocate for the humane treatment of people whilst institutionalized, and indeed both organizations joined forces to challenge the temporary cessation of an individual's disability grant for the duration of admission to a hospital, as has been the practice of the state.

Members of the activist organizations questioned about the contrasting nature of the public health measures that have been instituted with respect to HIV/AIDS and TB in South Africa did not see the differences as contradictory, despite the now extremely close association between the diseases. Co-infectivity in South Africa is very high, particularly with drug-resistant strains of TB, so the reality is that many of those people who have been forcibly institutionalized for TB in fact constitute a subset of HIV-positive people. The measures insisting on notifiability, institutionalization and directly observed therapy for TB in effect also become a way of controlling, in a traditional public health sense, the most epidemiologically dangerous group of HIV-positive people. Yet the separate measures for TB are justified by many on the grounds that the two conditions are very different, in that TB is more infectious and the means of spread by droplets ensures that members of the general public are exposed and can catch the organism unknowingly. The implication here is that since sexual intercourse is the usual behavioural precursor to contracting HIV, a measure of individual responsibility exists. In contrast, with TB there appears to be a general consensus that the rights of others need to be protected above those of the individual, as there is a sense of arbitrariness associated with droplet spread. A further reason given is that the stigma associated with HIV is greater than TB, so that people should not be singled out in any way and confidentiality has to be protected by all possible measures.[21]

These observations raise interesting implications given the current plans to integrate HIV and TB services in state health facilities. The tensions about the degree of coercion that is acceptable to ensure drug adherence are far from resolved. As the discussions about models to ensure drug adherence continue, it will be interesting to see whether the HIV/AIDS strategies will influence TB policy, or vice versa. However, the extent to which the exceptionalist talk will be maintained explicitly in documents and planning discourse, whilst new spaces are created and utilized behind the surface for alternatives to be implemented, remains to be seen.

Collective rights narrative

The notion of 'collective' rights provides the basis for another alternative to the exceptionalist narrative and may help justify the setting aside of exclusive concern for the individual in the context of hyperendemic illnesses. Such a collective rights-based narrative, which frames the epidemic in terms of responsibility associated with drug adherence and the need to protect the general public from highly infectious disease, has begun to be evident in public discourse. In a workshop discussion of rights-based HIV programming that I ran in the neighbouring state of Zambia, members of AIDS activist networks even put forward the view that considering first and foremost the rights of the 'community' and promoting socially responsible behaviour in the case of certain illnesses is part of an African notion of *ubuntu* (generally understood in Southern Africa to refer to a social mind-edness and way of behaving that foregrounds a common humanity).

In activist and legal circles in South Africa, the use of the terminology of 'collective' rights appears to be employed in other ways also as a means by which claims upon the state to enable the well-being of the population can be extended to the maximum. Thus there has been debate about the extent to which the constitutional rights are individual only, or incorporate a wider state responsibility. For example, the ALP and TAC became aware that many households were struggling considerably on a financial level when a grant recipient with TB entered hospital for an extended period of treatment: in such instances the state would stop a grant on the grounds that the patient was for this period being supported in a state institution. In mid-2008 the Department of Social Development was challenged on the withdrawal of the disability grants of those institutionalized for resistant TB, on the grounds that the right to social security in the constitution included the right to maintain dependents.[22] This argument contends that the relevant section 27 of the constitution is thus referring to a collective, not an individual right. The Department of Social Development will now review this policy, but on account of a legal technicality, namely lack of clarity as to whether a hospital constitutes a 'state institution'. Their position is vociferously that the section 27 right is an individual right. There is, however, evidence of a more general discussion in the Directorate of Social Security as to the extension of provisions such as the 'temporary relief of distress' grant into some form of household-level grant. There have also been renewed calls for a reconsideration of the need for a basic income grant and speculation in several quarters that more senior figures in the Department of Social Development might now be more in favour of such a measure. A press release in October 2008 (Musgrave and Brown, 2008) reported that the ANC is committed to costing a range of extensions to the social welfare system, which seems to depart from past tendencies to dismiss calls for a basic income grant. The new Minister for Social Development in the Zuma cabinet has received a cautious welcome, with the Black Sash calling on her specifically to implement the proposals for a chronic illness benefit and the HAT (*South African Mail and Guardian*, 2009). She in turn is reported as saying that, unless a better model for poverty alleviation can be instituted, the government's significant outlay on social grants[23] will not be reduced. This kind of perspective might begin to address the huge challenges of inequality and unemployment in a more comprehensive way and start to mitigate the factors responsible for the equity concerns that have been generated with respect to policies devising social security for HIV/AIDS in particular.

Case Study 2: Voluntary counselling and testing and the changing use of lay counsellors

The privileging of counselling

Psychological techniques have been prominent in WHO best practice guidelines from the outset of the epidemic, as encapsulated in the '3 Cs' of the WHO, a commitment to counselling, confidentiality and consent. Just as the provision of grants described in the first study has been largely based on an exceptionalist and rights-driven narrative about the epidemic, the principles relating to counselling also derive from an exceptionalist approach to HIV/AIDS that foregrounds the rights of those affected and includes special measures for the preservation of 'dignity'. 'Voluntary counselling' has therefore been central to the testing procedure aimed at encouraging people to determine their HIV status. The inclusion also reflects the adoption of assumptions in mainstream psychology practice about the need to be supported through a potentially adverse event.

The introduction of a cadre of workers designated as lay health providers and, specifically, the subset of this group made up of lay counsellors, could be viewed cynically as a cost-cutting measure or one response to the human resource shortage faced by health systems in Southern Africa in the context of expanding ARV treatment programmes through task shifting (see van Damme et al, 2008). However, it could also be viewed as an acknowledgement by the South African Department of Health of the value of psychological perspectives and an endorsement of the privileging of the individual rights of patients. In the Western Cape Province,[24] where the material for this case study has been collected, the health department has outsourced the training and supervision of lay counsellors to a number of NGOs, such as Lifeline, but is ultimately responsible for their salaries. Yet the terrain of HIV-testing protocol is certainly far from uncontroversial, and the shift in perspective to a chronic illness and the focus on treatment programmes has complicated the debates further. In the midst of the policy debates are the lay counsellors themselves, with specific concerns about their professional position and the burdens placed upon them.

Alternative testing approaches

The response of public health professionals and policy-makers to the role of lay counsellors has been mixed from the outset. On the one hand there are misgivings about the effect of this particular manifestation of an exceptionalist narrative and in particular the cost of the special measures it entails: there is a belief that the imperative to provide an in-depth counselling component has hampered the provision of testing (thus compounding the documented problem of large numbers of infected individuals remaining ignorant of their status and potentially spreading the virus).[25] Consequently, they argue, enrolment into treatment has also been negatively affected,[26] because of the challenge to train and supervise enough counsellors. Indeed, the city of Cape Town is piloting a scheme to supplement the conventional walk-in 'voluntary' testing with a streamlined 'provider initiated counselling and testing' (PICT). In an effort to increase the numbers tested, individuals attending a health centre (in this case a clinic for sexually transmitted infections (STIs)) for another reason are encouraged to receive on-the-spot HIV testing. This scheme shortens the pre-test 'counselling' intervention and 'task shifts' a condensed and more mechanized version to nurses, whilst the lay counsellors do group education (Naidoo, 2006). However, the vigilant ALP (Richter, 2006) has already expressed concern about the violation of patient rights to informed consent because of the potentially coercive nature of 'routine' schemes where patients have to explicitly 'opt out' of testing, such as those introduced in Botswana.[27]

The official responsible for lay counsellors in the Western Cape provincial HIV/AIDS Directorate,[28] believes that pilots such as this one to explicitly introduce PICT will not be instituted more widely, due to concerns over consent.[29] However, discussions with him of the plans in the Western Cape to expand the role of lay counsellors suggest that a reconceptualization of their role is in fact implicitly introducing a very different model to that envisaged in the WHO directives. Indeed, it appears quite possible for the language surrounding an issue like this one to remain untouched and thus for the official discourse to appear to remain in keeping with dominant exceptionalist narrative, whilst the actual practice is quietly being transformed behind the scenes. Thus an interview with a manager of the AIDS Training and Counselling Centre (ATICC)[30] brought to the fore the concerns from the side of psychologists regarding the nature of practices that are now referred to as 'counselling'. ATICC provides the training for all the lay counsellors currently employed in the Western Cape, and a programme has been developed over the past 15 years that takes 30 days to complete. In contrast, the nurses who were involved in the PICT trial were trained for three days. The manager is concerned that increasingly what is referred to as 'counselling' in the pre-test setting is nothing more than information giving or the mechanical running through of a checklist. She is vehemently resistant to any 'watering down' of what HIV/AIDS counselling should ideally be, but acknowledges that there is little control over the practices that might evolve once the trainees leave ATICC and adapt to the real life world of the clinic. The pressures that she pinpoints are threefold:

- to dilute what constitutes counselling;
- to reduce the time allocated for counselling;
- to cut short the length of training.

The situation of lay counsellors

A visit to Lifeline in Khayelitsha, on the outskirts of the Cape Town metropolis, revealed the challenges of providing lay counsellor services. The NGO is contracted by the Western Cape government to select and manage the 70-odd lay counsellors working in clinics in the township. All these individuals have passed through the ATICC training, and Lifeline is also responsible for organizing fortnightly group supervision sessions by a government-approved professional. A coordinator of the Lifeline programme in the area gives an account of the work that foregrounds the dominant place of statistical collection in the day-to-day work of counsellors in the clinic. It is evident that the 'uptake index' (the number of individuals that agree to an HIV test after pre-test counselling) recorded monthly in each clinic is seen as an extremely important measure of the quality of the counselling in terms of the motivational success of individual counsellors. These 'stats' are seen to indicate to the clinics where additional input is needed from the coordinator. The counsellors are explicitly presented as agents of behavioural change and also as community educators. Until recently in fact, more experienced counsellors could choose to do an additional ten days of training at ATICC to become adherence counsellors. These positions have been seen as more skilled and still attract a higher salary.

  In considering the work of lay counsellors in a setting like Khayelitsha, it is important to recognize the enormous expectations placed on these individuals. Rohleder and Swartz (2005) document the lack of adequate supervision for those put at the emotional coalface of the HIV/AIDS epidemic. In addition, they at present have no professional position within the structures designating state healthcare workers. Nationally their conditions of service and pay vary enormously. In some parts of the country, lay counsellors are officially considered 'volunteers' and are paid as little as R400 a month ($50), or do not receive any of the promised remuneration. The ALP has embarked on a project to collect accounts of such instances in order to launch a legal case proving that their conditions of service do constitute formal employment and thus are covered by employment legislation.[31] In the Western Cape the salaries start at R1400, and the HIV Directorate is exploring possibilities to agree nationally the placing of lay counsellors into a professional structure at the level of nursing assistants. This in many ways is proof of the increasing emphasis placed upon their role not only as voluntary counselling and testing counsellors, but more importantly adherence counsellors. In the Western

Cape, all counsellors are now to be trained in adherence work so that this becomes a core as opposed to an additional skill.[32]

This increasing emphasis on treatment adherence[33] in HIV programming parallels the conceptualization of HIV/AIDS as a chronic illness and intersects with exceptionalist narratives in interesting ways. A WHO task team report contends that psychological intervention can encourage enrolment in treatment programmes as well as treatment adherence, and points to the value of various counselling strategies in group and individual sessions in terms of motivating for behavioural change (Freeman et al, 2005). As treatment 'roll-out' progresses in South Africa, 'adherence counselling', 'treatment assistants' and facilitated 'psychosocial support groups' and measures to promote 'treatment literacy' are being advocated and different models compared.

The regulation of antiretroviral treatment has become a crucial and contentious issue amidst concerns about the effectiveness of adherence and drug resistance in settings of poverty, such as township areas where the incidence of the illness is greatest. Results from an ARV treatment initiative in the township of Khayelitsha in Cape Town have been used to argue strongly that a detailed programme involving counsellors in treatment preparation and adherence support has been a crucial factor in the high adherence levels and the very successful reduction in mortality in this locality (Coetzee et al, 2004). This programme is part-run by Medicins Sans Frontières, with strong ties to the TAC and its agenda to promote treatment literacy and encourage the emergence of 'expert patients'. There have thus been additional suggestions that the 'conscientizing' of the patient population through contact with the TAC has led to the positive results.

These perspectives underlie a belief that certain kinds of educational and psychological interventions can have significant success in creating a particular kind of patient to enter a treatment programme: doctors are concerned to develop and promote procedures that create patient-citizens who will behave in ways indicating an understanding of the risks to other citizens. Medicins Sans Frontières has called this a 'responsibilized' patient (Robins, 2006).

The emphasis on promoting individual responsibility is evident in the account of the ATICC trainers[34] of the adherence counselling strategies taught during the training. A Lifeline coordinator in Khayelitsha further detailed the way in which the lay counsellors are taught to encourage adherence in this setting.[35] Emphasis is placed on the fact that only two ARV regimes exist, and that the second line of drugs has considerably more side effects. Patients are warned that non-adherence will leave them with only this second option. They are also reminded that being immuno-compromised puts them at risk of a range of infections. Indeed, accounts indicate that patients on ARV programmes display considerable fear about returning to a level of illness experienced prior to initiating ARVs, and very much wish to remain on drugs for their own well-being. Maintaining a regime of adherence and managing the side effects of the medication have become a central part of their narratives of being chronically infected with HIV (see for example Mills, 2008). This fear of becoming ill again and having no further drug options must encourage people to respond to a discourse of individual responsibility and individual benefit related to adherence. However, whilst adherence issues might be framed in individualized terms at the clinic level in the language of the strategies to promote adherence, it can be argued that, behind the scenes, the public health discourse is one of achieving a certain moral compliance of large groups of affected people, an epidemiological responsibility. Individualist language is thus shadowed by an urgency to address population level concerns and achieve control of the dual epidemics of TB and HIV. Lay counsellors are seen as crucial to mediating this process and it appears that their practice will be pragmatically transformed in the service of implicit alternative narratives that highlight pressing public health challenges even if the exceptionalist narrative emphasizing 'counselling' continues to be prominent.

The fluid use of the terminology around counselling to cover a range of practices is worrying to the management at ATICC, as is the reduced emphasis on forms of counselling not linked to motivational interviewing to achieve behavioural change. There is concern that the fluidity of use of psychological discourse has created spaces to undermine the ideological basis of the 'Three Cs'. As an organization who see themselves as having a long and distinguished history in honing quality counselling services for HIV, they are also alarmed by intimations from the Western Cape Department of Health that in future they will have to shift their work beyond only HIV, in order to provide training in counselling with a behavioural change emphasis to a broader range of lay health counsellors. These individuals would then also be employed in clinics focused on chronic conditions like diabetes and hypertension. Such a vision on the part of the government might suggest a shift from a dominant exceptionalist narrative to one in which AIDS gradually takes a place alongside other chronic illnesses.[36]

Conclusion

In South Africa, the tenets of AIDS exceptionalism found fertile ground in the post-apartheid rights discourse. The material presented here suggests that in the South African arena these exceptionalist narratives and the applicability of the pathways of response they support have not been directly challenged. Shifts in practice, though they may be implicit and less overt, may have significant effects on the landscape of AIDS treatment.

It is evident that the language of rights and discussions about the intricacies of legal interpretations remains a strong feature of AIDS activism and of legal challenges to press the state to provide in particular for people with HIV/AIDS. However, the sheer numbers of people requiring these provisions are hugely challenging in the context of a hyperendemic area where ARV programmes are transforming the idea of HIV as a terminal illness to a conceptualization of chronic illness. This transformation has the potential to erode the official discourse of exceptionalism, not least by challenging it on equity grounds. In addition, the real public health challenges introduced by the prevalence of dangerous opportunistic infections has created public alarm and raised questions about when it is justifiable to limit individual rights in the collective interest. The case studies presented in this chapter suggest that these pressures are leading to a gradual redefining of what exceptionalism might mean in actual practice and a pragmatic shift to strategies that are considered possible in the local setting. Even if pragmatic measures do not explicitly challenge an enduring official narrative of AIDS exceptionalism, practice might be slowly transformed in revealing ways, with implicit alternative narratives privileging adherence and equity above individual rights.

In the case of grants, the exceptionalist narrative is prominent in activist circles and the framing of arguments for a grant is very much in terms of the necessity of special provisions. However, at the level of government, the measures being developed are gradually placing HIV on a level with other chronic illnesses, even if the political moment might not yet have arrived to implement a more explicit policy in this regard in terms of implementing a chronic illness benefit. It is possible that the close connection between HIV and TB does create a space for activists to articulate certain public health concerns that require more coercive responses: it appears that fears about resistant TB are more readily acknowledged than public health concerns about HIV, and AIDS activists have adjusted to an acceptance of more coercive public health measures in the former case. Accepting limitations upon the rights of those with drug-resistant TB in many cases provides a way of isolating the most epidemiologically threatening cohort in the HIV-positive population. The greater focus on TB infection, for example in the case of forcible institutionalization, de-emphasizes the likelihood of HIV co-infection and might enable actors to acquiesce to some limitation of the rights of HIV-positive people without explicitly doing so.

In the case of lay counsellors, a shared set of counselling practices and principles has gradually been eroded, whilst the official discourse of the 'Three Cs' has persisted. Public health concerns with increasing testing and human resource limitations on the numbers of highly trained counsellors have clearly contributed to this situation.

More recently it is adherence concerns that are reducing the counsel-ling dimension to a potentially narrow emphasis on achieving behavioural change through the individualization of responsibility. Whilst framed in individualist terms, the underlying concern is the creation of epidemiologic-ally responsible citizens who would maintain a moral compliance to treat-ment regimes in order to address population-level public health concerns.

These examples illustrate how a rights-based narrative can dominate discourse even if quite substantial shifts occur in what happens in practice. They suggest that spaces of practice can be created to deal pragmatically with the enormous challenges faced by the policy-makers in hyperendemic areas. A politics of representation maintains the rhetoric of policy as a front, obscuring a more varied range of practices that are in fact able to emerge and be tolerated. These redefinitions attempt to address not only the classic public health challenges posed by acute epidemics, but also the realities of grinding poverty and of inequality that ensure that Farmer's (1999a) notion of 'structural violence' remains a very relevant factor in the analysis of this long-standing epidemic that has become chronic.

Notes

1   The heads of state of African Union countries convened a special summit in Nigeria in April 2001 devoted specifically to addressing the 'exceptional chal-lenges' of HIV/AIDS, TB and other related infectious diseases'. Point 13 of the resultant Declaration (2001, p3) states: 'We recognise that the epidemic of HIV/ AIDS, Tuberculosis and other related infectious diseases constitute not only a major health crisis, but also an exceptional threat to Africa's development, social cohesion, political stability, food security as well as the greatest global threat to the survival and life expectancy of African peoples.'

2   See Elbe (2005) for an in-depth discussion of the shift to the framing of the pandemic as an international security issue and an analysis of the danger of perni-cious social practices being enabled through such securitization of the discourse. Whiteside et al (2006) argue that the claim that HIV/AIDS can destabilize security within states, and regionally, remains speculation.

3   Piot (2005) certainly stresses the need to have a response in keeping with the scale of the epidemic and was a big advocate for the setting up of the Global Fund. De Waal, however, takes issue with the disjuncture that he perceives between the tone of exceptionalist rhetoric and principles that have governed the practical outworking of responses.

4   For example, Dionisio et al (2006) outline the obstacles to providing equit-able access in poor countries and the challenges associated with attempting to encourage domestic production of generic drugs.

5   Garrett (2007, p14) has warned of the risk that large sums directed in a 'largely uncoordinated' fashion at high-profile diseases might worsen circumstances on the ground (for instance by deflecting attention from other diseases of poverty,

weakening health systems and enticing scarce health personnel away from the public sector coalface). Farmer (2007) on the other hand, whilst agreeing with some of her points, has responded to advocate for a more hopeful picture.

6   A recent review in the *Lancet* (Piot et al, 2009) has attempted to survey data on the cumulative effect of high-profile disease programmes on general in-country health services. In balance these data in fact suggest a picture of mixed influence, positive in some areas, negative in others.

7   England (2007, p344) claims that too much money is spent proportionately on HIV/AIDS globally if one considers the burden of overall disease in low and middle-income countries. He points to the undermining effect on health systems, and asks: 'Why has this happened? One factor surely has been the success of HIV lobbies and activists in promoting HIV as exceptional.' He has subsequently declared that 'the writing is on the wall for UNAIDS' (England, 2008, p1072).

8   The most recent population-based survey (HSRC, 2009) estimates that HIV prevalence amongst all age groups is 10.6 per cent. Thus 5.2 million people are thought to be HIV positive. Comparing this result to the previous two surveys by the same organization, the authors contend that South Africa's HIV epidemic is stabilizing. There are also signs of a decline in prevalence amongst children (attributed to prevention strategies like preventing mother to child transmission) and for the first time a decline has been suggested in incidence in adolescents aged 15–19 years. Prevalence figures vary considerably between provinces, with five out of nine provinces in fact showing increases in prevalence. A further worrying factor is persistently high prevalence levels in young women (peaking at 32.9 per cent in the 25–29 year age group). UNAIDS/WHO (2008) estimated prevalence in South Africa to be 18.1 per cent at the end of 2007.

9   Sub-Saharan Africa remains the part of the world most significantly affected by HIV. In 2007, 67 per cent of all people living with HIV/AIDS were from the region. Some 72 per cent of AIDS deaths occurred here. Countries in Southern Africa in particular demonstrated the highest levels of HIV prevalence globally (UNAIDS, 2008).

10   See Swartz and MacGregor (2002) for an analysis of the ideological drivers of this change.

11   The nine provincial governments are in contracts with 1600 non-profit organizations utilizing lay workers (Schneider, 2009).

12   The Treatment Action Campaign notes how difficult it is to determine accurately the number of people in South Africa on ARVs, due to poor data collection. They quote (with caveats) the Department of Health UNGASS Report (2008) that claims that 371,731 people had initiated treatment by the end of November 2007 (www.tac.org.za/community/keystatistics, accessed 6 December 2009). Other estimates put the figure now at upwards of 650,000 (Hanefeld, 2009).

13   1 South African Rand = GBP0.07; US$0.13

14   It is significant that the debate on measures to address the increase in the burden of chronic illness globally is usually focused on non-communicable disease (see for example Horton, 2007) and TB has not been foregrounded in this way as a key chronic illness. This suggests that it is the association to HIV infection that has attracted the attention in this instance.

15   Interview Paul Booth, AIDS Law Project, 21 October 2008.

16   The Department of Social Development is very cautious of such a measure on the grounds of their violating constitutional rights.

17   Leclerc-Madlala (2006) argues that her findings suggest that some people would rather die than lose a grant as they maintain that they are unable to eat without a grant. Other research suggests that people on ARVs do not leave treatment programmes when a grant is stopped (Venkataramani et al, 2008). De Paoli et al (2008) report that people in ARV programmes maintained that they themselves would rather lose a grant than risk their health, but claimed that others were stopping their medication to ensure that they remained eligible. Anecdotal reports exist which claim that the sale of blood by HIV-positive individuals for the purposes of obtaining a grant does occur.

18   Indeed, it is claimed that a comprehensive social security system that includes a basic income grant would improve food security and 'have a direct impact on reducing new TB and assisting adherence in TB and HIV treatment' (Achmat and Roberts, 2005, p4).

19   Interview Paul Booth, AIDS Law Project, 21 October 2008.

20   It is estimated that one-third of South Africans infected with HIV will develop TB in their lifetimes. The total number of TB cases reported in 2006 was 316, 863 (669/100,000). It is estimated that 55 per cent of these TB patients are in fact HIV positive. Unfortunately not all know their HIV status and in 2006 only 40 per cent of all TB patients received testing for HIV (National Department of Health, 2008).

21   In an address to the media in October 2008, the Minister of Health appointed in the place of Tshabalala-Msimang stated that the co-existence of the TB and HIV epidemics was one of the most significant problems faced by the health sector, referring to the challenge relating to 'the multitudes of people living with Tuberculosis as well as those affected by the extreme drug resistant strains, MDR-TB and XDR-TB'. The incidence of TB in the country remains one of the highest in the world. She emphasized the importance of ensuring drug 'compliance' and explained that '[i]n the interests of public health, those with MDR-TB and XDR-TB are hospitalized for a defined period of time, until they no longer pose a threat to their families and communities.' The emphasis on threat was balanced by commitment to a compassionate service and she concluded that 'we wish to make it clear that health is a human right and this is the principle that should continue to guide us' (Barbara Hogan, 2008).

22   See the SANAC briefing document for an outline (Booth and Silber, 2008).

23   The SANAC briefing document (Booth and Silber, 2008) quotes figures that the social welfare system supports over 12 million people, which amounts to 10.8 per cent of government expenditure (R70.7 billion).

24   In actuarial estimates generated for the provincial government, Dorrington (2005) predicts that the population of the Western Cape will reach 5.5 million by 2025, taking into account the effect of HIV/AIDS. Overall HIV prevalence is expected to peak at 6 per cent, which translates into 250,000 infected people in total. Furthermore, he predicts that given treatment, 65 per cent of these infected people will be asymptomatic by 2015, whereas 15 per cent of them will be AIDS sick. He worked on the assumption that ART is only expected to increase life expectancy on average by 5 years. In a report for the provincial government (Myers and Naledi, 2007, p9), the burden of diseases for the province in order of decreasing

magnitude in terms of contribution to early mortality (calculated as percentage Years of Life Lost) is recorded as the following ranking: infectious diseases, injury, mental disorders, cardiovascular disease, childhood diseases.

25   The UNGASS Report indicates that in the last 12 months of data collection, 1.3 million people (aged 25–49) received an AIDS test (National Department of Health, 2008). The Human Sciences Research Council (HSRC) (2009) claims that over the period 2002–2008, the number of people (aged 15–49) who reported an awareness of their HIV status doubled, success which the authors attribute to campaigns promoting, and increased availability of, voluntary counselling and testing services.

26   In 2007 the estimated number of people in South Africa in WHO Stage 4 of HIV/ AIDS and thus in need of ART was estimated at 889,000. However, only 55 per cent of these enrolled in a programme, and only 42 per cent initiated treatment (National Department of Health, 2008).

27   UNAIDS policy in fact endorses PICT in all health settings in areas with generalized HIV epidemics but with caveats and conditions that reinforce the primacy of the 'Three Cs' and practice that stays in line with WHO guidelines: 'In light of the need for individuals to have earlier access to treatment, care, support and prevention, UNAIDS and WHO are supporting a major expansion of access to HIV testing and counselling through the scaling up of client-initiated testing and counselling services and through the expansion of provider-initiated testing and counselling services in health care settings ... UNAIDS does not support mandatory testing of individuals. All testing, whether client or provider-initiated should be conducted under the conditions of the "Three Cs" ... Where there are high levels of stigma and discrimination and low capacity to implement testing and counselling under the Three Cs, these issues should be addressed before expansion of access to provider-initiated testing and counselling in health facilities.' (www.unaids.org/en/ PolicyAndPractice/CounsellingAndTesting/default.asp, accessed 30 June 2009.)

28   Interview 30 October 2008.

29   However, the most recent prevalence report from South Africa (HSRC, 2009) recommends that HIV testing be routinely offered to all patients at health centres. In a recent budget speech (June 2009), the new Minister of Health, Dr A. Motsoaledi, noted the findings and, whilst not committing outright, stated that the recommendation to implement PICT would be considered by the ministry.

30   Interview 28 October 2008.

31   Interview with S'Khumbuzo Maphumulo, 21 October 2008.

32   Interview with official in Western Cape HIV/AIDS Directorate, 30 October 2008.

33   Unfortunately the Department of Health has no data as yet to indicate how many of those who initiate ARV therapy are known to still be on treatment after 12 months, as figures have not been accurately collected (National Department of Health, 2008).

34   Interview 28 October 2008.

35   Interview 30 October 2008.

36   See Standing et al (2008) for a discussion of the range of potential roles for a cadre of lay health workers beyond disease-specific interventions.

Chapter 7

Fighting the Flu: Risk, Uncertainty and Surveillance[1]

Ian Scoones

Introduction

The state of knowledge about the swine flu pandemic is a curious mix of the certain and the unknowable. It is a very uncomfortable place for a government predisposed to confident prediction to find itself. On the one hand it risks being accused of scaremongering, on the other of a lack of preparedness ... At the heart of the government response to the flu pandemic is what is becoming a central preoccupation of authority – the management of risk ... Risk management, it is emerging, carries risks of its own. Trying to grasp as slippery a subject as epidemiology and then present it with certainty is a recipe for controversy. (Editorial, *The Guardian*, 18 July 2009).

As this excerpt from a UK newspaper editorial entitled 'Swine flu: known unknowns' highlights, the current swine flu pandemic has presented many dilemmas for global health policy-makers. While the dangers of scaremongering – and the associated panic or hoarding that can result – are very real, so too are the risks of a lack of preparedness when dealing with an unpredictable virus with the potential to mutate into something worse. Risk management, a set of quantitative tools for calculating risks and calibrating responses, has provided some shelter in the storm for governments and international organizations seeking to justify and order their responses. But, as the financial crisis has demonstrated, seemingly robust tools for measuring risk (often based on quantitative models), are frequently underpinned by unquestioned assumptions and may mask dangerous systemic vulnerabilities. When linked with the science of epidemiology, risk management presents an alluring vision of control that can mask a landscape of uncertainty and even ignorance which, while disconcerting, may be better acknowledged than covered up. These dilemmas, so well encapsulated in the ongoing swine flu case, are faced more generally in the response to epidemics from any source.

With the world confronting a pandemic H1N1 swine flu during 2009 and 2010, the lessons from the global response to H5N1 avian influenza – a different virus, from different origins, but with many similar characteristics – are particularly pertinent. Drawing on extensive interviews with key policy-makers at both national and international levels, this chapter examines the dilemmas faced by those attempting to respond to H5N1 avian influenza who are confronted with deep uncertainties and sometimes plain ignorance in the face of a potential pandemic threat. The chapter focuses in particular on the challenges of effective surveillance. This is at the heart of the international response strategies to influenza and other emerging or re-emerging infectious diseases. Early warning systems, control-at-source strategies and effective containment are at the core of the WHO's approach, for example, and are replicated within government pandemic preparedness plans across the world. Yet these are painfully inadequate given the challenges. In a comment piece in 2009, *Nature* argued that 'Surveillance of human diseases that originate in animals remains in the nineteenth century' (*Nature*, 2009, p889; see also Butler, 2006).

Over the last decade, and particularly on the back of the global avian influenza response, substantial resources have been invested in surveillance systems (see Dry, this volume). These are at the centre of risk management approaches that aim to gather information systematically on potential outbreaks, assess the risks associated with each and then deploy resources around a response, hopefully to eradicate or at least contain the disease. A whole information management and risk response chain is envisaged, whereby the latest information technology combines with highly tuned logistics operations to ensure that medical expertise and technology is delivered to the right place and at the right time.

This chapter explores the challenges in designing surveillance systems, and identifies a number of problems with a narrow 'risk management' approach. Such a response, the chapter argues, is often justified by a narrative focused on 'outbreaks' (see Leach and Hewlett, this volume), rather than on responding to the complexity of context-dependent social–ecological dynamics of human–disease interfaces. Avoiding such complexity, and all the attendant uncertainties, and reducing the assessment to one of probabilistic risk, it is argued, is highly problematic, even dangerous. Equally, assuming a neat, unproblematic flow of information through a logistics chain to a response system must be challenged when real-world settings are taken into account (Calain, 2007b). Such well-functioning bureaucratic systems exist nowhere, especially in a crisis. And politics and the assertion of authority in the face of uncertainty always come into the picture to disturb any neat plan.

But why does this matter? As discussed in the introduction, the only certainty is that humanity will be confronted, at some point, from somewhere, with a major pandemic with significant impacts, probably from an animal source (Jones et al, 2008). Avian influenza and now swine flu are perhaps just dress rehearsals for the inevitable 'big one'. We have of course missed emergent pandemics before. Where was the effective surveillance that would have picked up the transfer of the human immunodeficiency virus (HIV) from apes to humans, at sometime during the early 20th century, probably in the forests of Central or West Africa? Once HIV had established itself in human populations it was too late, and the subsequent history is well known (see Edstrom and MacGregor, this volume).

Global public health and security policies are therefore justifiably focused on preparing for and responding to pandemics, and surveillance is legitimately at the centre of this, its prominent place reinforced by the revised International Health Regulations. But do such efforts miss key elements, and so fail to acknowledge alternative sources of information, more diverse knowledge bases and the complexity of emergent disease socio-ecologies? With a design determined by risk management concerns, this chapter argues, mainstream surveillance approaches centred on outbreak responses need rethinking, adapting and extending if they are to be truly effective in responding to emerging disease threats. Fighting the flu – whatever the exact virus – requires a set of skills and resources beyond risk assessment, information processing and logistics management. Rethinking surveillance requires new skills, alternative sources of knowledge and expertise and a radically different design of response systems, as discussed below (see Table 7.1, p155).

Lessons from the international response to avian influenza

Over the last decade H5N1 avian influenza has spread dramatically across the globe. It has become effectively endemic in a number of countries in Asia, and presents a regular threat to avian populations in different parts of the world through bird migration and marketing links. While H5N1 has caused hundreds of millions of poultry deaths globally (much through culling), the feared human–human spread has so far not occurred. This does not mean that this will not happen in the future, especially through re-assortment with other influenza viruses that spread more effectively through human populations, such as H1N1 swine flu.

The dominant outbreak narrative has, over the last decade, shaped the international response in three overlapping 'outbreak narratives', which define the problem and suggest the solutions (Scoones and Forster, 2008; Scoones, 2010). The first is a strong narrative linking veterinary concerns with agriculture and livelihood issues: 'it's a bird disease – and affects people's livelihoods'. The responses have centred on veterinary control measures and industry 'restructuring', with the World Organization for Animal Health (OIE) and the Food and Agriculture Organization of the United Nations (FAO) being at the centre of the debate. Second, there is a human public health narrative that has dominated media and political concerns: 'human–human spread is the real risk, and could be catastrophic'. Here a combination of drugs, vaccines and behaviour change dominates the response, one very much centred on the WHO, with UNICEF (the United Nations Children's Fund) and a number of NGOs being important players too. And, finally, there is a narrative focused on pandemic preparedness: 'a major economic and humanitarian disaster is around the corner and we must be prepared'. Responses focus on civil contingency planning, business continuity approaches and containment strategies. Here, a much wider network of industry players and consultants are concerned, linked to different branches of government, notably prime ministers' and presidents' offices and finance ministries with concerns about the economic fallout of any pandemic. The humanitarian community – United Nations agencies, the Red Cross, development NGOs and others – is also important.

These three outbreak narratives have driven a massive global response. Over US$2 billion of public funds have been allocated through a series of pledging conferences in Beijing, Delhi and Sharm-el-Sheikh. At the centre of the response is the design of surveillance systems, sitting alongside capacity building of national veterinary and public health systems, interventions in poultry marketing systems, drug and vaccine production and stockpiling, and pandemic preparedness planning. Across the three narratives surveillance is seen as the key: spotting what is happening on the ground and monitoring changes will help the global response to be nimble and effective.

What does the current global surveillance system look like? A complex network of information gathering and processing efforts combine together across a range of organizations and groups. For zoonotic diseases, such as avian influenza, a key element is the integration of information and alert systems from animal and human disease surveillance. For human disease surveillance, hospital reporting is reasonably accurate and widespread, especially for more acute influenza cases, and diagnosis is straightforward if samples are sent to a laboratory. But of course not every case of human infection with avian influenza presents at a hospital, and not all hospitals and clinics will send samples. Thus inevitably the surveillance system picks up the acute, visible, accessible cases and misses altogether other cases, especially in more endemic situations where disease symptoms may be relatively mild. The focus is therefore on major outbreaks, where human mortality and morbidity are high.

The WHO is the main international public body responsible for human health surveillance. As mandated by the new International Health Regulations, this allows for intervention in sovereign states to enforce the sharing of information and the generation of an adequate response (Fidler, 2005), although in practice there are limits to such top-down interventionism in the name of global health security (Calain, 2007a). The current system involves data collection from a wide range of sources, including official reporting from government health authorities, as well as media and civil society reports. The GLEWS network (the Global Early Warning System for Major Animal Diseases, including zoonoses, a WHO-FAO-OIE partnership) includes scans of media reports and websites for early indications of animal outbreaks or human cases of many animal and zoonotic diseases, including avian influenza. They make use of the Canadian Global Public Health Intelligence Network (GPHIN), which includes media and internet searches across several languages, and the ProMed reporting system, along with the Global Infectious Diseases Epidemiology Online Network (GIDEON) database and country and regional offices of the partner organizations. In addition, there are 'outbreak hotlines' that people can contact – an email address and a phone number. There are also inputs from informal reports by WHO and FAO field officers, members of the GOARN (Global Outbreak Alert and Response Network) teams and others who are contacted when suspicions are aroused (Heymann and Rodier, 2001, 2004). Information is one thing, but verification is another. Formally this has to be through notification by national governments' health ministries – or designated WHO contacts – confirmed by laboratory tests, initially locally, and then in WHO reference labs. But such verifications can be slow in coming, and WHO personnel, particularly specialists in influenza, must make their own assessments as to the importance of a particular outbreak. Daily meetings at the WHO emergency centre – a well-equipped converted cinema, the SHOC room (the Strategic Health Operations Centre)[2] – provide the opportunity for assessing information from surveillance efforts.

On the animal side, official reporting of outbreaks of notifiable diseases goes through the OIE. Chief Veterinary Officers are obliged to report to the Paris headquarters which compiles regular information bulletins on disease incidence. At FAO, resources for the global avian influenza response have boosted capacity for surveillance through the Emergency Prevention System (EMPRES) for Transboundary Animal and Plant Pests and Diseases and its new information platform, as well as establishment of the Crisis Management Centre (CMC)[3] at FAO headquarters in 2006 which provides a counterpart to the WHO's facility. For veterinary public health, and for avian influenza in particular, the overall plan for avian influenza offers a vision of an integrated, joined-up cross-agency response (FAO and OIE, 2008).

In many respects, the system is impressive: the facilities are often brand new, the professionals involved are well qualified and the array of institutions involved (and so the list of acronyms) is often overwhelming. However, those working within the global surveillance system are realistic about what can be done. An FAO informant observed:

> *We quickly reach the limit of our system. We need expertise in the corridor to recognize what is going on. Surveillance is very different between countries: Indonesia and Nigeria for example. For the latter, there were no reports in September. In Indonesia they are looking and finding it. But again we are tracing events, not the situation in the country. Reporting in [X] is very poor. If they report, it's because everyone already knows. The key question, when it gets serious, is the high level of expertise we need in the corridor. It is more and more difficult to find good people.*[4]

Thus professional judgement always remains important; the data are never truly comprehensive or reliable. Reluctance by veterinary services to report outbreaks, or farmers in fear of the consequences; the lack of field staff in country and poor understanding of underlying epidemiological dynamics, all add to the layers of uncertainty, despite the impressions of precision given by the multi-coloured risk maps and interactive websites.

A central challenge raised by zoonotic diseases is coordinating surveillance across animal and human populations. Disparities in information quality and accuracy make this difficult, but across the international system there is a working attempt. This involves daily morning tele/videoconferences between the WHO and FAO emergency centres (the SHOC room in Geneva and the CMC in Rome), with interactions intensified with OIE and others when new outbreaks are defined. There is clearly an effective, collegial interaction across the agencies. In many people's eyes this represents unprecedented coordination and integration, assisted by donor funds for the avian influenza response and a committed set of professional individuals.

But how effective will this impressive and growing infrastructure be in the face of a pandemic? The risk management framework presents a neat, phased unfolding of a pandemic that may be wildly unrealistic.[5] Surveillance is key to the overall strategy, and the WHO pandemic preparedness documents show how early detection results in rapid containment, and a slowing of the pandemic in Phases 3 and 4, allowing time to get ready for the major consequences of the outbreak in the full global pandemic phase. Such neat risk management plans offer an aura of certainty. Yet deep uncertainties remain – about information accuracy, prediction possibilities and response strategies – and no one knows quite what will happen when. Will we be faced with a 'slow-burn' epidemic or a global catastrophe? A UN official candidly observed that behind the neat plans, a more complex, contingent and uncertain reality lurks:

> It is accepted ... that containment will not work. In all countries with humanitarian crises, governance tends to be weak. How can such strategies be implemented? Even in Europe. We are already moving to the next step – response. But what realistically can be done? Some basic capacity issues, yes. Keep the electricity functioning, ensure some basic services. This is important. But vaccines and so on? No. Basically you are on your own. Sit indoors and hope for the best![6]

So despite the very substantial investments in risk-based surveillance and pandemic response systems, many insiders recognize the gross disconnect between the theory and the most likely reality. The real world is not one where pandemics follow a linear, phased sequence or where information will be captured early and responded to according to the risk assessment and management guidelines. Contingency, chance, politics, bureaucratic fumbling and real world complexity will all enter the picture. Yet, often rather simplistic, risk-focused, managerial understandings are at the centre of each of the three outbreak narratives that have driven the international avian influenza response – and because of the resources invested and the institutional commitments made – all subsequent responses to other emerging infectious diseases.

Each narrative is framed by particular, institutionalized, professional concerns. Thus in the veterinary narrative, the identification of outbreaks, followed by rapid laboratory testing and then stamping out control measures are at the core. The focus is on bird populations, and particularly poultry. The veterinarians who are responsible for articulating this narrative place little emphasis on the bird–human interface, perhaps the critical control point for any pandemic concern, instead focusing on more standard veterinary interventions. For many veterinarians who had been starved of public funds for years, avian influenza was a good excuse for doing things that should, in their view, have been done much earlier. Restructuring marketing systems, for example, to improve biosafety has been a central concern. This has often favoured larger scale poultry operations, and cast backyard and small-scale poultry outfits as unsafe and a potential source of infection. In the same way, avian influenza funds have been used to boost the capacity of veterinary services through the OIE's 'performance of veterinary services' approach,[7] again with a vision of modernization and effective risk management at the centre. With the focus squarely on disease and animals, wider social, ecological, economic and political dimensions have been often left off the core agenda.

In the human health outbreak narrative, the focus is on public health concerns, often framed in terms of 'health security'. With the spectre of the 1918 influenza pandemic firmly in people's minds, the big fear is a major human pandemic and substantial human deaths. Epidemiological risk modelling of avian influenza spread has been especially influential. A pair of papers published in *Nature* (Ferguson et al, 2005) and *Science* (Longini et al, 2005) had a huge influence on the debate. These highlighted the importance of 'at source' containment when human-to-human infection occurs. This reinforced the emphasis on containment efforts, using the control of movement, including the deployment of military force if necessary, as well as the focused use of antivirals to reduce infection and spread. Alert systems, based on networks of laboratory testing, are emphasized, combined with an armoury of technical measures, sometimes requiring the use of compulsion and force. The language of security and the perceived urgency of public health issues are used to reinforce the message. At-source interventions in the fast-changing and unstable regions where outbreaks are most likely to occur are needed, it is argued, to protect the world – or at least those places where economic wealth and power reside.

Finally, in the pandemic preparedness outbreak narrative, a classic logistics-focused managerialism is evident. Here, the development of risk management plans is the central feature. These are to be developed at national levels, but also in public organizations and businesses. Armed with a plan, the necessary responses can unfold in a coordinated and effective manner, bringing together different agencies in a management response to expected disease risks, it is argued.[8] In support of this pandemic planning narrative, different sources of expertise are drawn upon, including contingency planning, disaster risk modelling, military logistics and emergency-response approaches.

Knowledge, expertise and biopolitics

Throughout the last decade this dominant trio of outbreak narratives, and their associated advocates, have competed for attention and resources, with different players deploying a variety of arguments to justify prioritizing their set of solutions. All focus on outbreaks and deploy risk management tools. Thus, through a complex combination of professional expertise, bureaucratic processes, and commercial and political interests, knowledge and policy are co-constructed, with a resulting focus on particular approaches to risk assessment and management (Stirling and Scoones, 2009). Through this process, alternative framings – of risk and response – are downplayed, obscured or ignored. Yet, as discussed later in the chapter, such alternative framings suggest a different set of narratives about the nature of the problem and the potential solutions, with significant implications for how surveillance is thought about and practised.

The trio of outbreak narratives fit neatly into the scientific and policy cultures that promote them. Policy solutions and policy knowledge are co-constructed in particular institutional settings, all with long histories. The scientific knowledge that informs policy, as we have seen, has been dominated by a particular type of medical and veterinary expertise, reinforced by emergency and humanitarian response approaches. This response emphasizes disease events in particular places, with an implicit imperative to control and eradicate disease. Policy then responds in particular ways that are well suited to existing bureaucratic routines and funding protocols. These narrow risk management approaches act to black-box uncertainty and deny forms of ignorance, and other perspectives, that are difficult, awkward or just do not fit. Instead, the mainstream risk management tools, such as surveillance, early warning systems and treatment and control strategies, concentrate on situations where outcomes and likelihoods are known, or at least assumed to be knowable.

The nature of expertise and the authority it carries have huge consequences for the way public policy is designed. Evidence-based policy is the contemporary mantra, but what evidence is used, and what is ignored, in the development of public policy? And in what ways is such knowledge and evidence framed? A more critical look at the underlying basis of arguments that influence policy is required. How do particular narratives – in the case of avian influenza focused on the trio of outbreak narratives discussed above – come to dominate the way things are done, and the way resources are deployed? Answering these questions requires turning to the heart of science for policy: the framing devices used, the way data are presented and the technologies and practices used (Jasanoff and Wynne, 1998). As discussed, in the avian influenza case, some perspectives have not been prominent in the policy debate, while others have taken centre stage, linked with powerful people, organizations and money. Thus a study of knowledge in policy is also a study of power – and the construction of discourses and practices in particular contexts. Following Foucault (1997), we can see the unfolding of the avian influenza response as a study in biopolitics and biopower, where actors and associated networks exercise power and control through processes of framing, and practices of categorization, ordering and governmentality (Rose, 2006).

The framing of all three of the dominant outbreak narrative responses has been around probabilistic notions of predictable, manageable risk – with an emphasis on risk assessment and control. Nowhere, except in more unguarded informal commentaries, is a more central admission of uncertainty and ignorance made. This is deeply problematic, and possibly even dangerous. Look at virtually any policy statement or position paper on avian influenza and the well-used statistics on potential mortalities are trotted out. For effect these tend to be at the high end of the spectrum. Despite the qualifications and conditions attached, these statistics are the ones that get picked up in the media and in popular treatments – in the growing library of books, magazine articles and op-eds on the issue – as well as in ministers' briefings and policy proclamations. This is natural and not surprising. There is no conspiracy involved – and indeed the doomsayers may be right. Better to be cautious and plan for the worst than use uncertainty or ignorance to do nothing: 'if you accept the premise that some things are beyond the reach of science, that doesn't prevent us from taking actions', argued one commentator.[9]

How then do such framings arise? As we have seen, there have been intense political and bureaucratic pressures – with commitments from international agencies and powerful politicians, from the US President downwards, pushing the process. There has been a jockeying for position and funds in the policy debate that followed, with headline grabbing an important tactic. And there have been the workings of science advice itself within and between organizations involved in the avian influenza response. For, in the processes ongoing within the main policy actors at the international level – the WHO, FAO, OIE, UNICEF, UN System Influenza Coordination (UNSIC), the World Bank and the rest – science and policy are inevitably co-constructed. Science does not neatly feed into policy in an unproblematic and linear way, nor do politics and policy simply dominate science. There is a two-way traffic. But sometimes technical 'truths' are not fully questioned. One commentator observed:

> *The major technical premises on which the [global] strategy was developed, were never clearly articulated or well explained. That's true for things like culling, vaccination, compensation ... no one seems to ask stupid but hard questions, like why are we doing this in this way when before we were told that vaccination is no use? Or why are we culling in countries where the virus is endemic, because that hurts a whole load of small farmers and doesn't stop the infection spreading? So why are we sticking to a system that doesn't seem to make a whole lot of sense?*[10]

The organizational politics of the international avian influenza response have often undermined the design of effective surveillance. Different organizations, with different mandates and different professional and disciplinary foci, compete for funds and parallel systems emerge. Each is rooted in a particular outbreak narrative, and biases against a broader view become entrenched.

Risk, uncertainty and ignorance: Reframing the response

Much of this knowledge politics hinges on definitions and interpretations of risk. The neat plans and policy frameworks that have garnered so many resources usually assume a knowable, predictable and manageable world. But what happens when we don't know outcomes or likelihoods? What happens when there are alternative framings of impacts and their consequences? For avian influenza this is most of the time, for most situations. Here a narrow version of risk assessment is grossly inadequate.

Figure 7.1 offers a diagrammatic representation of contrasting approaches to dealing with incomplete knowledge in policy contexts. It distinguishes knowledge about likelihoods and outcomes, identifying four 'ideal types' – risk (where the probabilities of specified outcomes are known), uncertainty (where the possible outcomes are known but there is no basis for assigning

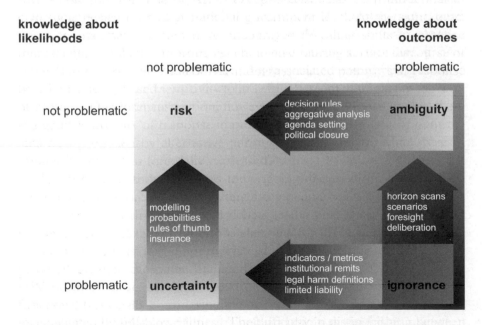

Source: after Stirling, 1999, 2008

Figure 7.1 Four responses to incomplete knowledge

probabilities), ambiguity (where there is disagreement over the nature of the outcomes, or different groups prioritize concerns that are incommensurable) and ignorance (where we don't know what we don't know) (Stirling, 2008; Leach et al, 2010). In addition, the figure highlights (with the arrows) some of the potential cognitive, procedural and institutional pressures that influence a move towards the top-left-hand corner, and so a focus on a narrow approach to risk assessment, and away from a more plural response to different types of incomplete knowledge. In later sections of this chapter I argue that these tendencies to close down around risk assessment and management exclude alternative responses that embrace uncertainty, ambiguity and ignorance. In the context of the response to avian influenza – or indeed any other epidemic or potential pandemic – this creates problems, and potential dangers. A more open, pluralistic response – and particularly one that addresses these concerns in the context of surveillance systems – is urgently needed.

Let us consider the two axes in this diagram: knowledge about outcomes and likelihoods. When considering outcomes, the potential impacts of avian influenza can be looked at in diverse ways. Very often the framing focuses on particular risks: to human lives (estimates of potential mortalities) or to the global economy (impacts on GDP). Thus for example, senior policy figures have estimated that up to 150 million human deaths might result from a major pandemic emerging from avian influenza.[11] Equally, models have defined a total cost of a major pandemic at US$1.5 trillion at a global level (Burns et al, 2006). These estimates define outcomes in terms of aggregate, quantitative impacts, usually at the global level. Cast in a different way, outcomes may be seen in terms of lost livelihoods and the impacts on poverty and well-being. Here the potential of a low-likelihood but high-impact global pandemic is played down in favour of a focus on the impacts on poultry and livelihoods. After all, avian influenza remains largely a disease of birds not humans and many of the impacts of the disease for humans are felt through the control measures implemented in order to reduce pandemic likelihoods – such as culling campaigns directed at backyard birds. The distributional consequences of such outcomes may also be part of the picture, as poorer people in rural areas, very often women, are the worst hit.

In terms of Figure 7.1 there is therefore much ambiguity. There is no neat definition of outcome available: it all depends on positioning and standpoint. Agenda setting by international agencies, influenced by political discourse in richer countries, however, acts to close down debate about alternative outcomes. Thus in most policy discussions around avian and pandemic influenza, global impacts (and particularly those that affect North America or Europe), even if of relatively low probability, are emphasized over higher likelihood consequences affecting poor poultry producers in urban Asia.

Aggregate analysis and dramatic quantitative figures of global impact act to encourage closure, shifting from a discussion of multiple potential outcomes in a context of ambiguity to an assumption of full knowledge about potential outcomes, defined in a narrow risk frame. Yet with wider deliberation and the examination of different outcomes through scenario planning, horizon scanning or foresight discussions, for example, a clearer definition of the possible array of outcomes, each with their distributional consequences outlined, would easily be possible. The lack of debate means that the default mode is that systems are narrowly designed using risk management tools, assuming that more is known or knowable than really is. Surveillance and response systems are, in turn, constructed based on the assumptions driving narratives about global risks and aggregate, unitary outcomes.

Turning to the second axis, as already discussed, knowledge about the probabilities of different impacts is very limited, indeed mostly absent. The debate about avian influenza is largely therefore in the realm of uncertainty and ignorance. A wide range of uncertainties exist – from the big unknown (will a catastrophic pandemic happen at all, and if so when?) to the specific unknowns, such as causal mechanisms (viral change, re-assortment and genetic dynamics), spread in animals (ducks, wild birds, trade), incidence (estimates of viral load, the cyclical, inter-annual and seasonal patterns, and the prevalence of 'endemic' settings), transmission (and the likelihood of human–human transmission), impact (on mortality rates of wild birds, domestic poultry and humans) and response (efficacy of bird culling, vaccination and so on in different settings) and many more. Yet, despite the wide recognition of this – even, as shown by the opening quote, in the public media – policy-making persists on the assumption that more is known about likelihoods than is really the case.

This grasping for certainty in the face of the unknown or unknowable is a perfectly understandable reaction, particularly in political-bureaucratic settings where firm, decisive action is expected. Accepting uncertainty can be seen as dithering, a failure to act when the world is in peril. No politician or bureaucrat wants to be cast in this light, and so be exposed to media ridicule or, perhaps later, damaging litigation. There is always a political imperative to be seen to be doing something in an era of anxiety, worry and perceived threat. So, through a range of processes, bureaucratic, funding and institutional imperatives mean that ignorance is denied. Even when uncertainty is accepted, there are always attempts to reduce this to risk.

A much favoured route to this reductionist thinking is the use of modelling. Here uncertainties are dealt with by making assumptions about likelihoods – of transmission, spread and impact – even when the figures are really just (relatively) informed guesses. Most models deployed in the policy debate about avian influenza have been, at their core, concerned again with an aggregate, global view of pandemic risk. Thus epidemiological models emphasize the importance of 'at source' containment and control, in order to reduce the risk of pandemic spread (Coburn et al, 2009). The risks are to global populations, not those arising from the immediate impacts on local populations of intensive containment measures.

Thus through a variety of processes, policy responses settle in the top-left corner of Figure 7.1. This is the comfort zone for many professionals and institutions, where knowledge about likelihoods and outcomes is deemed unproblematic, and amenable to narrow forms of risk assessment and management. All these moves are reinforced by a set of disciplinary cultures which value quantitative, disease-focused assessments over more complex analyses of social, economic, political and ecological dynamics. A reconfiguring of disciplinary expertise and an involvement of alternative forms of knowledge, including that of those directly affected by the disease, could, as suggested below, have a dramatic effect on the framing of the problem and the response, allowing alternative narratives, beyond the trio of outbreak narratives that have dominated the response to date, into the picture. This would help to bring to the fore real uncertainties, ambiguities and forms of ignorance, and push policy to respond to these explicitly, rather than wishing such awkward, troublesome dimensions away.

The following sections argue that a narrow risk framing that does not effectively acknowledge issues of uncertainty and ignorance – and the ambiguity of alternative interpretations of likelihood and outcome – can act to narrow our assessment and response in ways that may fundamentally undermine the effectiveness and resilience of responses. Incorporating alternative narratives about risk and response allows the debate to be reframed, and surveillance systems in particular to be rethought.

Alternative narratives: Reframing the debate

Looking across the three main outbreak narratives discussed so far, we have to ask what is missing, hidden or obscured? Is there a set of alternative narrative framings that emerge from the margins as critiques of the mainstream? Rosenberg (1992) has argued that epidemics can be explained in at least three radically different ways – contamination (focused on disease transmission), configuration (focused on disease context) and disposition (related to the individual carrier of the disease). Each is important, yet the contamination strand, and its emphasis on disease outbreaks, laboratory diagnosis and a treatment response, has dominated at least since the mid-20th century. As we have seen, this has certainly been true in the case of the avian influenza example.

In the welter of activity, funds, people and acronyms that the mainstream 'outbreak narratives' have generated, it is easy to ignore alternative framings. This section emphasizes the importance of two alternative narratives in offering a different perspective on surveillance. The first focuses on the causes of the disease and its dynamics, while the second focuses on poverty, livelihoods and equity outcomes of disease interventions.

True to their name, outbreak narratives focus on the outbreak event, not the underlying causes. Surveillance systems are thus based on reporting outbreak events, not shifting epidemiological dynamics, and responses hone in on the diseased organism with treatment measures, or the diseased area with disease control or eradication measures. Technological interventions – and models of different sorts in particular – act to reinforce this framing. For example, computer models of disease spread show clearly how localized 'at source' eradication or containment efforts are critical in preventing a global pandemic. This justifies cross-border intervention, and potentially draconian interventions. But of course models are just models and dependent on often quite heroic assumptions – such as diseases spreading in concentric circles, the relative insignificance of borders of countries and districts, and the easy prevention of people from moving. Surreptitiously these ideas have an impact on policy framing, such is the power (and simplicity) of modelling, pushing the diagnosis and solution towards one focused on risk (and so the top-left corner of Figure 7.1).

But – and no one denies this – it is not so simple. Complex disease dynamics mean that we do not know what is going to happen when, and when outbreaks do occur, their pattern and impact are highly context-specific. Uncertainty and ignorance prevail. Such complexity is not amenable to simple outbreak models, and requires a deeper understanding of changing ecologies, demographies and socio-economic contexts – and, in particular, their interactions and dynamics in particular places (see Slingenbergh et al, 2004). This field-level understanding of dynamic contexts is startlingly absent in much of the work on avian influenza. Yet quite a lot seems to be known, even if it appears rather anecdotally in research papers and conversations. The vivid descriptions of the situation in Qinghai lake in western China, where migratory birds that carry the virus gather, are startling. As one ecologist put it: 'There is a whirlpool of genes re-assorting… It's a dream for reshuffling of viruses. The lake is a soup of viruses.'[12]

But without an integrated understanding of disease dynamics the key to effective surveillance and control may be missed. One informant commented on the situation, making reference to physician John Snow, who famously deduced the source of contaminated water responsible for a cholera outbreak in London in the 19th century and removed the pump handle, thus halting the epidemic:

As an epidemiologist, I keep looking for that pump handle solution.
You know, what is that thing which is causing, mostly women, who
are mostly the ones who raise chickens, to become infected, and then go
on to die? What about the slaughter process? What about the habit of
picking the sickest bird in the group for the pot? And not being able to
seek medical advice. The control might not actually be with birds, but
at the human–animal interface that says how can I safely handle an
infected bird? That may be an area that has gone under-investigated.
Maybe we need to hit exactly where the ministries of health and agri-
culture meet.[13]

If the real dangers lie exactly where the ministries of health and agriculture meet, it may be that the response, focused as it is on separate narratives of human and animal health, may miss the 'pump handle'. And, surely,
understanding the underlying drivers of disease change – and the socio-
ecological dynamics of emergence – must be part of any international
response. Zoonotic diseases frequently emerge where natural reservoirs of
disease from wild fauna are found close to rapidly growing urban centres
with intensive human–animal contact, usually in settings where regulation
and human health and veterinary services are weak or non-existent (Bloom
et al, 2007). Southern China is an example – as are Indonesia, Vietnam
and much of South and Southeast Asia, as well as urbanizing Africa. The
risks may be further enhanced by certain practices – consuming bushmeat,
living with livestock, shopping in wet markets and so on – and certain
conditions – notably poverty, malnutrition and immune system suppression
(such as through HIV infection). These so-called 'hot spots' are not isolated
places far from anywhere as the term might imply, but encompass most
of the developing world where most of humanity lives. As one informant
explained:

With avian influenza there is a slow realization that it is no longer an
emergency. It is a deep rooted issue underlying the disease. But this is
very slow; and is resisted. It is more attractive to be doing something in
emergency mode rather than investing in strategic thinking… Avian
influenza to my mind is more a symptom of massive changes in the
poultry sector globally… there have been massive increases in poultry
and duck production. An avian influenza was bound to arise. The
question is how to improve the management of these sectors. Not just
about the disease. Overall, we should be aiming for a framework for
other viruses. If this one is not it, some other will be. But we are not
there yet. Far from it.[14]

An outbreak narrative is an appropriate framing for those who do not live in these places and who want, for perfectly legitimate reasons, to protect themselves from diseases that arise there. But it is perhaps less so when seen from another perspective. In many settings in the developing world, people are used to living with infectious disease. They have deeply embedded 'cultural logics' (Hewlett and Hewlett, 2008) that influence the way they understand and respond to diseases – of both animals and humans, and thus their constructions of risk. These may be at odds with standard medical and veterinary framings, resulting in disconnects between official programmes and local responses.

Such an alternative narrative, focused on the dynamics of disease and local responses, casts the agenda wider than the standard outbreak-treatment-eradication mode. Whole ecosystems and their complex interactions must be examined, and the social–cultural–livelihood interactions must be at the centre of both diagnosis and response. Given the way the current response has been framed, structured and financed, this may prove difficult. But, as discussed further below, such a perspective has important ramifications for surveillance approaches – in terms of disciplinary and professional skills, organizational arrangements and identifying the focus for funding.

A focus on local-level, socio-ecological dynamics also raises questions about the distributional impact of disease burdens. Outbreak narratives focus on diseases not people and livelihoods, but a shift in framing might point in particular to the impacts of diseases on different people, and also the impact of top-down, disease-focused, risk management interventions. To date, avian influenza mostly affects poultry keepers in the developing world, many of whom are poor. The responses geared at a 'global public good response' – which is often designed to protect richer countries – have a disproportionate negative effect on poor livestock keepers. For those framing the problem as an emergency – and focusing on pandemic threat to humans – mass culling of chickens is seen as a necessary evil, which if compensated for, offers a substantial public good benefit. But looked at from the perspective of those whose livelihoods at least in part depend on these poultry, such an intervention can be catastrophic.

As Farmer (1996, 1999a) points out, structural inequalities define health policy and intervention. Attention to the wider political economy of the international response to disease is therefore critical, and one that brings up sharp dilemmas and uncomfortable truths for narrower technical framings. Again, the debate about poverty and equity – and the wider political economy questions associated – highlights the division between those with essentially a disease-focused risk framing of the problem and solution, and those who adopt a broader livelihoods and development perspective. Such a perspective could, in turn, lead to surveillance tools that address questions not just of disease incidence and spread, but of poverty, livelihoods, and distributional consequences, opening up a diversity of new questions and perspectives.

Surveillance systems that are based solely on disease-focused risk assessment may therefore miss some important issues. A broader attention to the complex socio-ecological dynamics of disease systems from what might be termed systemic surveillance highlights the array of uncertainties and sources of ignorance at the heart of the surveillance challenge. Without explicit attention to these dimensions, we may, for example, miss important shifts in disease ecology, and so we may be caught by surprise, with serious consequences. Equally, opening up surveillance to a wider deliberation on outcomes (addressing ambiguity) and the distributional impacts on poverty and livelihoods shifts is vitally important. Recognizing the ambiguities, and inherent politics of choice, between different outcome scenarios may allow more concrete deliberation around alternative consequences for different options. In other words, asking who will be affected, where and with what implications for poverty? Such distributional questions associated with different disease responses should be seen as central to any discussion of policy, but get occluded from the analysis by a universalistic, 'science-based' risk framing.

Rethinking surveillance

What will it take therefore to move beyond the narrow risk assessment and management framing that has characterized the outbreak narratives guiding policies for avian influenza to date? How can alternative narratives of disease dynamics and response be incorporated, ones that embrace complexity and address uncertainty and ignorance? What would surveillance look like if such alternatives were made more central?

Table 7.1 offers a summary of some of the themes identified in the chapter so far, contrasting outbreak and systemic surveillance. Of course these are not binary opposites in reality: shades of grey exist across a continuum. However, by identifying the central contrasts, the aim is to emphasize the potential effects of a shift from a narrow risk framing – with a focus on outbreaks, and a centralized, planned response approach, rooted in probabilistic assessment and modelling of risks – to one that encompasses complexity, uncertainty, ambiguity and ignorance. An alternative framing, driven by a different conceptualization of dynamics and knowledge about the likelihood of different outcomes, emphasizes decentralization, flexibility, adaptation and responsiveness in design. Such approaches would draw on diverse knowledge bases, and particularly from those who live with disease

Table 7.1 *From outbreak to systemic surveillance*

Characteristic of surveillance system	Outbreak surveillance	Systemic surveillance
Approach to risk	Risk framing – probabilistic modelling, risk assessment and management	Risk plus ... uncertainty, ambiguity, ignorance: a focus on incomplete knowledge
Focus of intervention	Disease, outbreak focused – separation of animal and human diseases	Emergence, dynamics focused; diverse disease contexts; animal–human interfaces
Type of organization encouraged	Universal, centralized, blueprint, global	Context-specific, networked, flexible, adaptive
Type of knowledge prioritized	Science-driven, expert-led	Participatory, inclusive – multiple forms of knowledge
Disciplinary affiliation	Quantitative epidemiology and modelling	Participatory epidemiology with sociology, anthropology: located understandings of disease emergence and dynamics
Use of technology	Digital detection and databases	Diverse and appropriate technologies for recording, sending and collating information
Types of responses	Focus on outbreak alert and rapid response systems	Principles of precaution and high reliability
Framing of health security	Protection from external threat (to northern, rich people and economies)	Resilience in the face of uncertainty (especially in places where disease emergence most likely)

and inhabit so-called disease 'hot spots'. The shift represents a move from a reliance on 'hard', quantitative science and modelling, led by professional experts with particular disciplinary and institutional commitments, to a more diverse, plural conception of expertise, with an emphasis on participation, inclusion and deliberation. Thus with multiple sources of expertise, including from those with experience of a range of diseases, a greater deliberation on risk framings and on response priorities and options would result. Equally, rather than singular technical fixes, more diverse technological and organizational routes to similar ends can be sought, suggesting a more flexible design of surveillance infrastructures. Finally, this alternative framing of surveillance would affect how health security, that central mantra in contemporary policy discourse, is understood. An alternative surveillance would aim at generating resilience in the face of uncertainty (and ambiguity and ignorance) in order to secure the health and livelihoods of people, particularly in the most disease-prone areas of the world. This would replace surveillance tools which serve simply as mechanisms for detecting threats to the rich and powerful, and so secure narrow privilege rather than broader livelihoods.

There are examples of initiatives that offer a glimpse of the way forward. Here I identify four instances:

- First, advocates of a 'One World, One Health' approach[15] identify the importance of linking human and animal health in an integrated, holistic approach, breaking down the disciplinary, professional and institutional barriers which make little sense when dealing with zoonoses (Zinsstag et al, 2009).
- Second, arguments for the integration of climate change, ecology and health are similarly helpful in thinking through how efforts in one area – such as climate adaptation – must be integrated with interventions in another, such as vector or disease control.[16] Eco-health approaches emphasize both long-term dynamics, as well as shorter-term ecological change, and avoid focusing solely on the disease agent and its transmission, allowing an investigation of how and why diseases emerge and spread in the first place (Parkes et al, 2004; Kapan et al, 2006).
- Third, as part of pioneering work by the Viral Forecasting Initiative, there is increasing interest in monitoring what has been termed 'viral chatter': the continuous transfer of viruses between animals and humans[17] (Wolfe et al, 2005; Wolfe, 2009b). Focused on particular 'hot spot' sites, sentinel populations or animals and around particular transmission pathways – such among bushmeat hunters in the forests of West Africa or the informal wet markets of urban Asia – 'virus hunters' can look for novel material through a systematic testing programme which aims to pick up sudden changes in virus incidence, composition or genetic make-up, thus spotting diseases as they emerge. Looking for novelty offers a frontline response that, had it been in place before, might have prevented the spread of HIV.
- Fourth, approaches to information management, and particularly the integration of data from internet sources, represent another step forward in including diverse, non-expert knowledge in surveillance systems, as well as a more rapid tracking of events as they unfold (Galaz et al, 2009; Dry, this volume). The acceptance of non-official data, including reports from NGOs and others, in the WHO's surveillance system was a great step forward (Heymann and Rodier, 1998). Fast-developing web-crawling applications allow, for example, the spotting of Google searches for keywords such as 'high temperature' or purchasing patterns of thermometers, and can provide early warning long before any official reporting (Ginsberg et al, 2009).[18]

All of these approaches, or adaptations of them, offer much promise, and are tangible examples of what an alternative framing of surveillance might look like. But each of them, as currently proposed, does not go far enough. The same professional, procedural and institutional forces often push them back towards a risk framing, and so towards the top-left-hand corner of Figure 7.1. In order to achieve success, the One World, One Health challenge must be more than simply the integration of professional areas into a new technical super-discipline, where two outbreak narratives are combined more forcefully and with more resources. Old wine must not simply be placed in new bottles, without any fundamental change in the way things are done. A One World, One Health agenda must address some of the organizational challenges implied by getting serious about integrating different perspectives on health (Scoones, 2010).

The experience of swine flu is particularly instructive in this regard. Veterinary authorities were very quick to play down the role of pigs in the swine flu outbreaks of 2009, stressing that no pig–human transmission had been observed. The apex body, the OIE, argued successfully that swine flu should be dropped as a term for this outbreak, and instead the more accurate nomenclature of 2009/10 AH1N1 be used.[19] This of course reflected a wider politics of influence in the veterinary community, one that often results in slow reporting particularly of diseases with economic implications. Too often it is only when human cases start appearing that pressure increases to address the veterinary aspects. In the case of swine flu, a June 2009 *Nature* report lamented 'patchy pig monitoring', noting that 'public health experts are warning that a lack of surveillance may be allowing the 2009 pandemic H1N1 flu virus to go undetected in pigs, making it more likely to reassert into a deadlier strain' (*Nature*, 2009, p894). Clearly, inappropriate over-reactions, such as the mass pig culling in Egypt (see Tadros, this volume), are to be avoided. At the same time, systematic blindness to disease dynamics in animals for fear of trade-related impacts is also unacceptable. As genetics work has shown, H1N1 viruses have probably been circulating for years prior to the pandemic, and pigs are certainly an important host (Smith et al, 2009), yet there has been a failure in surveillance systems across the global pork industry. Similar reluctance has been seen with avian influenza, particularly in the early phases of the epidemic.

If we are serious about rethinking surveillance, we must consider the political economy of diseases. A simple merging of public health and veterinary concerns will do little if the underlying incentives and disincentives for transparent, clear and timely reporting are not dealt with. It makes sense to design organizational arrangements so that those who collect the disease surveillance information are not also those who respond to it. Currently veterinarians are often feared, for example, because they may return and cull animals, often without compensation. Separating commercial-industrial concerns from health interventions is also important. With surveillance of animal populations in the hands of those who must regulate the livestock industry, there is often not a clear separation of interests. The same may be argued for public health authorities who often have considerable pressure brought to bear on them by politicians and industry representatives. Surveillance is not a neutral, technical act, separated from politics.

As the virus sharing controversy has vividly shown, the even-handedness of international bodies such as the WHO, and its network of experts and laboratories, must be demonstrated and earned, not simply assumed (Fidler, 2008). As soon as trust is lost, institutional arrangements falter, and the idealized prospect of an integrated One World, One Health approach founders. The OIE/FAO network of experts on animal influenza known as OFFLU[20] has argued vociferously for joined-up coordination among laboratories working on the human–animal interface and for the sharing of virus samples internationally. There is a growing consensus about the need for an independent international body for research into human–animal disease interactions, one that would be broadly trusted and could not be accused of responding to vested interests (*Nature*, 2009).[21]

Beyond the integration of public health and veterinary functions, other areas of expertise are urgently needed. For example, ecologists are needed to understand the complex dynamics of diseases in different ecosystems: anthropologists and sociologists are required to incorporate cultural understandings of diseases by different people and understand how these shape behaviours and responses, and political scientists are needed to provide insights into the political and institutional dimensions of disease responses. Perhaps above all the network of expertise needs to be extended beyond formal, accredited sources to encompass local experiential knowledge. Diseases and their interactions with environments and humans are understood within particular cultural frames, rooted in particular, often very located, ways of knowing. Such 'cultural logics' (Hewlett and Hewlett, 2008; see Leach and Hewlett, this volume), can be vital in understanding local responses to diseases. This must go beyond the 'butterfly collecting' approach to indigenous ethno-medical or veterinary knowledge to a deeper engagement with local forms of knowledge and practices that might be the key to spotting early disease emergence. Such a system would depend on the ability to integrate and process such knowledge in myriad forms, not only standard scientific or medical classifications. A mutual appreciation of different ways of understanding is essential. Unfortunately this is largely absent in standard surveillance systems.

The case of the emergence of H1N1 swine flu in Mexico is a case in point. While diplomatic niceties have prevented much criticism of the

Mexican authorities, it is clear that there were big gaps in detection and reporting in the early part of 2009. It is also apparent that local people knew of the disease, and had some strong hypotheses about its origins. Anselma Amador from La Gloria, the village where the first known case of swine flu occurred commented to the *Guardian* newspaper:[22] 'We are not doctors, but it is hard for us not to think the pig farms around here don't have something to do with it ... The flu has pig material in it and we are humans, not pigs.' A large, industrial pig farm, owned by multinational company Smithfield Foods, is blamed. According to the *Guardian*, residents in La Gloria say the prevailing wind invariably blows the fetid air their way, where it gets stuck because of the hills that rise just behind the village. These explanations were dismissed out of hand by the Health Minister and the company, but why are such leads not being tested and followed up? And, perhaps more importantly, why are such early warning approaches, based on local knowledge about disease incidence and its dynamics, not part of the standard surveillance system? Why is such knowledge of the 'not doctors' so easily dismissed? As discussed in earlier sections of this chapter, the lessons from the avian influenza outbreaks in Southeast Asia and beyond point to the vital importance of local understandings of disease and its spread, as well as the significance of engaging with the local cultural understandings of people living with disease. Medical doctors, epidemiologists, virologists, veterinarians and other specialists need to work hand-in-hand with local people in order for surveillance to be truly effective.

How might such embedded, systemic surveillance be realized? Who might do it and how? Again, there are pilot cases which offer some useful pointers. The work of the Global Viral Forecasting Initiative, for example, envisages a global network of scientists able to monitor viral change, focusing on particular 'sentinels' and 'hot spots' in different parts of the world. Currently 100 scientists are involved across six sites. Systemic surveillance is focused on particular animal–human disease pathways, for example looking at influenza viruses in domestic poultry and wild birds, especially in Asia or a range of RNA viruses in simians in forest areas of West Africa. This effort is primarily focused on identifying and documenting the viruses through scientific assessments. It is based on a precautionary approach which recognizes uncertainty and ignorance, and potentially offers a major head start in what will always be an ongoing battle between humans and emerging diseases. But the focus on virus monitoring and characterization only goes so far. What about a wider understanding of the socio-ecological changes that produce so-called 'hot spots' in the first place? How can systemic surveillance identify drivers of disease emergence and their potential tipping points? What factors allow new diseases to emerge? This is a much bigger task and requires a deeper understanding of the socio-ecology of disease emergence: patterns of demographic and land-use change, for example, interact with shifts in settlement patterns, and eating habits change both the types of outcome and their likelihood.[23] Broad, open-ended disease vulnerability mapping may help identify current, and potentially future, hot spots, and allow a more honed, focused surveillance system.

It must also be asked, who is the best placed to run such monitoring systems; who already has such systemic understandings? Is it white-coated 'virus hunters' arriving with gung-ho bravado in a remote forest site, or is it local people – the 'sentinels' themselves – who might offer the key to understanding? Working with local people – say market traders in a Southeast Asian market – not with the goal of enforcing some form of externally defined 'behaviour change' or 'market restructuring' but of understanding disease risks, uncertainties, ambiguities and sources of ignorance – may create the foundation for more effective, systemic surveillance. The 'technical fix' approaches that might work in the US or Europe based on web-crawling and internet search cataloguing, may not be appropriate in rural Africa or Asia. But other cheap, decentralized information technologies might allow for the capturing, relaying and integration of local knowledge systems at very low cost. Text messaging or hand-held computers and satellite-based location devices, for example, might allow regular recording, as well as alerts from key sites. Integrating such information through geo-referenced databases might allow a wider picture of evolving change. Such a picture, based on a set of meaningful and useful criteria, mutually decided upon by those working along the surveillance chain, could then form the basis of a more broad-based surveillance, allowing more detailed analysis of viral dynamics to be effectively targeted. Clearly such systems would not be zero cost, and they would have to be backed by organizational support and incentives in order to avoid the problems of information withholding for fear of exposure, backlash or heavy-handed intervention.

In sum, such approaches all centre on responses that accept and address incomplete knowledge, and move substantially beyond the risk assessment and management framing of conventional surveillance. Because uncertainty and ignorance prevail, a systemic, integrative approach is required which adopts a precautionary stance, and deploys less precise, but ultimately more useful, methods and tools. Rather than reducing system complexity to a single aggregated value or prescriptive recommendation (as is normal in risk assessment), the prudent and rigorous approach is to acknowledge the variability in possible interpretations (Stirling, 2008). Sensitivity, scenario and interval analysis, used alongside a range of decision heuristics, are well-established approaches that avoid the pitfalls of conventional risk assessment (Stirling and Scoones, 2009). None justifies a singular decision, but each reveals options and choices in a rigorous and transparent manner.

In the end, judgement calls are necessary. Despite the paraphernalia of risk assessment and its assumptions of science-based decision-making, such judgements are always required. As a senior official involved in global surveillance in the WHO commented:

> *The internal risk assessments are heavily based on expert opinion. We don't have the data to say these are valid variables. Our experience is what matters. We look at anecdotal things – the likelihood of reporting and so on; stories about the hiding of information – people who went to the doctor but did not say they had poultry. There is more risk where people are hiding. It cannot be quantified though. The long term goal is to validate the variables, ideally with FAO. But now it is expert opinion and many uncertainties...*[24]

This is the sensible, mature approach, but in this case taken without formal recognition, and dressed up as risk assessment, rather than recognizing the importance of anecdote, uncertainty and opinion. The system again pushes the formal procedures to the top-left-hand corner of Figure 7.1, even if the actual practices are centred on grappling with incomplete knowledge, often in the absence of methods and tools for making such assessments more rigorous and transparent.

Conclusion

As the opening quote made clear, the governance of risk is always open to controversy; something increasingly realized in public and media debate. Making uncertainties and sources of ignorance clear, and deliberating explicitly on the judgements made, must be part of any future systemic surveillance system. We must examine closely the assumptions that drive the outbreak-dominant narratives shaping the response to influenza. Involving more people – extending the disciplinary range and including those living with disease – allows a more inclusive approach, where more diverse forms of knowledge are brought to bear on a complex problem. Addressing the inherent ambiguities in disease control choices requires such inclusivity, along with a more bottom-up, participatory and deliberative approach to surveillance. This does not mean that such systems must be cumbersome, slow and painfully participatory at every turn. Information technologies can streamline data collection, and strategic sampling allows focus and targeting.

Thus to bring surveillance from the 19th to the 21st century, and from outbreak to systemic approaches to surveillance, some major shifts are required – in knowledge, expertise, organization and technological application. The case of avian influenza has provided some important lessons, and perhaps some breathing space in which to experiment, reflect and design alternatives. Rethinking surveillance is thus vital – for fighting the flu, as well as any other emerging infectious disease – and must be an urgent priority for international public policy.

Notes

1   This chapter draws substantially from Scoones and Forster (2008) and Scoones (2010). This work was supported by the ESRC STEPS Centre epidemics project, as well as the FAO Pro-Poor Livestock Policy Initiative (www.fao.org/ag/againfo/programmes/en/pplpi.html, accessed 6 December 2009), the DFID-funded Pro-Poor Risk Reduction Project (www.hpai-research.net/index.html, accessed 6 December 2009) and the Chatham House-led work on the global governance of the livestock sector, supported by the World Bank and the UK Department for International Development.

2   The J. W. Lee Centre for Strategic Health Operations, www.who.int/bulletin/volumes/ 84/10/06-011006/en/, accessed 1 October 2009.

3   www.fao.org/EMPRES/default.htm, accessed 1 October 2009; ftp://ftp.fao.org/docrep/fao/011/i0346e/i0346e.pdf, accessed 1 October 2009.

4   Interview, Rome, 1 February 2008.

5   See: www.who.int/csr/disease/influenza/pandemic/en/, accessed 6 December 2009, for the Global Pandemic Preparedness Plan.

6   Interview, Geneva, 5 March 2008.

7   www.oie.int/eng/OIE/organisation/en_vet_eval_tool.htm, accessed 1 October 2009.

8   www.un-pic.org/web/documents/english/About%20PIC.pdf, accessed 1 October 2009.

9   Interview, New York, 9 June 2008.

10   Interview, Washington, DC, 12 June 2008.

11   http://news.bbc.co.uk/1/hi/world/asia-pacific/4292426.stm, accessed 1 October 2009.

12   Interview, Rome, January 2008.

13   Interview, Washington, DC, 13 June 2008.

14   Interview, UK, 11 March 2008.

15   See www.wcs.org/conservation-challenges/wildlife-health/wildlife-humans-and-livestock/one-world-one-health.aspx and also www.oneworldonehealth.org/, accessed 1 October 2009. For more recent explorations in the context of the avian influenza response, see FAO et al (2008)

16   See the recent ILRI initiative on this theme: www.google.co.uk/search?sourceid=navclient&ie=UTF-8&rlz=1T4SKPB_enGB260GB260&q=climate+change+animal+health+ilri, accessed 1 October 2009.

17   www.gvfi.org/, accessed 1 October 2009.

18   www.google.org/about/flutrends/how.html, accessed 1 October 2009.

19   www.oie.int/Eng/press/en_090427.htm, accessed 1 October 2009.

20   www.offlu.net/, accessed 1 October 2009.

21   www.nature.com/nm/journal/v15/n3/full/nm0309-227a.html, accessed 1 October 2009.

22   www.guardian.co.uk/world/2009/apr/29/swine-flu-outbreak-mexico, accessed 1 October 2009.

23   Long-term demographic and health change monitoring already occurs as part of the INDEPTH network (www.indepth-network.org), but this does not extend to wider socio-ecological dynamics.

24   Interview, Geneva, 7 March 2008.

Chapter 8

Multidrug-resistant Tuberculosis: Narratives of Security, Global Health Care and Structural Violence

Paul Nightingale[1]

Introduction

Of all the diseases analysed in this book tuberculosis (TB) is one of the most tragic. The *Mycobacterium tuberculosis* pathogen has evolved to take advantage of weaknesses in the bodies of its victims, and the emergence of multidrug-resistant TB (MDR-TB), and now extensively drug-resistant TB (XDR-TB), reflects the pathogen's capacity to take advantage of new evolutionary niches created by ineffective health systems and HIV co-infection. The emergence of drug-resistant TB helps highlight the dynamic interactions between pathogens, technology and society. It highlights particularly starkly how different narratives about disease and associated pathways of response can help change the social distribution of disease and its consequences. In a dynamic world, technologies and responses that shift risks away from the rich can unintentionally create new evolutionary niches among the poor where new epidemics, that threaten rich and poor alike, might emerge.

Part of the tragedy of the current TB and MDR-TB epidemics is that they were potentially avoidable. For patients with well-functioning immune systems, control over their lifestyles and access to well-organized health care, treatment is very effective and relatively cheap. Unfortunately, such conditions are not found everywhere. As a result, TB has become the second leading cause of infectious disease mortality worldwide.[2] In 2004, 9 million people developed the disease and about 2 million died, generating approximately 4400 deaths a day (WHO, 2006). TB is the leading cause of death both for HIV-infected individuals and for women of childbearing age. It is strongly associated with poverty. Twenty-two high burden countries account for 80 per cent of the total number of cases and so-called developing countries account for 98 per cent of TB deaths (Dye et al, 1999). In industrialized countries infection rates are much lower, but growing, reflecting both immigration and pockets of poverty where the disease can more easily establish itself and spread. In the UK, for example, changes in TB infection rates are strongly stratified by income. Between 1980 and 1992 the poorest 10 per cent of the population saw its infection rates increase by 35 per cent, the next poorest 20 per cent increased by 13 per cent and the remaining 70 per cent of the population saw no change (Bhatti et al, 1995).

The resurgence of TB in industrialized countries in the 1990s, driven in part by increased levels of social exclusion creating pockets of infection among the poor, has increased its public prominence. One of the UN Millennium Development Goals is to eliminate TB by 2050. The Stop TB partnership targets, for example, are for the global rate of TB to be reduced by 50 per cent (compared to 1990) by 2015, and the global incidence to be less than 1 case per million by 2050. This increased attention to TB represents a substantial shift in policy. In 1989 the WHO employed only two TB specialists and in 1992–1993 had a total TB budget of US$10 million (Raviglione and Pio, 2002). This lack of attention can be seen in the relative amounts of money spent on aid. Today, by contrast, there is a substantial global infrastructure of research, treatment and advocacy focusing on TB. This shift reflects changes in how TB has been seen: from a 'disease of the past' (or less charitably, a disease of the poor) to a new, potentially destabilizing and global epidemic.

This chapter tracks some of the shifting narratives about TB in play from its recognition in the 19th century, through to more recent phases in which MDR-TB and XDR-TB have become concerns. In this respect the chapter provides a recent history of the disease, although a very selective and partial one based on a range of carefully identified secondary literatures. The aim – in picking out particular events, episodes and dimensions – is to draw attention to the interrelationships between narratives, health policies and interventions, and their feedback effects on the social–microbial dynamics of disease – including conditions that have shaped epidemic re-emergence.

The chapter begins with some background on the biology of *Mycobacterium tuberculosis* to highlight how its origins as an environmentally robust bacteria have given it, or more specifically its surface, properties that make it cause atypical epidemics: the TB epidemic is slow rather than rapid and for most people infected with the bacillus the disease remains latent, surviving outside the reach of the immune system. In this context, the chapter then explores early narratives about TB, highlighting the rise of a biomedical narrative out of a socially and historically particular way of understanding a complex phenomenon in which pathogens dynamically interact with a diverse population of victims in complex social and technological settings. The chapter then outlines how versions of a biomedical narrative became interlocked with particular approaches to diagnosis, treatment and management of TB during the 20th century. It goes on to track key processes in the late 20th century when TB re-emerged as an epidemic, along with the rise of the new spectre of MDR-TB. The chapter then explores three distinct, though overlapping, narratives about MDR-TB, which consider the problem respectively in terms of security, of global health care, and of structural violence, rights and context. Each narrative frames the relationships between pathogens, people and their settings differently, justifying different emphases in approaches to managing disease. The final section of the chapter shows how mismatches between the pathways which have become dominant, and diverse, dynamic settings, have helped lay the ground both for new problems of social marginalization, and for new evolutionary niches for the emergence of XDR-TB – and with it a host of further challenges for understanding and policy.

TB – background

Mycobacterium tuberculosis evolved to survive for long periods of time in desiccated soil by augmenting and strengthening its cell walls (Bates and Stead, 1993). To do this about 30 per cent of its genome is devoted to lipid synthesis and metabolism. As a result, the pathogen is environmentally robust and can survive in the air for several days. In 1920 Corper and Cohn inoculated a culture bottle and left it at 37° for 12 years, after which they were able to culture bacterium from the sediment. The pathogen's robust cell wall also pre-adapts it for a complex parasitic relationship with its host's immune system. Specialized lipids in the pathogen's cell wall down-regulate its host's immune response, allowing the pathogen to protect itself from attack by the immune system and thus to survive in a latent state for decades. As a consequence, the host's body does not generate a sterilizing immune response that clears the disease and makes the host immune to infection. This environmental robustness also makes TB resistant to a range of standard disinfectants and antibiotics, makes diagnosis difficult, and makes treatments long and complex (Blower et al, 1995; Kaufmann, 2007). Even producing a vaccine is complicated because vaccines would need to produce an even stronger immune response than the pathogen itself in order to confer sterilizing immunity.

The complex relationship between *Mycobacterium tuberculosis* and the human immune system has evolved over long periods of time (Daniel, 2006). Tuberculosis is an ancient disease and has been identified in the remains of Neolithic humans. It probably originally existed earlier as a disease of lower mammals. The ability of the pathogen to exist in a latent state makes evolutionary sense as it enabled the pathogen to maintain itself within a population, while only causing disease and transmitting from a smaller subpopulation. For most of history it was uncommon, and only became epidemic with the ecological changes generated by increased urbanized living from the 16th century, until by the 18th century it was responsible for about 25 per cent of all adult deaths in Europe. The link to urbanization connects the disease to modern institutions such as factory production, high-density housing and imperialism. As a result, its global diffusion occurred in waves that generated multiple organ failures in susceptible populations. These waves eventually waned and left resistant individuals with chronic lung infection. In industrialized countries, where the disease emerged earlier, social changes that drove declines in mortality happened sooner, leaving the current situation where the disease burden falls most heavily on poorer nations.

Overcrowded urban living is an important contributing factor to the transmission of TB because it is caught through inhalation of infected air. Roughly a third of those exposed to the disease develop an infection. The infection generates an immune response in the form of activated T-cells and macrophages that migrate to the mycobacteria in the lungs and form granu-lomatous lesions. These isolate the bacteria and prevent primary disease in over 95 per cent of cases.

As previously noted, *Mycobacterium tuberculosis* has evolved a range of immune evasion strategies to survive immune-mediated destruction. In many instances the immune system does not kill the mycobacteria, and it survives with limited oxygen or nutrients. In about 90 per cent of cases the mycobacteria remain in this dormant state, do not get transmitted and TB does not develop. In a small number of cases TB is reactivated and the person becomes contagious. This risk is roughly 2–23 per cent over a person's lifetime – although with HIV infection it is substantially higher at about 5–10 per cent a year, highlighting the importance of maintaining a healthy immune response to keep infection at bay. Once the immune response is weakened 'the protracted course of trench warfare is trans-formed into an aggressive assault allowing for massive growth of bacteria, exceeding a trillion (10^{12}) organisms, which are then transmitted through the air to other individuals' (Kaufmann, 2007, p891).

Kaufmann's metaphor of trench warfare is particularly apt for a pathogen that evolved to survive hostile conditions in soil for long periods of time, and then rapidly re-emerge to over-run its hosts' immune systems, spread, infect others and then settle down again in a new latent state. The reactivation of latent TB is still poorly understood, but is clearly associated with factors that weaken immunity such as poor nutrition, drug use, alco-holism and HIV infection as well as with poverty, poor housing, social class, unstable lifestyles and immigrant or second-generation immigrant status. A study of 224 TB patients in a New York hospital, for example, found that 70 per cent were homeless or had unstable living conditions, and of the 178 discharged on medication, 99 per cent never returned (89 per cent had no follow up care) (Griffith and Kerr, 1996, p242).

TB – early narratives

Narratives about epidemics and the threats they pose typically connect a particular framing of the biological, social and other elements of the 'system' involved with a disease, to a causal mechanism and to moral concerns. Narratives then provide a guide to organizing a response. TB is no exception.

Before the late 19th century there was no general, robust understanding of how the diverse forms of TB were linked, or in many instances even if they were linked. Instead, illnesses of various kinds were understood in general descriptive terms based on fitting symptoms and empirical regularities such as links between illness and sites of infection (e.g. 'jail fever') into shared frameworks (Rosenberg, 1992). Understanding remained fluid as the disease and its symptoms progressed. In this context, the interpretation and treatment of TB reflected local idiosyncrasies, diverse cultural models of disease, and the diverse sites and symptoms of infection – giving rise to a variety of narratives and responses. TB was known as consumption, King's Evil, lupus vulgaris and phthisis, and the complex, slow and varied impact of TB produced a variety of responses including 'Bleeding, purging, bed rest, horseback riding, the mountains, the seashore, cod liver oil, castor oil, chaulmoogra oil, phrenic nerve interruption, thoracoplasty, and pneumothorax' (Yamey, 2003).

One such localized narrative, associated with a particular cultural model of disease, can be seen in 19th century England where consumption was associated with Gothic creativity.[3] John Keats, D. H. Lawrence, Anton Chekhov, Emily Bronte, Charlotte Bronte, Franz Kafka, Amedeo Modigliani and Frederick Chopin all suffered from consumption and helped link the disease to ideas about romantic creativity and the notion its victims were consumed from within by their passions (Mathema et al, 2006). Meanwhile, the global sanatoria movement emerged and drew on environmental narratives of TB as a disease of the dirty city that could be cured by fresh air, following Herman Brehmer's 1854 thesis describing the curative properties of the Himalayan mountains. The movement increased in popularity in the late 19th century with Edward Livingston Trudeau (1848–1915) establishing his Saranac Lake retreat in New York's Adirondack Mountains as a treatment and research centre in 1882. Sanatoria provided a place where the sick could be removed and treated by specialized phthisiologists, thereby reducing the risk that they might infect the healthy.

By the late 19th century radically new ways of understanding disease in general were emerging. As Rosenberg (1992) has described, these were based on proposing or identifying a specific mechanism that would produce an ideal-type clinical case. Rather than disease being identified from the symptoms of the patient, disease was 'imagined outside their embodiment in particular individuals and explained in terms of causal mechanisms within the sufferer's body' (Rosenberg, 1992, p242). This involved a major cognitive change, as real-world illnesses were seen as imperfect manifestations in particular times and places of abstract diseases. Rather than the symptoms defining the disease, now the disease defined the symptoms and patients whose very real illnesses deviated from these ideal types were referred to as atypical and seen as suffering from 'complications' (Rosenberg, 2002, p243).

This general scientific and societal shift in understandings of disease had a profound effect on understandings of TB. It involved more than simply thinking in terms of pathogens – Benjamin Marten, for example, had proposed *A New Theory of Consumption* in 1720 in which it was caused by 'minute living organisms' – but did not think of diseases as manifestations of abstract ideal types. Within the new cognitive framework, diagnostic models enabled the diverse outcomes that emerge from the complex interactions between different pathogens, hosts and environments to be seen as expressions of a mechanism that follows a classic case history (Morgan and Morrison, 1999) which gives the disease its prognosis and (later) helps define its treatment. In formulating a particular diagnostic or cultural model, a subset of causes is selected as important for understanding the disease. In the case of TB, this prioritized the pathogen as at the time the full extent of latent TB where the pathogen existed without generating disease was unknown. This directed attention away from other causal factors such as poverty, overcrowding and poor ventilation, and in so doing shifted the emphasis from TB as a multi-causal stress on society, to TB as a mono-causal shock. Further transformations in social and moral dimensions of TB narratives followed.

Once TB began to be associated with a pathogen, it lost its romantic edge. When TB was defined by its symptoms, and those symptoms were understood in terms of being consumed by creative Gothic passions, the disease posed little risk to others. But once it was established that the disease was contagious, in the 1880s, the *Spes phthisica* of well-being and the euphoria of the creative poet were displaced by a view of the victim as a danger to the rest of society and the disease became notifiable.

TB – biomedical narratives and responses

This broad-based biomedical narrative about TB, informed by its particular cultural-diagnostic model of the disease, in turn shaped particular pathways of response. As this section outlines, during the 20th century mechanism-based diagnostics for TB informed a range of particular treatment, clinical and public health practices, linking medical understandings to particular scientific tools and techniques, institutional arrangements and ways of dealing with incomplete knowledge.

Within this broad biomedical narrative, scientific instruments came to translate knowledge between the lab and the hospital bed. Koch's 1882 lecture, in which he showcased his discoveries about the bacteriology of TB, drew on his microscope, the culture dish invented by his colleague Petri, and the new dyes being developed in the German chemical industry. New technologies such as X-rays (1895) and sputum staining and micro-scopy (1882) could be used to inform diagnosis and prognosis. Even today, however, diagnosis remains a problem: X-rays involve cumbersome machinery and are subjectively interpreted, while sputum microscopy is dependent on the patient being able to produce a sputum sample, which may be difficult for small children and impossible if the infection is outside the lungs, as well as a trained technician being available to stain the sample and read the slide. As a result, it is estimated that only one case of TB is diagnosed for every eight to ten infections (Grange and Festenstein, 1993). The certainties generated by an abstract diagnostic model do not match the uncertainties of day-to-day medical practice.

Diagnosis also informed changes in hospitals as sites of treatment (Rosenberg, 2002). Mechanisms provided a clearer prognosis and a shared way of understanding a treatment regime. By writing down the case notes of a patient on printed forms, their individual experience could be related to the textbook course of the disease in a standardized way. This allowed for institutionalization and bureaucratic support for structured diagnosis, prognosis, research and treatment. It also structured the relationship between patient and doctor, giving patients a new identity, a sense of the future course of *their* disease, and expectations about the behaviour of the institution (Rosenberg, 2002, p245).

Mechanism-based diagnostics also framed TB as preventable and encour-aged public health authorities and scientific researchers to act. In the early 20th century educational, fundraising and research associations were set up to produce books, posters and stamps, with the International Union Against Tuberculosis and Lung Disease (IUATLD) set up in 1920. These organ-izations played a major role in fundraising and changing health policy, with important results. A year after the formation of the IUATLD, Albert

Calmette and Camille Guérin began to administer their Bacillus Calmette-Guérin (BCG) vaccine which provides protection against severe disease in children. However, the vaccine does not prevent latent TB or its reactivation in later life, and the closer to the equator one goes the less effective the vaccine becomes. It provided no, or very little, protection in India for example (Tuberculosis Prevention Trial, 1979). Since it makes diagnosis through skin testing difficult it was abandoned in the US in the 1950s. Other treatments that were developed in the early 20th century included surgically collapsing the lung so that it could heal, and removal of infected parts of the lung.[4]

The big breakthrough in treatment came in the 1940s with the development of antibiotics. Selman Waksman purified streptomycin from *Streptomyces griseus* in 1943 and his graduate student Albert Shatz showed it to have antibiotic properties against *Mycobacterium tuberculosis* in vitro and in animal models. In 1944 it was administered to a human patient and then successful large-scale clinical studies were conducted (Medical Research Council, 1948, 1955; Pfuetze et al, 1955). In 1944 the Mayo Clinic in Minnesota was using streptomycin to cure TB and its governance was successfully extended through the use of contact tracing. In the same year para-aminosalicylic acid (PAS), a modified form of aspirin, was produced by Ferrosan at the behest of Jörgen Lehmann, a Swedish chemist who had noted that the bacteria took up aspirin and could therefore be killed by a similar molecule. It produced dramatic results and was less toxic than streptomycin. In the late 1940s both drugs began to be used together and cured some 80 per cent of patients. Later still the sulphonamides, and particularly isoniazid (1952), followed by rifampicin (1970), were developed. The drugs were used together because the *Mycobacterium tuberculosis* bacterium quickly developed resistance to individual drugs (Ryan, 1993).

These anti-TB drugs are limited in number and efficacy, have side effects and need to be taken for six to nine months because of the low tissue concentrations of the drugs and their need to target the small subpopulation of dividing bacteria. Because of the long treatment times and the high rates of drug resistance the initial use of chemotherapy was to prepare patients for surgery. In the 1950s John Crofton developed the 'Edinburgh method' that avoided drug resistance and improved prognosis using streptomycin, PAS and isoniazid. This drug regimen aimed for a 100 per cent cure rate. Today the standard short course for TB treatment is a modified version of Crofton's regime: two months of isoniazid, rifampicin, pyrazinamide and ethambutol followed by four months of isoniazid and rifampicin, although ethambutol can be removed if the pathogen is fully susceptible. Given the problems with resistance it is recommended that patients are observed taking their medication, in what has become known as Directly Observed Treatment, Short Course, or DOTS (see Bayer and Wilkinson, 1995, for a history).

The re-emergence of TB and the growth of MDR-TB

With the clinical value of the multidrug treatment method established, the treatment pathway became a victim of its own success. Sanatoria were shut down as the scourge of TB in industrialized countries declined. For example, in 1952 there were 50,000 TB cases in Britain, yet by 1987 the number was reduced to 5500 (Thorpe, 2008). Today the numbers are still small: 8417 in the UK in 2007, with 72 per cent of cases originating from outside the UK (HPA, 2008). Arguably, this decline was under way before the introduction of modern treatments and may reflect the natural course of the epidemic. Nevertheless, by the 1970s the belief that infectious diseases were a problem of the past coincided with changing political priorities and TB services were reduced (Espinal, 2003, p45). The British Medical Research Council tuberculosis unit, for example, was shut down in 1985–1986 and treatment shifted from hospitals to outpatient settings.

This scaling back of the dominant biomedical narrative and treatment pathway in industrialized settings brought particular social and biological consequences, however. The deterioration of public health programmes for TB and weaker compliance in outpatient settings, especially amongst marginalized groups, combined with the rise of HIV infection and poor infection control in prisons, created the conditions for both increases in TB and for the growth of MDR-TB in the 1980s (Farmer, 1999b).

The social distribution of the new TB reflected its ecological niche among the most marginalized in society. In a major outbreak in New York City, for example, overall incidence rose from 23 to 50/100,000. It rose from 90 to 220/100,000 in Harlem, and was 469/100,000 among black men aged 35–44, a figure 45 times the national average (Bureau of Tuberculosis Control, 1991; Coker, 1998). Similarly, Coninx et al (2000) show that over half of the new cases of TB in Russia occur in prisons. Prison epidemics tend to follow prison 'caste systems', with low caste prisoners marginalized further and often denied healthcare treatment or forced to give up or sell their drugs.

These outbreaks increased the public prominence of TB in industrialized countries. They also increased awareness that the improvements in TB treatment in Europe and the US were not being matched globally. As a result, from the late 1980s onwards there was a significant shift in international health funding and resources back to TB. In 1989 the US Centers for Disease Control (CDC) announced its intention to eliminate TB by 2010. Soon after, in the 1991 World Health Assembly, new data were presented on TB infection rates which highlighted that 8 million people a year would be infected and several million would die despite there being very cost-effective treatments. In 1993 the World Bank published its *Investing in Health* report, which stressed the cost-effectiveness of TB controls (see Murray et al, 1991), and the WHO declared a Global Health Emergency (WHO, 2006; Cox et al, 2008). During the 1990s a series of global and often well-funded initiatives emerged (Brown, 2000). In 1994 the WHO, IUATLD and other partners launched the Global Project on Drug Resistance Surveillance (DRS) to monitor and assess the extent of drug resistance. This improved further as the WHO Model List of Essential Drugs encouraged generic production of TB drugs, with major falls in costs (Yong Kim et al, 2005, p850). In 1998 IUATLD and WHO came together to form the Stop TB Initiative, which later became the Stop TB partnership, with a focus on expanding DOTS, addressing TB-HIV, MDR-TB, developing new drugs, diagnostics and vaccines, and advocacy. By 2000 the G8 meeting proposed to halve the rate of TB from its 1990 levels by 2015, and provided political support for the WHO to expand its TB programmes.

A central part of many of these schemes involved the five measures in the DOTS programme:

1   national TB programmes;
2   detection through sputum smear microscopy;
3   a supervised standardized short-course chemotherapy using first-line drugs for all smear-positive cases when they are first detected;
4   a regular supply of all essential drugs;
5   a monitoring and evaluation system.

The DOTS approach was developed in the context of evidence suggesting that detecting 70 per cent of infectious (smear-positive) patients and curing 85 per cent of them could reduce the incidence of TB by 6 per cent per year, which would translate into halving TB within a decade (Elzinga et al, 2004). A key target was therefore to raise treatment success rates to more than 85 per cent at six months. By 1995 DOTS was being implemented in 187 countries to 4.9 million patients (covering 89 per cent of the world's population) (Cox et al, 2008, p1) with relative success (Frieden et al, 1995).

In line with the single, generic diagnostic model of TB on which it is based, the DOTS strategy promotes a TB response pathway based on standardized provision in healthcare facilities. Yet the potential for mismatches between such a generic programme, and the diverse needs, social and medical circumstances of patients in particular settings, is great, and only magnified as DOTS was extended globally. Not surprisingly then, DOTS strategies generated diverse effects when applied 'on the ground' in varied local contexts. Cox et al (2008), for example, found substantial heterogeneity in post-treatment relapse rates under trial conditions, ranging from 0 to 14 per cent at 18 months suggesting that 'all other things may not be equal'. Indeed, DOTS drew on pilot studies in nine countries, of which Senegal, Mali and Yemen were regarded as failures (Cox et al, 2008). In Uzbekistan only 65 per cent of patients who had completed treatment were alive and free of disease at 18 months (Chiang and Riley, 2005). In the 13 provinces of China that introduced DOTS the TB prevalence rate was cut by 30 per cent in a decade (1990–2000), but a similar programme in Vietnam produced little impact (WHO, 2005). In Cox et al's review (2008) HIV infection and level of resistance were the main influences on poor cure rates, but others have pointed to lack of resources and infrastructure, poorly governed private sector treatment, decentralized health reforms and lack of political commitment (MSF, 2007).

As we have seen, the robust nature of *Mycobacterium tuberculosis* makes chemotherapy difficult in all settings and this has made drug resistance a major problem. While drug treatment can be very effective, it needs to be continued for a long period of time to ensure compliance with the regimen. Given the side effects of the drugs such compliance can conflict with the immediate needs of patients. As Crofton noted: 'People feel better in three or four weeks, and say "I'm cured and I don't need to go on taking this stuff"… they have other priorities, especially poor people – like where the next meal is coming from' (Thorpe, 2008). Such problems are important because within the dominant biomedical narrative, the clinical course of the disease is based around a series of assumptions about the pathogen (it is susceptible to antibiotics), the patient (that they have a reasonably typical, working immune system) and the treatment regimen (it will be followed to completion by the medical profession, the patient and the support infrastructure). Under these conditions the treatment works extremely well, hence the successes in the reduction of TB cases noted above. However, when these assumptions do not hold conditions are created for the emergence of drug resistance (primary MDR-TB) and its subsequent spread (secondary MDR-TB) (Medical Research Council, 1948).

MDR is technically defined as resistance against at least two first-line drugs – isoniazid and rifampicin. However, almost 80 per cent of new MDR cases are resistant to three or more drugs (Shin et al, 2004). Resistance complicates treatment and increases its cost approximately 100-fold (Kaufmann, 2004). This is because second-line drugs are more expensive, more toxic and less effective. This in turn increases treatment times that can extend to 18–24 months, with four to eight medications typically including a course of daily injections for six months (Farmer et al, 2000). The costs of bringing the New York City MDR-TB outbreak under control were

LIVERPOOL JOHN MOORES UNIVERSITY
LEARNING SERVICES

estimated at US$1 billion and helped shift resources back to public health and TB control (Garrett, 2000). Since MDR-TB is a particular problem for patients with compromised immune systems, its combination with increased HIV infection rates poses a severe public health risk (Cahn et al, 2003). Since high levels of HIV and TB infection are mainly found in the world's poorest settings, the costs fall disproportionately on the poor.

Early experience of clinical failure produced an infrastructure of surveillance for drug resistance. In the 1960s the Pasteur Institute developed the 'critical proportion method' for drug susceptibility testing and regular surveys found substantial outbreaks of drug resistance, particularly in developing countries. France, however, ceased monitoring resistance in the 1970s as the overall TB infrastructure was wound down, and the US and UK followed in the 1980s. The re-emergence of TB and the emergence of widespread MDR-TB in the 1980s increased the surveillance of resistance. Surveys were published by the WHO in 1997, 2000, 2005 and 2008. The first report in 1997 was based on data from 35 countries and showed that drug resistance was ubiquitous (Espinal, 2003, p46). The latest report covers tests for 91,577 patients in 81 countries and two Special Administrative Regions of China. The extent of drug resistance to one drug varies from zero in two Western European countries, to 56 per cent in Baku Azerbaijan, with MDR-TB rates from 0 per cent to 22.3 per cent in Baku and 19.4 per cent in Moldova (WHO, 2008d, p11). MDR is highly concentrated, with 14 of the top 20 regions in the former Soviet Union and four in China. In total just under half a million cases emerged in 2005, with about half in China or India and 7 per cent in Russia, and other hot spots in Estonia, Latvia, the Dominican Republic and Côte d'Ivoire (WHO, 2008d). In European countries MDR-TB is not a mainstream public health concern and is limited to marginalized groups such as the homeless, refugees and immigrants (Lillebaek et al, 2001). MDR-TB is not yet a major problem in many poor rural settings because the poor are often unable to buy enough drugs for resistance to emerge – although they would be at severe risk if secondary MDR-TB began to spread.

MDR-TB – diverse narratives

As people and institutions have come to acknowledge and make sense of MDR-TB, a variety of narratives has arisen. These frame the problem, its causes and possible consequences in different ways, and suggest different kinds of response. They are united, however, by a shared sense of a threat which involves many unknowns – it is not observable, delayed in its impact, and new and poorly understood by science – and many dread factors – such as being global, fatal, unfair, future orientated, uncontrolled, involuntary and increasing; factors which Slovic (1989) has associated with an amplified perception of risk. It is therefore of no surprise that the dramatic change in public policy noted in the introduction occurred.

Security

A first narrative about MDR-TB, promoted especially by global health agencies and by European and US governments and media, casts it as a threat to personal and societal security. This security narrative is characterized by a number of features: it takes social structure as given and therefore not in need of change, and focuses on contagion, attributing blame and risk to outsiders, that is, foreigners or immigrants. Security has a powerful appeal. This appeal can be seen in the WHO (2007a) report *A Safer Future* with its subtitle of *Global Public Health Security in the 21st Century*. It can be seen as the 'Out of Africa' rhetoric about newly emergent diseases in the UK Foresight documents. Although in this case the direction is reversed: a disease that came out of Europe and is destroying Africa does not fit a 'Southern threat to the North' model well (compare Leach and Hewlett, this volume).

There is also an East–West security framing reflecting concerns in Europe about immigration from the East. Within this narrative, it is emphasized that Europe has a particularly high incidence of drug-resistant strains (13 countries with MDR-TB rates in excess of 10 per cent), low detection rates and poor treatment success rates partly because 'Europe' is defined to include Eastern Europe and central Asia. The approximately 450,000 TB infections and nearly 70,000 deaths each year disproportionately reflect HIV/AIDS co-infection in Russia and Ukraine and the socio-economic collapse of Eastern Europe and the Russian Federation where TB cases almost tripled in the decade after 1989. Given differences in global health provision, immigrants can make up disproportionate numbers of cases of infectious diseases. In the UK they made up three-quarters of cases of TB, HIV and malaria reported in 2004 (HPA, 2008). Migliori et al's (2007) data suggest that Russian and other ex-Soviet Union immigrants are the main victims of MDR-TB in Germany. Gaining little attention within this narrative are those contrary data that suggest that immigrants do not represent a major health risk. For instance between 2001 and 2005 more than 30,000 former Soviet citizens arrived in Norway but only four were diagnosed with MDR-TB on arrival, and their infections were not transmitted (Dahle, 2005).

In the US in the 1980s concern about MDR-TB was trumped by security concerns about the 'war on drugs' that focused on putting large numbers of petty dealers and drug users, rather than money launderers, in prisons. However, the resulting explosion in the prison population, without an increase in the funding needed to deal with increased HIV infection, led to major MDR-TB outbreaks and a 1500 per cent increase in TB rates among African American men between 1985 and 1990 (Farmer, 2003, p184). The European response was fundamentally different, reflecting a very different approach to the penal system. MDR-TB generated a public expression of a belief in the potential of science and technology combined with a willingness to provide relatively modest amounts of aid.

One marginalized group that is seen as representing a particular threat in Europe is ex-prisoners from Russia. In this respect, the security narrative, with its triple whammy of illegal immigrants, criminals and disease, offers the potential to provide rhetorical power to broader human rights concerns. Paul Farmer, for example, notes, 'This epidemic is only briefly local. It will not remain within borders. Forty two per cent of the Russian problem is in prisons. Prison bars and national borders are inadequate to stop transmission' (quoted in Tanne, 1999). The Russian prison system contains some 100,000 prisoners who had TB in 1999 when Farmer was writing, and of those, some 40,000 had MDR-TB, of whom 12,000 are released back into the community each year (Meek, 1998; Tanne, 1999). This is part of a wider problem as prisons are a particular high-risk, poor-treatment setting. Kimerling et al (1999) highlighted a treatment failure rate of 35 per cent in a Siberian TB referral prison in the Kemerovo region despite the implementation of what should be an effective treatment regime. Given the extremely poor conditions within the Russian prison system where large numbers of prisoners are crowded into poorly ventilated cells, it is unsurprising that their infection rates are so high and they do not match the treatment model underpinning DOTS. The security narrative suggests that Russian prisoners should be treated – but this is largely to protect Western Europeans, rather than – as a human rights framing would suggest – to help them because they are sick.

Neglect of health care

An alternative narrative about the MDR-TB problem treats it as a much more systemic problem. This 'neglect of health care' narrative has a number of features. It blames configurations of social and institutional arrangements – and imbalances in these, taking social structure to be in need of change to either restore or create effective health care. And it attributes blame to structural changes, often driven by political choices, and sometimes personified in politicians. For example, in the context of cutbacks and declining funding for TB services and public health a major element of the framing of the 1990s New York City outbreak was as a 'Payback for Reagan'. President Reagan had cut social programmes and public health, and the 1980s saw increases in social poverty and homelessness. As a consequence, TB got out of control, and was made worse by the failure properly to treat patients in socially marginalized groups – including, as we have seen, prisoners. Examples of such arguments about the price of neglect include CDC (2006) information which states: 'In the 1970s and early 1980s, the nation let its guard down and TB control efforts were neglected. The country became complacent about TB, and many states and cities redirected TB prevention and control funds to other programs.' Similarly, the WHO report that 'Tuberculosis control is being neglected in most countries worldwide, and … MDR-TB is a manifestation of this global neglect' (Tanne, 1999).

In this narrative, therefore, the global spread of MDR-TB reflects failures in global health care. Sixteen countries in Africa, for example, experienced drug stock outs during 2005, 14 with first-line drugs, creating conditions where resistance can emerge. With the system framed in global terms, this narrative about healthcare systems failure has much in common with the 'world out of balance' narratives found in the work of Laurie Garrett (Garrett, 1994) and others. While powerful and widely communicated through the media, these do raise unanswered questions about what the world was like when it was in balance. Nor, in this narrative, is it clear whether the problem lies with the diagnostic model and its treatment regimen, or with its implementation. Taking the diagnostic model as given and seeing the emergence of MDR-TB in terms of non-compliance could direct attention to the patient. Or it could direct attention to the healthcare system where the majority of non-compliance problems emerge (Chintu and Zumla, 1995), and have done through the history of TB treatment (Lerner, 1997).

In any case, the key policy prescriptions to flow from this narrative centre on greater investment in well-structured global healthcare systems that can extend DOTS and ensure its effective, controlled application. In some versions, this narrative is associated with a rejection of market-based forms of coordination in favour of more publicly controlled and hierarchical ones. Tang and Squire (2005), for example, argue that market-oriented reforms to the healthcare system in China since the 1970s had created perverse incentives for doctors to over-prescribe antibiotics and have weakened coordination between acute and chronic care. Wallace et al (1995, 1999) develop similar ideas and suggest that neoliberal policy creates an ecological niche for TB.

A related concern is the lack of shorter and simpler TB treatments because of structural problems in the research system. Orbinski, for example, suggests that:

> *Governments have a political responsibility to promote, protect and ensure peoples' right to health care. In the face of a major public health emergency like TB, governments must either intervene in the market or*

> *establish public capacity for new drug development ... To date, govern-*
> *ment has failed, the pharmaceutical industry has failed, and market*
> *forces alone will fail to respond to TB. TB is a social and political*
> *problem and a failure to act today will have incalculable consequences*
> *for generations to come around the world.* (MSF, 2000)

Similarly, the Global Alliance for TB Drug Development involves attempts to reconfigure the drug development system and control the TB and MDR-TB epidemics through technology. Gro Bruntland has proposed that a new partnership between the WHO and industry would help develop drugs that reduce the duration of the treatment to less than three months. This mixture of innovation and activism has considerable political support. In the UK, for example, an all-party group for TB has been created and has helped double the UK government's grant to the Global Fund to Fight AIDS, Tuberculosis and Malaria to £100 million (Moszynski, 2006, p938).

While it is clear that improved treatment is needed, others argue that the focus on technical solutions does not address future problems with their implementation, nor the fact that effective drug regimes already exist but cannot be effectively implemented. There is therefore a potential risk that 'science becomes a substitute for social action' (Sarewitz, 1999). Funding research for future cures provides a politically convenient way of turning a current, politically difficult problem, that requires making political choices today, into a problem for the future.

Structural violence, rights and context

A third narrative about MDR-TB, promoted particularly by a range of civil society organizations and activists but increasingly embodied in global health agencies too, sees the problem and possible solutions in terms of 'structural violence' (Farmer, 1995) and rights in particular contexts. Like the previous narrative, it is configuration focused, but suggests that social and institutional structures need to be radically changed rather than merely extended or returned to a prior 'balanced' state. Blame is attributed to wider societal inequalities, as when Yong Kim et al (2005, p848) note: 'Tuberculosis is not a matter of infection; it is a reflection of patterned resource distribution.' Thus for instance, MDR-TB infection is particularly likely in prison, so infection patterns are shaped along the racial, income, age and gender lines that strongly pattern who goes to prison. In keeping with this narrative's concern with equality and inequality, there is more emphasis on an individual rights-based approach to intervention rather than the top-down, hierarchical public health approach supported by the previous narrative. As a consequence, the emphasis is on pathways of response that are more bottom-up, flexible and attuned to local contexts. Rather than coordinating activity through bureau-cracies or markets, coordination is more alliance and network-based.

Indeed, the rights-based approach justified by this narrative can clash with the public health ethos behind the DOTS programme. The prime concern of the latter is to prevent further infection, so the focus is on infectious patients. To ensure effective treatment within a resource-constrained environment DOTS divides patients into four categories from high-priority smear-positive patients (Cat. I) to low priority (MDR-TB) and chronic cases (Cat. IV), aiming to treat 'at least all' Category I patients. However, DOTS detection technologies can miss the 15–20 per cent of patients with non-pulmonary TB. Previously this was not a major public health issue as smear-negative patients were considered unlikely to die. Today this is not the case. With MDR-HIV co-infection, non-infectious extra-pulmonary MDR patients are almost certain to die without treatment. From a rights-based perspective they have just as much need for treatment as Category I patients even if they are less of a threat to public health.

Similar clashes emerge over resource allocation. While standard public health narratives have focused on value for money and aggregate measures of cost-effectiveness, proponents of a structural violence perspective draw attention to major inequalities in resource allocation. Farmer et al (2006) argue that value for money can falsely assume costs to be fixed, when they can be very successfully reduced. The same trade-offs exist in all healthcare choices.

Elements of a structural violence narrative have influenced the global response to MDR-TB. Global public health bureaucracies such as the WHO initially sought to implement standardized DOTS programmes to reduce primary MDR-TB, but had to move to DOTS-plus, including two or more second-line drugs (Iseman, 1993). Second-line drugs can now be procured at reduced prices through the Green Light Committee of the WHO, following the coordinated actions of the NGOs successfully working with international health organizations to push rights to treatment amongst poorer populations. The treatment is either individualized (after drug susceptibility testing), or given as a standard regimen for patients who fail supervised re-treatment. In 2006 DOTS-plus had a 60 per cent success rate in WHO Green Light Committee projects, although the cure rate for MDR can be as low as 5 per cent in Russia (WHO, 2008d). As a result, studies now suggest that on the grounds of both equality and cost-effectiveness, DOTS-plus is a reasonable investment for low-income countries (Mukherjee et al, 2004, p478).

While the initial treatment of MDR-TB focused on hospital settings because of the complexities of drug treatment and potential toxic side effects, recent work by Farmer et al (2000) and Shin et al (2004) has shown that community based MDR-TB treatment can be both effective and cost efficient. Within Peru, cure rates have approached over 80 per cent, which is comparable with US HIV-negative cohorts (Shin et al, 2004, p1530). This community-based MDR-TB treatment emphasizes approaches that respect the needs of individual patients, and are attuned to local contexts. It involves integrated teams, trained community health workers and volunteers who build close rapports with local patients and their families (Espinal and Dye, 2005). They monitor drug treatment and contacts, note side effects and provide considerable non-medical support with back-up from nurses, physicians and ancillary staff.

This approach is more flexible than the standardized DOTS model which was developed for a world without MDR-TB, when drugs were expensive and financial resources more limited. While its early introduction was largely top-down, this has softened and Mario Raviglione, director of the WHO Stop TB department has said that 'The statement in the early 1990s that DOTS was the only solution was a great mistake. We now accept that we need both DOTS and new tools, that it is not a competition between these two approaches' (MSF, 2007). Put another way, this is a recognition that MDR-TB response pathways need to integrate effective public health programmes and interventions with a careful attuning to the needs and rights of patients in particular local contexts.

This more flexible approach should have been relatively successful at getting MDR-TB back under control (Dye et al, 2002). However, it coincided with increasing levels of HIV infection and the emergence of XDR-TB, as the *Mycobacterium tuberculosis* bacterium found a new evolutionary niche (Marston and Miller, 2006).

The emergence of XDR-TB and HIV co-infection

XDR-TB is defined as infection that is resistant to the best second-line medications: fluoroquinolones and at least one of three injectable drugs (amikacin, kanamycin or capreomycin). It remains relatively uncommon in industrialized countries with only 49 cases being reported between 1993 and 2006 in the US (CDC, 2006). It is, however, becoming a major concern in Eastern European, former Soviet countries and a range of African and Asian countries. WHO (2007a) data from 35 countries suggest that 301 of 4012 cases of MDR (7 per cent) were in fact XDR. South African data, for example, suggest that 996 of 17,615 MDR cases were XDR (2004–2007), with the majority (656) of cases in KwaZulu-Natal. This follows on from data gathered between January 2005 and March 2006 which found 221 (41 per cent) of 536 TB sputum samples in Tugela Ferry (SA) to be MDR-TB, of which 53 were XDR (Ghandi et al, 2006). Fifty-two of those infected with XDR-TB died, with an average life expectancy of 25 days.

The emergence of XDR-TB has been driven by HIV co-infection (Chretien, 1990; Ghandi et al, 2006). The standard biomedical cultural and diagnostic model for TB made assumptions about the drugs, pathogen, patient and treatment regime. With MDR-TB, as indicated in earlier sections, the treatment regime assumptions failed. However, with HIV co-infection, additional assumptions about drug action, pathogens and patients' immune systems all need to be rethought (De Cock and Chaisson, 1999; Del Amo et al, 1999). Indeed Nunn et al (2005) suggest that without HIV, TB would be in decline almost everywhere. With HIV, however, TB infection is increasing and some 15 million people are now co-infected, with 2 million new cases being added each year (Kaufmann, 2007, p891). As a result, conditions have emerged for the evolution of XDR-TB and TB deaths have doubled in Africa from 42/100,000 in 1990 to 84/100,000 in 2004 (MSF, 2007, p11).

Molecular genetics studies suggest that like MDR-TB, XDR-TB occurs regularly and can disseminate relatively easily when care and disease control are poorly managed. Poor prescribing practices, low drug quality, disrupted supply and failure to adhere to treatment subject the bacteria to intense selection pressures that allow them to accumulate resistance mutations to mono-therapies. Like MDR-TB, XDR-TB can also occur though secondary infection. The mutations that cause antibiotic resistances generally reduce the virulence of the pathogen and make it less likely to cause secondary infection in people with well-functioning immune systems. However, people with weakened immune systems can be infected easily. This is why there is so much concern about the epidemiology of HIV-TB co-infection (Nunn et al, 2005).

In this context, outbreaks of XDR-TB have the capacity to generate major fear, often being interpreted and responded to within security-focused narratives. Thus even though the outbreak of XDR-TB in South Africa generated only a limited number of deaths (74 by 2006), by 2006 'its virulent nature and mortality of nearly 100 per cent is starting to cause panic in southern Africa. Doctors in the region fear that it threatens to overwhelm Africa's fragile health systems, which already face the world's highest AIDS burden' (Moszynski, 2007). Resource-poor countries are faced with increases in case loads as TB infections rise, which can lead to increased drug resistance as treatment programmes become overwhelmed and fail (Sidley, 2006). As a result, extreme measures for the control of XDR-TB have been proposed including forced confinement (Singh et al, 2007), overriding concerns about patients' rights and social justice (which contrasts with the English case described in Welshman, 2006).

With grim predictability the burden of HIV-TB co-infection and XDR-TB falls disproportionately on the poorest countries and on the weakest within those countries. Roughly one-third of new TB cases in the

African region are attributable to HIV co-infection (Cobertt et al, 2003; Espinal, 2003). South Africa, for example, has 0.7 per cent of the world's population but had 19 per cent of all cases of TB in adult HIV-positive people in 2005. The rest of the African region accounted for a further 61 per cent with 10 per cent in India. Of the XDR-TB deaths at Tugula Ferry, all 44 that were tested for HIV were positive. Approximately a quarter of pregnant women in Zambia are HIV positive, with the result that TB has become the leading cause of pregnancy-related mortality (Ahmed et al, 1999; Gandy and Zumla, 2002, p388).

HIV-TB co-infection does not just increase infection; the diseases are synergistic. HIV infection of CD4+ cells helps transform latent TB into active TB, while latent TB promotes the activation of immune cells and increases the replication of HIV, bringing the onset of AIDS forward and creating conditions in which TB can kill the patient (Kaufmann, 2007, p891). To make matters worse, HIV is also a complicating factor in vaccination, as the BCG vaccine, which protects against TB in newborns, is a live vaccine that can cause BCGosis in immune-compromised patients. It is therefore not recommended for HIV-positive children (Kaufmann, 2007, p892). HIV infection can also lead to malabsorption of drugs, and therefore increase the prevalence of acquired rifamycin resistance (Wells et al, 2007). In addition, rifampicin can reduce the uptake of ARV drugs making AIDS more likely. Furthermore, antiretroviral therapy and highly active antiretroviral therapy (HAART) can disrupt the 'trench warfare' between latent TB and the immune system to either promote outbreaks of disease or make existing disease worse (Nunn et al, 2005; Colebunders et al, 2006). As a consequence there are major technical problems in developing treatments for co-infection (Pepper et al, 2008).

The problems that co-infection raise for treatment have pushed Médecins Sans Frontières and other organizations to argue that the two separate vertical regimes for HIV and TB set up by the WHO are now out of date and make treatment more difficult. An alternative narrative is emerging which argues that HIV-TB co-infection needs to be understood as a disease in its own right. Pathways of response need to be developed accordingly, rather than as an overlap between two separate, vertical programmes. Thus, treatments need to be combined: a Thai study showed 88 per cent of patients with both HIV and TB who received ARVs were alive at year 3, compared to 9 per cent who only received TB treatment (MSF, 2007, p13). Similarly, diagnostics need to be rethought – sputum microscopy is a poor test for co-infection and picks up less than 50 per cent of cases (many HIV-infected patients are likely to have extrapulmonary TB and therefore do not produce sputum). While culture and X-ray techniques can be used, cultures take time, both are often not available in resource-poor settings, and X-rays are often atypical for co-infected patients. HIV tests by contrast are fast and accurate and arguably give a better picture of TB infection than TB tests.

In many settings HIV treatment is well funded but good quality TB care is lacking, so co-infected patients face a service that differs in both its quality and in the sites at which it takes place. As MSF argues 'the best way to ensure good care for co-infected patients is to provide care for both TB and HIV at the same site – an integrated service' which builds on 'similar needs for monitoring, funding, staffing, community support, nutritional support, drug supply, and training' (MSF, 2007, p25). A programme in Khayelitsha, South Africa, where the HIV-TB co-infection rate is 70 per cent, has integrated HIV-TB care since 2003. From December 2007 it launched a pilot community-based management of drug-resistant TB on top of the existing networks developed for its community-based HIV treatment programme (Zachariah et al, 2004; MSF, 2007). Combining HIV and TB treatment in this way is part of the gradual emergence of a new diagnostic model with explicit causes related to TB and HIV, scientific mechanisms, a research programme producing diagnostics and new drugs, new sites of treatment, new bureaucratic structures, and new relationships between healthcare professionals and patients. Community-based approaches also draw on the perspectives of 'structural violence, rights and context' narratives of the MDR-TB era, suggesting that its lessons – about the importance of attuning approaches to particular needs and contexts – will need to be part of the repertoire for coping with the challenges of XDR-TB and HIV-TB that the world now faces.

Conclusions

The emergence of MDR-TB provides a case study of the progress of an epidemic and the diverse ways in which social groups attempt to understand and respond to the complexity and randomness associated with epidemics through constructing selective, simplified narratives and pathways of response. The case of MDR-TB also highlights how the successful generation of a treatment regimen for one disease – in this case standard TB – can nevertheless create an environmental niche for the emergence of a new epidemic. For cases of TB that closely approximate the standard model, DOTS-based chemotherapy provides highly effective treatment, neatly fitting a narrative about global public health care and the need to roll it out and scale it up. For cases that diverge from the assumptions underpinning the standard model, treatment can be ineffective, and resistance can emerge and spread to produce new infections. Under these conditions a new diagnostic model and treatment regime is needed. DOTS-plus adapts the older model to the pathogen through different drugs, and – when delivered through a more rights-and-context attuned lens – to the patient through community support.

With XDR-TB the patient and the pathogen (and often their environments) differ further from the original diagnostic model to the point that questions can be asked about whether a new treatment regime is needed or if the standard model is flexible enough to adapt. It raises important questions about whether conceptualizing MDR-TB as a single infection is the most useful approach. As argued in an alternative narrative, rapidly gaining ground amongst NGOs, frontline health workers and a growing number of scientists, the real disease may now be HIV-MDR-TB co-infection, with HIV-negative patients increasingly atypical.

Intersecting with the dynamic interplay of narratives documented in this chapter are the dynamics of the pathogen itself, and the social-ecological-technological systems with which it has been co-evolving. These dynamics reflect the way *Mycobacterium tuberculosis* as a pathogen has readily found ecological niches among the most marginalized. MDR-TB emerged among groups whose social exclusion made their treatment regimens ineffective, while XDR-TB has emerged as a major problem for HIV co-infected patients and marginalized groups, such as Soviet prisoners. The emergence of XDR-TB highlights the interactions between pathogens, treatment, scientific understanding and medical practice in the context of changing patterns of healthcare provision and social interactions. The pathways of TB response rooted in 20th century biomedical narratives proscribed technology, bureaucracy, sites of treatment, relationships between patients and medical professions, drugs and precautions. Their success helped address a major societal stress in industrialized countries and turn it into a much smaller feature of public health. However, the emergence of MDR-TB in the 1990s was a shock. With MDR emerged a new treatment regimen and new sites of treatment and bureaucratic support. However, with the increased overlap between HIV and TB infection, these pathways too began to founder as bureaucratic structures, designed for a single disease with a single pathogen causal mechanism, failed to cope with the emergence of a 'new disease' caused by two pathogens acting together. In both cases the TB pathogen found an ecological niche at the margins of the pathways among patients and healthcare systems that diverged from the underlying assumptions that made the narratives and their associated pathways so effective in their original settings.

As noted in the introduction, the tragedy of TB is that the niches in which new pathogens develop resistance to drugs have so often been among the most marginalized people and places. The pathogens, the patients and their environments failed to match the assumptions of the dominant narratives, and as a result the treatment regimens failed. The social distribution of risks and rewards of narratives and associated interventions does not fall equally on everyone and that very fact has been exploited by *Mycobacterium tuberculosis*.

Notes

1 The author would like to thank Melanie Newport for her comments on this paper.
2 WHO data suggest that the global TB incidence rate peaked between 2000 and 2005 (WHO, 2006). However, population growth has meant that the number of new cases is increasing in Africa, the eastern Mediterranean and Southeast Asia.
3 This Gothic element (and link to vampirism) emerged as infected individuals wasted away, went pale, avoided light but managed to maintain a will to live and a clear mind.
4 Surgery remains important for the treatment of MDR-TB and is widely used in Russia.

Chapter 9

Epidemics of Obesity: Narratives of 'Blame' and 'Blame Avoidance'

Erik Millstone[1]

Introduction

Once a relatively minor health issue, over the past 20 years obesity has rapidly become a significant public health policy issue that affects an enormous range of countries, from the richest to the very poorest. The US was the first industrialized country in which it was categorized as a public health challenge, when in 1985 the National Institutes of Health drew attention to the increasing scale of the problem (Brody, 1985; Burton et al, 1985; NIH, 1985). By 1996, the US National Center for Health Statistics reported that, for the first time, overweight people outnumbered other Americans (Lawrence, 2004). Recent evidence indicates that the incidence of obesity in school-aged children has doubled over the past ten years in many European countries, a fact which has provoked high levels of concern amongst health professionals and policy-makers.

In the last few years, reports of rapidly rising rates of overweight and obese populations have emerged from a striking array of countries, including those with large numbers of people who are hungry living in them (Delpeuch et al, 2009). There are many ways to measure overweight and obese people. Current definitions used by the WHO are based on the body mass index (BMI), a ratio of a person's weight (in kilogrammes) to the square of the person's height (in metres). According to this measure, European and Caucasian adults with a BMI of greater than 25 are considered overweight. Those with a BMI over 30 are considered obese (WHO, 2000b). Different figures are used as benchmarks for different population groups.

The purpose of this chapter, however, is not to document the changing socio-geographic incidence of obesity but rather to map the competing ways in which the phenomena have been described and addressed, with a predominant focus on analysing how policy debates have developed and evolved in the highly industrialized countries of Europe, North America and east Asia (such as Japan and Singapore). Those countries have been selected not because they have a monopoly of obesity, or because they are the only interesting examples, but because their debates have been documented and are available in English. In order to provide such a map, I will describe competing narratives for characterizing the changing incidence of obesity, with an aim towards understanding why some narratives have become relatively dominant in public discourse while others are less prominent. At the same time, I will assess the gap between rhetorical dominance of a given narrative and its efficacy in enacting concrete changes in policy, behaviour or obesity rates.

The bulk of the public debates about possible policy responses to the rising incidence of obesity focus on identifying the cause of the epidemic and attributing responsibility for addressing the problem. Even actors with very different opinions on these points nonetheless generally agree that unhealthy weight gain is a consequence of what physicists and physiologists might term 'thermodynamic dis-equilibrium': an imbalance between energy intake (from food and drink) and energy expenditure (in metabolic and physical activity). Excess intake over expenditure is normally stored in the body as fat. The question that shapes much debate is which side of the exercise/food equation is responsible for the problem. Or, as Jebb and Prentice put it: 'Should obesity be blamed on gluttony, sloth, or both?' (1995)

While the competing narratives examined generally share a broad framing of obesity as an epidemic, they differ substantially on how they answer this question and on how, in turn, they justify particular pathways of response. Some feature protagonists, such as public health professionals and consumer organizations, who argue that the main determinant of the occurrence and incidence of obesity is the overconsumption of rich foods and drinks and therefore that reversing trends entails significant changes in dietary habits. Others, especially in the food and advertising industries, argue that the main determinant of obesity has been a decline in levels of physical activity and energy expenditure, and therefore that reversing obesity trends will require significantly higher levels of physical activity. Most commentators argue, however, that obesity is a consequence of important changes to both dietary habits and levels of physical activity, and therefore that both need to be changed, which shifts the focus of debate onto how such changes can and should be achieved (Jebb and Prentice, 1995). Key axes in those debates revolve, unsurprisingly, around the relative responsibilities of individuals, governments and the food industry, and where the main responsibility for making constructive changes should be located.

A broad range of debates about obesity has arisen in the medical, social scientific and policy literatures as well as in policy networks. Within the scholarly literature those debates often focus on identifying the causes of rising rates of obesity and designing responses, while in policy circles debates focus on attributions of responsibility for past developments and future initiatives. Positions taken in those debates vary across time, social and cultural settings, and interests, and they are compounded by macro-social changes and culturally diverse perspectives. One important axis in the debate is marked by two competing narratives: one that attributes responsibility for rising rates of obesity to individual choices and actions versus a contrary perspective that grants primary blame to features of the social and economic environment. A second axis is concerned with competing views on the potential role for governments: one narrative suggests that governments might have to intervene actively and extensively, while a contrary view argues that governments should play only a very limited role.

Should governments intervene? If so, along which lines, and how far?

Although at the margin there are a few individuals and groups who maintain that governments should take no measures to intervene to change the incidence of obesity, there are very widespread agreements in numerous jurisdictions that it is not just appropriate but also necessary for governments to introduce public policy measures to diminish the incidence of obesity. Almost no one, in the UK and in much of the European Union (EU), argues that nothing needs to be done about either food consumption or about levels of physical activity. There are, however, enormous differences about what actions should be taken, by whom, and to what extent. These are rarely 'all or nothing' debates; they are, rather, complex arguments between those favouring maximalist and those favouring minimalist approaches along the numerous dimensions of debate.

The distinction between 'individualistic' and 'systemic' or 'environmental' framing narratives influences the types of possible policy measures, or pathways of response, that individuals and organizations deem appropriate. Those favouring an individualistic framing often argue that, if any measures are to be taken, they should be ones that strengthen individuals' abilities to make well-informed choices. Consequently they are often far more willing to support improved educational provision for school children and improved labelling of food products in retail outlets and sometimes also on menus in commercial catering contexts than to support the creation of new government bodies (which are often disparaged as bureaucracies) or regulatory controls on the composition of processed foods. Similarly, representatives of the food industry are often keener on measures to encourage and facilitate higher levels of physical activity than on measures to change the supply of, or demand for, foods.

In practice, however, there is evidence indicating that stakeholder groups, such as representatives of food companies or consumer organizations are not always reliable predictors of policy framings, and that within particular stakeholder groups there are significant variations within and between countries. For example, while representatives of British consumer organizations are enthusiastic about the introduction of mandatory and improved nutrition labelling on the fronts of pre-packaged foods, their French counterparts have disparaged such initiatives as reflecting a narrowly Anglo-Saxon approach that was inappropriate for France where the cultural significance of food and meals was radically different (Holdsworth et al, forthcoming).

The position in the EU is complicated because European legislation already specifies some issues that are matters of pooled sovereignty, while others may be decided by individual countries. For example, to facilitate a single European market, rules on the labelling of food and drink products are set at an EU-wide level, but each EU member state can decide separately whether to regulate the provision of school meals. Since measures to combat obesity clearly cross these jurisdictional lines, the policy landscape is quite complex.

Before these axes of responsibility and intervention are explored, it is worth considering the extent to which obesity qualifies as an epidemic at all.

Obesity as a global epidemic

One slightly tangential debate, about the terms in which the changing incidence of obesity has been discussed, concerns the question of whether or not the term 'epidemic' should be applied to obesity even though it is not an infectious disease. Since at least the 1970s several non-infectious diseases such as coronary heart disease, cardiovascular disease, asthma and cancer have been characterized as epidemics (Lawther and Aldridge, 1979). In 2008 the British Prime Minister referred to obesity as a 'lifestyle' disease and as a modern 'epidemic' (Brown, 2008).

One occasionally encounters a few individuals arguing that the phenomenon of people being overweight and/or obese is being exaggerated, and that a 'moral panic' is being deliberately manufactured for cynical political reasons. Campos, for example, has argued that there is a cultural hysteria about body weight in the US, supported by a collusive conspiracy between health puritans and the diet industry for which there is no evidential justification (Campos, 2004). A similar narrative is articulated by the self-styled Center for Consumer Freedom, which portrays itself as 'a nonprofit organization devoted to promoting personal responsibility and protecting consumer choices' (Center for Consumer Freedom, 2009). That organization has a web page entitled 'An Epidemic of Obesity Myths', which denies that obesity is an epidemic in the US or that it is a significant health or public policy problem (see www.obesitymyths.com). According to the Center for Science in the Public Interest, however, the Center for Consumer Freedom is a coalition of restaurant, catering, food industry and tobacco corporations rather than a genuine consumer-based organization (Center for Science in the Public Interest, 2008).

On behalf of the WHO, and by implication its member states, a report was issued in 2000 entitled 'Obesity: Preventing and Managing the Global Epidemic' (WHO, 2000b). None of the WHO's members publicly complained about the title of that volume, and so accept that obesity can properly be characterized as an epidemic.

In 2002, two leading Australian public health epidemiologists, Egger and Swinburn, went beyond portraying obesity as an 'epidemic'; they characterized it as a 'pandemic' (Egger and Swinburn, 2002). That usage has not been widely adopted in official policy discourses, but a simple Google search on 'obesity pandemic' on 20 October 2008 instantly located some 539,000 hits, suggesting that the expression is being widely used.

A further debate about obesity hinges on its capacity to cross borders in the same way that infectious diseases do. Most epidemics, such as avian flu, Ebola, HIV/AIDS, and tuberculosis are microbiological infections, with specific pathogenic agents that are transmitted between animal and human hosts (see Scoones, Leach and Hewlett, Nightingale, Edstrom and MacGregor, this volume). Although obesity is not caused by a pathogen, it has been characterized (somewhat controversially) as a contagious disorder spreading from individual to individual through social networks (Christiakis and Fowler, 2007; for an article challenging this view, see Cohen-Cole and Fletcher, 2008). More broadly, obesity is widely interpreted as a side effect of industrialization in developing countries; as populations move away from subsistence farming and become urbanized, they develop increasingly sedentary lifestyles and eat cheap foods that are high in fat and sugar. In this sense, it may be argued that obesity crosses borders in the same way that infectious pathogens do.

In recent years, evidence has emerged of a rapidly rising incidence of obesity in all Organisation for Economic Co-operation and Development (OECD) countries as well as many non-OECD countries. The latter include China, where the number of overweight people jumped from less than 10 per cent to 15 per cent in just three years; Brazil and Colombia, where around 40 per cent of people are overweight; and sub-Saharan Africa, where most of the world's hungry people live, and which has seen an increase in obesity especially among urban women (Randerson, 2006; FAO, 2009). Consequently obesity is rising up the policy agendas in many parts of the world, including countries such as Sudan, in which undernourished people far outnumber the overweight and obese (personal communication, 20 February 2008). As a result, Sudan and other developing countries are facing a double blow, with rates of obesity rising among adults simultaneously with high rates of undernutrition among children (Doak, 2002; Randerson, 2006). While it is difficult to obtain reliable statistics on nutrition and body mass index, some analysts have suggested that overweight people now outnumber hungry people globally, with 1 billion of the former and 800 million of the latter (Patel, 2007). As the prices of internationally traded foodstuffs have risen sharply in recent years, the relative preponderance of undernutrition and overnutrition may have shifted, but the claim that the two problems are of similar magnitudes remains striking. It is clear that obesity is becoming globalized and, in turn, that globalization may be contributing to its growing occurrence as the availability of cheap, nutritionally inadequate foodstuffs increases. Delpeuch and colleagues now refer to the challenge as 'globesity' (Delpeuch et al, 2009).

Nonetheless, while the diffusion of obesity from OECD countries to non-OECD countries resembles the transfer of infectious disease across borders, no corresponding narrative describes obesity as coming 'out of America and Europe' in the same way that infectious diseases are often figured as coming 'out of Africa ' (see Hewlett and Leach, this volume). In addition, the fact that obesity is not transmitted by a pathogen has institutional implications for the role of the World Health Organization. While the WHO may claim a role in managing cross-border transmission of infectious diseases, with respect to obesity the role of the WHO is restricted to producing reports and recommendations, and to organizing international conferences, limiting its ability to meaningfully intervene in this epidemic.

While the causes and ramifications of this spread of obesity from OECD to non-OECD countries are significant and worthy of detailed analysis, my focus here will be on policy debates unfolding in fully industrialized countries which are currently grappling with high levels of the disease. Similar debates may be expected in non-OECD countries as their rates continue to rise, with the added complexity of high numbers of hungry people in some of those settings.

Narratives of obesity

As mentioned above, narratives about obesity can be helpful grouped according to how they map against two spectra: the degree to which they attribute individualist versus systemic causes to obesity and the degree to which they advocate government intervention versus non-intervention. In the following sections of this chapter, I will analyse four competing narratives that demonstrate different combinations of these characteristics, with reference to specific countries in which these narratives have been most dominant. The first narrative, which may be termed individualist and interventionist, finds its strongest articulation in Singapore and Japan. The second narrative, individualist and non-interventionist, has been most prominent in the discourse of the US food lobby and was prevalent under the administration of President G. W. Bush. The third narrative, systemic and interventionist, finds broad articulation in several European countries characterized by strong welfare states, such as Finland and the UK. And finally, the fourth narrative, systemic and non-interventionist, is dominant among a few other EU countries. This analysis is based on several decades of research into food and health policy in European and North American settings, as well as a 30-month EU-funded nine-country comparative study of obesity policies (Millstone and Lobstein, 2007).

Individualist/interventionist narratives: enforcing healthy lifestyles

Individualist and interventionist narratives represent the obesity epidemic as a result of individuals failing to eat healthily and stay active and they typically advocate a highly interventionist response in which citizens are required to participate in government programmes aimed at improving diet and lifestyle. Privacy and freedom are sacrificed in favour of an attempt to effect dramatic changes in obesity rates. The food industry remains outside the circle of blame, while pharmaceutical companies – and targeted biomedical solutions – are not considered appropriate. Rather, traditional public health campaigns emphasizing diet and exercise are applied directly to overweight and obese people. Social pressure and sometimes outright stigmatization are considered useful tools in the most extreme version of this narrative, which views obesity as too harmful and too expensive in a highly industrialized nation to be left to less-targeted solutions. Government ministries, schools and employers are the main actors in this narrative, charged with designing and implementing programmes for behaviour change in a target population.

So far, only one country has slowed, if only briefly, the rate of rise in the incidence of obesity: namely Singapore. In 1992 the Ministry of Health launched a national programme to promote healthy lifestyles in order to target common risk factors for chronic diseases, including obesity, lack of physical activity and smoking. This undertaking included a 'Trim and Fit' programme aimed at improving fitness levels among school children. Overweight children were singled out for special physical exercise regimens, while obese children were referred to school health services for further assessment, treatment and follow up with doctors and dieticians. The 'Trim and Fit' programme reported a decline in rates of obesity of approximately 2 per cent for children aged between 11–12 and 15–16 between 1992 and 2000 (Toh et al, 2002; Soon et al, 2008). However, the measures that the government imposed to achieve that result were unsustainably draconian, even in that notoriously authoritarian state, and in March 2007, the *Washington Post* reported that the Singapore government had decided to end the programme after parents complained that overweight children were bullied and stigmatized. The targeted programme was replaced with a more holistic plan aimed at all school children, not simply the overweight or obese (*Washington Post*, 2007).

Three observations are relevant at this stage:

- First, no other country has yet succeeded in slowing down, let alone reversing, the trend in the incidence of obesity.
- Second, Singapore only achieved that change by imposing measures that stigmatized individual children deemed overweight or obese.
- Thirdly, those measures were socially and politically unsustainable in a country where the citizenry is not noted for its disobedience but for its compliance.

If the combination of a highly interventionist and highly individualistic approach proved unsustainable in Singapore, it may be unsustainable everywhere.

A somewhat less severe version of the individualist/interventionist narrative can be identified in the backdrop to a Japanese government programme to combat obesity. This narrative emphasizes again the importance of a public education campaign focusing on diet and physical exercise and, like the harsher version evident in Singapore, also focused specifically on obese and overweight individuals. In March 2006, the Japanese government introduced its 'Health Japan 21' programme, which included a specific focus on individuals deemed too heavy and a set of health targets to be reached by 2010 (McCurry, 2006). After just two years, the government transformed its approach to a far more interventionist one. In April 2008, a national law was introduced requiring companies and local governments to measure the waistlines of people between the ages of 40 and 74 as part of their annual health check-ups. Accounting for nearly half of the population, those middle-aged and senior citizens found to have waistlines exceeding set limits would be given dieting instructions if they had not lost weight after three months. Further guidance would be provided again after six months to those who still had not achieved a target waistline. It is too soon to assess the impact of these measures on the incidence of obesity (initial findings indicate that the prevalence of obesity among male adults had increased since the start of the programme, while the mortality from cardiovascular disease had fallen) or on social harmony in Japan (Matsuda, 2007).

The approach of the Japanese and Singapore governments is, by European standards, remarkably interventionist, and directly attributes responsibility to individuals to change their behaviour. The focus of these approaches is on food intakes and physical activity, but also on individual choices rather than on environmental conditions, such as provision for exercise and outdoor recreation facilities or subsidies for healthy foods. The pathway of response justified by this individualist/interventionist narrative places almost the entire burden of compliance on overweight and obese individuals, using social stigmatization and targeted public health campaigns to encourage those individuals to lose weight, either through exercise or healthy eating. In contrast, the food industry and the pharmaceutical industry remain relatively absent from this narrative, neither acting as promoters of it, nor being subject to government pressure themselves to change. At the same time, government is very active and the gap between policy statements and policy interventions appears to be minimal.

Individualist/non-interventionist narratives: Reductionist accounts and pharmaceutical fixes

Two versions of an individualist/non-interventionist narrative are forcefully articulated in the US, where the approach to obesity has involved a high level of official recognition and quantification alongside individualistic and non-interventionist narratives. The first narrative is one that places the blame for obesity on individuals and grants them responsibility for changing their behaviour to address the problem. In this narrative, the government is expected to intervene sparingly, if at all. The second narrative, voiced by the medical and pharmaceutical industries, argues that obesity can be reduced to biological causes alone, and is therefore susceptible to biomedical interventions alone. These narratives will be discussed in turn below.

The first narrative has the force of history behind it: most efforts to design public health interventions to combat obesity have failed (Kersh and Morone, 2002). At the same time, the food industry has long been successful at lobbying for subsidies or other sources of aid from federal, state and local authorities. Producers of the three main sources of fat in the American diet – red meat, plant oils and dairy products – have all been able to mount long-running and successful lobbies in Washington to block legislation that might end those subsidies or otherwise damage their business. Indeed, until 2004 the Bush administration resisted calls to treat obesity as a challenge for public policy, preferring instead to characterize it solely as a problem for individuals, to which the appropriate response was changes in personal choices and behaviours. The Bush administration focused on individuals, and on increasing their levels of physical activity, rather than on reducing their calorific intakes (HHS, 2005). That policy was strongly supported by the US House of Representatives, which in 2004 and 2005 approved a bill for the Personal Responsibility in Food Consumption Act, though it failed to be adopted by the Senate. The Act was designed to protect food and beverage companies from civil litigation that might be initiated by disgruntled, overweight or obese consumers (Delpeuch et al, 2009, p1). Subsequently it has come to be known as the 'Cheeseburger Bill'.

Representatives of the food, beverage and advertising industries endeavour to focus as much attention as possible on the choices and actions of individuals. For example, the US food trade association called the Grocery Manufacturers of America maintains that: 'Individuals need to develop appropriate lifestyle plans that allow them to make small improvements in eating and physical activity patterns that over time add up and move them closer to meeting the recommendations of the Guidelines' (GMA, 2008). In its view, the changes that are needed are changes to the behaviour of individuals, and those changes may well consists of 'small' shifts, implying that radical changes are unnecessary and inappropriate. Food industry representatives also often suggest that its role is just to respond to whatever consumers demand, although occasionally they acknowledge their efforts to stimulate demand.

This industry-driven narrative is captured in the slogan that 'there are no bad foods, only bad diets', suggesting that while the industry markets products, diets are constructed by consumers. Another narrative favoured by many large food companies has emphasized the importance of physical activity to de-emphasize the consumption of food. For example, when discussing obesity in Europe, Coca Cola's EU Group Nutritionist explained in 2005 that the EU's food and drink industry contributed to over 300 events per day in: 'Our commitment to sustainable physical activity' (Cunningham, 2005). Of course, the food industry never says explicitly that it emphasizes physical activity to divert attention away from the input side of the energy balance, but it would be bizarre if that were not the case. One further narrative offered by the food industry highlights its efforts innovatively to provide low-sugar, low-calorie and low-fat products, although Egger and colleagues have pointed out that 'the widespread availability of reduced-fat, low-calorie and sugar-free foods does not seem to be sufficient to influence the increase in obesity worldwide' (Egger et al, 2003).

In the face of this powerful lobby, US government initiatives have been paltry. In April 2005 the US Department of Health and Human Services launched its main anti-obesity initiative, which was specifically targeted at African American children and was supported with relatively modest funding of just US$1.2 million (HHS, 2005). That remarkably poorly funded initiative aimed at African American youngsters was presented in a way unlikely to elicit enthusiastic engagement from the intended target audience. Bush administration policy, justified according to a strongly individualist and non-interventionist narrative, resulted in meagre outcomes. The particular pathway of response it justified focused narrowly on racially characterized children, and emphasized individuals making more informed choices (which should include in particular increased levels of physical activity,) with no explicit indication that there were any particular categories of food that should be consumed in smaller quantities, or that the physical, economic or social environment of those citizens should be changed.

The Bush administration's response to obesity never extended beyond encouraging voluntary action focused on changes to individuals' choices. Since the Obama administration has repudiated many of the policies of the previous administration, it may yet come to regard obesity as requiring a public policy response, but at the time of writing in April 2009, such initiatives have yet to emerge. Were the Obama administration to do so, it would entail a shift of the US from the anti-interventionist and individualistic ends of the policy spectrum.

Reductionist accounts of obesity

A second set of narratives propounded by the medical and pharmaceutical industries in the US suggests that obesity is a biological disorder that is amenable to being treated by medicine and science. While the causes of obesity are seen to lie with the individual according to this narrative, they are not due to individual choices or behaviours, but rather to a reductionist account of human physiology and biochemistry. Drawing both on general analyses of scientific culture in the US, and specific evidence from debates about obesity, Lawrence observed that: 'Obesity is often framed ... by the medical and pharmaceutical industries, as a *biological* disorder that can be understood – and potentially cured – by science. This 'medicalized' understanding of obesity emphasizes impersonal causes that may only be rendered controllable through further scientific discovery' (Lawrence, 2004, p61).

These reductionist accounts, most commonly articulated either by representatives of pharmaceutical companies or by laboratory investigators, portray obesity as a consequence of either a deficiency problem (such as a lack of some pharmacologically active therapeutic agent) or as a consequence of excessive levels of some dietary ingredient or contaminant. In the UK, such reductionist narratives are more prevalent in popular science and commercial trade journalism than amongst scientists themselves. For example, the food industry's information service FoodNavigator.com reported in September 2008 on a study that had identified a protein (SH2-B), which can act as a 'signal' molecule and mediate the response of cells to the hormone leptin, which in turn influences 'satiety' or feelings of digestive fullness and subsequent food intake with the headline: 'Specific protein the answer to rising obesity?'('Specific protein', 2008). That report derived from a study showing that SH2-B had an effect on leptin levels, but the authors acknowledged that many other proteins would exert similar effects, and never claimed SH2-B was on its own decisive (Ren et al, 2005). They never suggested it was either the cause of, or a potential solution to, the problem of obesity. Journalists, however, have well-deserved reputations for exaggerating the significance of individual fragments of evidence.

Other types of biochemical-based reductionist narratives are also artic-ulated. For example, a paper emerged in 2008 reporting the results of a study that examined the association between consumption of MSG (or monosodium glutamate, also known as E621) and overweight in some 750 healthy Chinese women aged 40–59. The paper provided evidence indi-cating that: 'With adjustment for potential confounders including physical activity and total energy intake, MSG intake was positively related to BMI' (Ka et al, 2008, p1875). Those results seem to imply that a single chemical compound, when used as a food additive, may have a significant adverse effect on the weight of adult consumers. To argue that the consumption of dietary ingredients such as MSG may be contributing to the incidence of obesity is, of course, not to portray obesity simply as a result of consuming MSG. It also leaves unaddressed the issue in industrial economics of why the food industry makes such liberal use of MSG. Since, however, MSG acts by enhancing the apparent flavour of processed foods to which it is added, it would not be surprising if it were an appetite stimulant.

In the same reductionist vein, there is, most prominently in the US and the UK, but probably elsewhere as well, a conspicuous group of geneti-cists, molecular biologists and pharmaceutical company representatives who suggest that obesity is fundamentally a problem of genetics, arguing that our bodies are not adapted to eating contemporary diets, or at any rate to controlling intakes in urbanized sedentary lifestyles ('Insect study', 2006; Froguel, 2007; Wilding, 2007; Wardle et al, 2008). They typically recommend heavy investments into research on genetic predispositions for obesity, and envisage effective drug therapies for those who are obese, and prophylactic drugs for those not yet overweight or obese. Since human genes have barely changed in hundreds of thousands of years and the inci-dence of childhood obesity has more than doubled over the past ten years in most European countries, public policy-makers in Europe tend to discount genetic framings of the issue, and focus on eating, drinking and physical activity; nonetheless the genetic and pharmaceutical narratives continue to be articulated. These narratives are notable for the pathways of response that they shape, driving the development of pharmaceutical solutions to obesity, which, if successful, could potentially create a world of thin 'haves', who can afford the medication, and obese 'have-nots' who cannot.

Systemic/interventionist narratives: Blaming an obesogenic environment

In direct opposition to those who proffer reductionist accounts of the cause of obesity, the Australian public health epidemiologist Boyd Swinburn and colleagues have articulated the concept of the 'obesogenic environment' as the primary cause of obesity, with the clear implication that if obesity trends are to be reversed, environments need to be changed, for example in terms of the prices and availability of differing kinds of foods and beverages, controls on the commercial promotion and marketing of calorifically dense foods and the socio-economic and physical factors that inhibit, discourage or prevent physically active lifestyles (Swinburn et al, 1999). From that perspective, responsibility for obesity is attributable not simply to individual preferences, choices and decisions, or to individual genes or molecules, but to the industrial, technological, commercial and cultural environments in which people live. Correspondingly a response to obesity might involve changes to our physical, cultural, economic and commercial environments. An approach of that sort was endorsed by the UK Prime Minister, who in January 2008 said: 'We must do nothing less than transform the environment in which we all live. We must increase the opportunities we all have to make healthy choices around the exercise we take and the food we eat' (Brown, 2008).

Many commentators have provided evidence that there are income, ethnicity and gender gradients to the rates of prevalence of obesity in numerous countries (Lobstein et al, 2004; National Centre for Social Research, 2004). Delpeuch et al have shown that while the very poorest people in non-OECD countries may suffer undernutrition, amongst those who can afford sufficient calories, obesity is most prevalent amongst those least well-off (2009). In the face of that evidence, it is difficult to avoid the conclusion that such environmental factors may be very influential.

In practice, in the context of debates about obesity, the concept of the 'obesogenic environment' has been interpreted rather broadly to encompass a wide range of different environmental categories. Those categories have included, for example, physical features such as buildings, towns, cities and transport systems, as well as economic features such as prices, taxes, subsidies, stocks and flows. Commercial features such as the extent and characteristics of marketing and product innovations have been discussed as well as cultural features such as educational curricula and culinary practices. As a result, discussions about environmental causes of obesity – and responses to it – tend to be much more varied than those about individual behaviour.

This set of narratives can be seen to be most dominant in Finland, the only country with a track record of successfully introducing and sustaining a national public nutritional health policy regime. Finland's uniquely successful large-scale initiative was developed in the 1970s in response to a widespread national consensus that the prevailing rate of cardiovascular disease in Finland was conspicuously higher than in any other European country, was avoidable and unacceptable. That initiative came to be known as 'the North Karelia Project' ('North Karelia Project', undated). The policy regime included both supply- and demand-side initiatives. It both changed dietary practices and raised levels of physical activity. It involved compulsory physical education in schools, but for all children, not just for some. It included the promotion, by the mass media, of healthier choices and diets, and subsidies for the purchase of vegetables and salads. On the supply side, financial incentives were also given to farmers to shift their production away from meat and dairy products towards vegetables, fruits, berries, nuts and seeds. Over a period of some 25 years, starting in 1972, the initiative served to bring the cardiovascular disease rate down by about 75 per cent, to the European average. Finland is, however, now experiencing rates of increase in obesity that are similar to those elsewhere in Europe (Borg and Fogelholm, 2007).

As Borg and Fogelholm observed in 2007:

> *It has been only recently that obesity as a topic rose to mainstream media discussion [in Finland] which has readied both citizens and politicians to the idea that new obesity prevention policies and tools may need to be implemented in order to ensure the health of the present and future generations ... discussions on new strategies are emerging and have risen into public discussion ... large scale discussions on political level are still lacking ... (2007, p48)*

Finland is, however, uniquely well placed to draw on its own experience with a portfolio of public health nutrition initiatives of the sort that characterized the North Karelia Project.

The UK is another country in which an interventionist narrative that places heavy emphasis on nutritional public health is strong. While it is not as forcefully articulated as it is in Finland, Japan or Malaysia, it is more forceful than in several other EU countries and the US. The UK government considers obesity to be both an individual and an environmental issue (Brown, 2008, piii). At the start of the 21st century there were few suggestions that obesity was a serious problem to which a public policy response was required; within six years it was widely accepted that obesity had become a serious problem, to which public policy-makers required a strategic response.

In February 2004, Wanless argued that investments of public resources in preventative health measures should be 'evidence based', by which he meant measures should only be taken if the value of anticipated benefits can be shown to exceed anticipated costs (Wanless, 2004). By May 2004, however, the Commons Health Select Committee had adopted a more precautionary approach. Though they acknowledged that more evidence was needed about the cost-effectiveness of public health and preventive policies, they argued that existing programmes should be evaluated as a 'series of natural experiments' and that there was no 'excuse for inertia'. Strikingly, they emphasized that the problem of obesity should be addressed 'at the highest levels across government' and recommended that a Cabinet public health committee, chaired by the Secretary of State for Health, be appointed. They encouraged official action, urging the government to 'resist inaction caused by political anxiety over accusations of "nanny statism"', especially since the government would ultimately be liable for some of the huge costs that would accrue if nothing were done (House of Commons, 2004, paragraphs 155, 56 and p5).

The reference to 'nanny statism' highlights an issue of considerable political sensitivity in the UK. While the government may be very keen on the idea that individuals can and will change their patterns of behaviour, especially in relation to food consumption, ministers are fearful of being portrayed as telling people what they should and should not eat. On the other hand, the cost implications of failing to reverse the trend in obesity frighten them at least as much (Millstone et al, 2007).

In response to the high salience of the obesity policy issue, and the UK government's stated intention to combat the problem, firms and trade organizations in the UK food and drink industries joined the public debate. Food industry representatives articulated narratives to the effect that the government should not tell the public what they should and should not eat, nor should it impose any further regulations on the food industry, which was already heavily regulated. The UK food industry's trade association, the Food and Drink Federation (or FDF), and many of its member companies, engaged with the topic of obesity. The FDF established a website and distributed a CD-Rom both called 'Join the Activators', aimed at parents, teachers and school children.[2] The primary emphasis was on increased levels of physical activity, since the FDF argued that obesity occurred because levels of energy expenditure had fallen more rapidly than its estimates of calorific intakes.

Subsequently, the British government decided not to follow the approach preferred by the FDF and its members; at least in relation to young children if not to the wider adult public. The implicit logic was straightforward – children need and deserve special protection, since they may not be in a position to make well-informed choices, so governments should act to protect them. The UK government was persuaded that there was an urgent need to reintroduce minimum nutritional standards for school meals, which had been abolished in the early 1980s by the Thatcher government. Much of the credit for that change belongs to the makers of a set of television programmes, featuring the chef Jamie Oliver, and his revelations about the poor nutritional quality of school meals.[3] The knowledge base of school children about nutrition and physical health may have started to improve in the UK in recent years, but that has yet to be reflected in statistics for the incidence of childhood obesity. The UK government also decided that some restrictions needed to be imposed on the advertising of food and drink products high in fats, sugars and calories especially in television programmes that are specifically targeted at children.

Beyond those two children-specific sets of measures, the UK government has actively promoted one further informational reform; it agrees with the European Commission and a large majority of EU member states that EU-wide food labelling regulations need to be changed. Instead of only requiring nutritional information on labels of products that make a health claim, such information should be available on the generality of processed and packaged food and drink products. Moreover nutritional information should not be confined to the backs and sides of products; those labels should be supplemented with front-of-pack indications in relation to key nutritional variables, such as calories, fats and sugars.

In the UK and the EU, there has been a vigorous debate about which form of front-of-pack labelling will be adopted, with the food industry showing a clear preference for quantitative indications of percentages of 'guideline daily amounts', while consumer and public health interests generally favour a so-called 'traffic light system'. The axis of debate has been almost entirely confined to the form that such labels should adopt. The decision to introduce mandatory and more informative labelling was settled several years ago. Debates about the form of that labelling have, however, served to delay their eventual introduction.

In 2007, the overall approach of the British government to obesity was neatly captured in the slogan adopted by the Department of Health, namely 'small changes – big differences' (Department of Health, 2007). That phrase was remarkably revealing, as it highlighted the tension between the government's desire to make a big difference, but wanting to achieve it with changes small enough not to provoke social or political friction. But it is not obvious that that circle can be squared.

In January 2008, the UK Secretary of State for Health, Alan Johnson, launched the government's most recent shift in official thinking and policy on the challenge of obesity. On that occasion he repeatedly said that obesity 'is an issue of personal responsibility. We live in an obesogenic environment' (Cross-Government Obesity Unit, 2008, pvii). Those remarks were replete with ambiguities; are the overweight personally responsible for the obesogenicity of their environment?

The Prime Minister also tried to reconcile the individualist perspective with the systemic or environmental perspective, saying:

> *There should be no doubt that maintaining a healthy weight must be the responsibility of individuals first – it is not the role of Government to tell people how to live their lives and nor would this work [... but] to make sure that individuals and families have access to the opportunities they want and the information they need in order to make healthy choices and exercise greater control over their health and their lives.*
> (Brown, 2008, piii)

With uncharacteristic boldness, the UK government set a challenging quantitative target, namely: 'that by 2020 we will not only have reversed the trend in rising obesity and overweight among children but also reduced it back to the 2000 levels. And whilst our focus is rightly on children, we need to see progress on rates of obesity in adults as well' (Brown, 2008, piii). The government also made a commitment to publishing an annual progress report with indicators of behaviour change such as breastfeeding rates, food consumption, rates of physical activity and children's health (Brown, 2008, pxii). Setting a target and making a commitment to publish data showing whether or not progress towards the target is being made might be construed variously as bold and brave, or as recklessly giving a hostage to fortune. In practice, the gap between bold programmatic statements and the relatively modest measures that have so far been taken is becoming increasingly conspicuous.

Systemic and non-interventionist narratives: European consensus and dissent

Narratives suggesting that the rapidly rising rates of obesity can and should be attributed to macro-systemic factors have been articulated more frequently by scholars than by public policy officials. In the US, Schaffer, Hunt and Ray portray the epidemic of obesity there as a direct consequence of US agricultural policies (Schaffer et al, 2007). They argued that US agricultural subsidies, especially for crops like corn and soybeans, result in overproduction and lower prices. Those low prices encourage the food processing industry to increase its usage of, for example, high-fructose corn syrup and soybean oil to produce low-nutrient calorie-dense products. They argue that eliminating such subsidies would reduce the incidence of obesity. A similar analysis for the EU has been provided by Schäfer Elinder, who focused in particular on the way in which surplus butter, produced in the EU as a result of agricultural subsidies, has been sold at discounted prices to the cake, biscuit and ice cream industries, increasing the calorific density of European diets (Schäfer Elinder, 2005; see also Lobstein and Bauer, 2005 and Hyde, 2008b).

One of the most trenchant articulations of a systemic framing has been set out by Wells in 2008. Wells argued that:

> *What is really driving the obesity epidemic is not increased dietary intake, or decreased activity levels, but the web of economic strategies and commercial interests that cause individual people to change or maintain certain behaviours. The way industry understands and manipulates individuals' behaviour is fundamental to the growth of the obesogenic niche … there are enormous profits to be had from obesity. The foods that maximise profit just happen to be those high in sugar or fat. They are cheap to produce, easy to brand and market, and easy to stock in supermarket aisles.* (Wells, 2008)

That approach places almost all responsibility for obesity on macro-economic and political considerations, and portrays citizens as victims of commercial manipulation. A similar, but slightly more subtle line of argumentation has been developed by Tillotson, who attributes the US obesity problem to what he characterizes as 'supply-side factors' rather than to 'demand-side factors' (Tillotson, 2004).

This narrative has been articulated most strongly in the EU. Given the heated differences about policy responses to the challenges of obesity within and between European countries, the extent to which a rhetorical consensus has been established on so many aspects of obesity policy across the whole of Europe, from the Baltic to the Balkans, from the Urals to the Atlantic, is quite remarkable. Nonetheless, the rhetorical consensus on obesity in the EU has not been matched by a corresponding burst of effective policy. Indeed, the practical outcomes of this rhetoric have been limited.

In November 2006, an inter-ministerial meeting of the entire WHO European Region was held in Istanbul to discuss the challenge of obesity. The WHO's European Region includes a total of 46 countries, yet they all contrived to agree on a very wide range of propositions and proposals (WHO European Ministerial Conference, 2007). The conference issued a 36-page conference report and a five-page document entitled the European Charter on Counteracting Obesity (WHO European Ministerial Conference, 2006).

All 46 countries committed themselves to a Charter that said, among other things:

> *We declare our commitment to strengthen action on counteracting obesity ... and to place this issue high on the political agenda of our governments... Sufficient evidence exists for immediate action ... Obesity is a global public health problem ...* (WHO European Ministerial Conference, 2006, paras 2.3.1–2.3.2)

On the key issue of the tension between individualistic and systemic framings of the obesity problem, the Charter said that 'a balance must be struck between the responsibility of individuals and that of government and society. Holding individuals alone accountable for their obesity should not be acceptable.' Instead, vulnerable groups such as children and young adults should receive special attention to ensure that they are not unfairly targeted by food advertisers. The Charter also emphasized the need to support poorer people, who face 'more constraints and limitations on making healthy choices'. Making healthy choices accessible and affordable to all was considered to be a key objective (WHO European Ministerial Conference, 2006, paras 2.3.3–2.3.8).

Remarkably, all 46 countries endorsed a 'systemic' and 'environmental' framing of the challenge of obesity, seeing it not simply as an issue for individual citizens and households. The document also stipulated that a package of 'essential preventive actions' should be promoted (WHO European Ministerial Conference, 2006, para 2.4.9). Those packages might include restrictions on marketing, particularly to children, ensuring access to and availability of healthier food, economic measures to facilitate healthier food choices, access to affordable recreational and exercise facilities, including support for socially disadvantaged groups, reductions of fat, sugars and salt in manufactured foods, improved and adequate nutrition labelling, and the promotion of cycling and walking by better urban design and transport policies (WHO European Ministerial Conference, 2006).

Finally, the Charter also stipulated that comparable international core indicators should be developed so that obesity could be measured across nations. Monitoring progress over the long term was considered essential because it was expected that outcomes such as reduced obesity and related diseases would take time to manifest themselves. Initially, three-year progress reports were to be prepared at the WHO European level, with the first due in 2010. It is, however, too soon to tell, because although a richly comprehensive policy document was adopted in Istanbul in late 2006, very few new policy measures have yet been introduced, and no indication of the hoped-for trends has yet emerged.

The fact that such provisions were endorsed by all 46 countries is quite striking. The extent of the rhetorical consensus can most readily be explained by the fact that many governments were ready to assert that the costs of their failing to deal with obesity would substantially exceed the costs of doing so, and none of the administrations represented at the meeting chose to contradict that narrative. The European headquarters staff of the WHO had made extensive preparations for the meeting, to the extent that the only disputes were about how prescriptive the charter should be, and how far it would emphasize statutory measures as well as voluntary initiatives.

The decision to establish national surveillance systems using a set of agreed indicators to monitor both inputs and outcomes, and to review progress after three years, may have created the conditions under which European countries may start to make progress in combating the obesity epidemic.

Conclusion

The challenge posed by the rising incidence of obesity to public policy-makers is a difficult one in the sense that there are no easy answers, and it is not a problem that can be addressed without encountering powerful and entrenched interests, particularly in the food and beverage sectors.

Narratives that advocate differing pathways of response have been mapped onto two dimensions, one running from the most individualist to the most environmentalist, and the other from the most to the least interventionist. Singapore and the US have both adopted highly individualistic framings, but Singapore combined an individualistic with a highly interventionist approach while the US has intervened in only homeopathic doses.

In Europe, obesity is very widely portrayed as a challenge that demands effective public policy responses, although the detailed characteristics of those responses are still being negotiated. At the level of an agreed rhetorical narrative, there has been remarkably deep and wide agreement that action needs to be taken in response to obesity, and that highly individualistic framings, especially those entailing stigmatizing victims, have been explicitly repudiated. Forty-six European countries have all signed up to a document that tries to encompass and reconcile both individualistic and environmental considerations in support of a strong case for public policy measures. On the other hand, only very few measures have actually been taken, and so far no evidence has emerged that they have started to be effective, let alone sufficient. Governments are keen to see slowing or declining trends in the incidence of obesity in their populations, but they are reluctant to take on vested interests to achieve the changes that they wish to see.

Within the EU, there is a consensus that even includes most large food manufacturers and retailers that nutritional information will need to be provided on all packaged and processed food products, not just those making health claims, and that a front-of-pack summary indicator will also be required. It remains to be seen which format is adopted, or even if EU member states can reach a sufficient consensus, or whether for a few years at least individual countries will experiment with their preferred options. It also remains to be seen whether and how such front-of-pack labelling indications change purchasing practices.

While heterogeneous packages of measures are being proposed, debated and introduced in many countries, the only country that has managed to reduce the rate of rise in the incidence of childhood obesity, namely Singapore, was obliged to withdraw measures that were widely seen as draconian and socially unacceptable, perhaps because they were overly individualistic.

Policy salience is a significant factor in accounting for some of the differences between which narratives become dominant in a given setting. Obesity is a far more prominent public policy problem for EU governments and the European Commission, for example, than it has been for the US government. The salience of the obesity issue in poorer countries is also highly variable and rapidly changing (Delpeuch et al, 2009).

The main reason for the US–European contrast is that European countries have broader and deeper socialized provision of health care than is the case in the US. There are some important differences between the debates on policy responses to obesity, when comparing the US with Europe. Although the incidence of obesity started to accelerate in the US before doing so in Europe, and although the incidence in the US is higher than in much of Europe, obesity is not as high on the public policy agenda in the US as it is in Europe; but there is a straightforward explanation. As European countries have public health services, many of the costs of obesity fall on those public healthcare systems, and consequently the issue is highly salient for public policy-makers. In the US, where there is far less by way of public provision, most of the costs of obesity fall upon insurance systems and individuals' budgets, so federal government policy-makers have often not seen obesity as a problem that they need to address. In the UK, on the other hand, for example, pressure for effective measures to be adopted to slow and reverse recent obesity trends emerged in the Treasury before it arose in the Department of Health (Lobstein and Millstone, 2006). The debates in the UK and Europe are frequently about how public policy-makers should respond, and how they might induce behavioural change in individuals and organizations, while in the US the federal government often endeavours to avoid the issue or has just focused on how individuals can be better informed so that they act more appropriately.

Consequently many of the costs of rapidly rising rates of obesity in Europe are falling on public expenditure, rather than on insurance companies, 'health maintenance organizations' or individuals, as is the case in the US. It was striking that in a recent comparative study of obesity policy in nine European countries, the levels of concern about obesity were higher in finance ministries than in health ministries (Lobstein et al, 2007). The Obama administration in the US has indicated its intention significantly to extend public healthcare provision, and if it is successful in that regard the public policy salience of obesity could well increase.

Within not just the EU, but across the entire WHO European region comprising 46 countries, it has been widely accepted not just by governments, but also in the wider policy communities, that governments should introduce public policy measures in response to the rising incidence of obesity. There is, however, far less agreement as to what those measures should be. There are, moreover, differences within governments, and amongst the wider public policy networks, through which eventual decisions will be negotiated. The disjunction between rhetoric and action also remains conspicuous in the narratives at the non-interventionist end of the spectrum. Articulating general aspirations and issuing calls for increased individual responsibility have not produced any of the hoped-for changes.

The UK government's slogan 'small changes – big differences' can be said to represent the implicit view of many governments around Europe and in many other parts of the world too. They are hoping that one or several of their number will discover relatively modest and socially acceptable measures that will make a sufficiently big difference to either food intakes or expenditures of energy, or to both, to solve the obesity problem without their having vigorously to confront entrenched interests or practices. Hyde has argued, however, that to overcome the obesity epidemic in the UK, the government would need to 'have the junk food industry for breakfast' (2008a). There are few indications that the UK government, let alone the European Commission or other governments, are prepared at this stage to adopt such a confrontational posture *vis-à-vis* the food industry. On the other hand, if such actions are not taken it is quite likely that the incidence of obesity will continue to rise and the epidemic will be more deeply entrenched and increasingly widespread. Ultimately such a trajectory may become unsustainable, but in the interim alternative and more sustainable pathways have been signposted but not yet effectively pursued. In the US, the Obama administration is (at the time of writing) endeavouring to persuade Congress to enact legislation to provide publicly supported health care to the vast majority of those that have not been covered by commercial insurance schemes or by Medicare or

Medicaid. If such legislation is enacted, the healthcare costs of sustaining and treating obese and overweight citizens will add to public expenditure, and under those conditions it is quite likely that the approach of the US authorities might become more interventionist; but it remains to be seen whether it adopts a predominantly individualistic framing or a more systemic one.

As far as developing countries are concerned it will be very interesting to see whether or how they develop epidemiological and policy narratives on issues of diet and health. With simultaneous challenges of 'undernutrition' and 'overnutrition' within their jurisdictions, their policy narratives are hard to predict; but it would not be entirely surprising if their narratives became even more ambiguous and equivocal than those articulated in the industrialized world.

Notes

1   The author would like to thank Sarah Dry for extensive editorial revisions.
2   See www.jointheactivaters.org.uk/, accessed 20 October 2008.
3   See www.channel4.com/life/microsites/J/jamies_school_dinners/, accessed 6 December 2009.

Chapter 10

Scapepigging: H1N1 Influenza in Egypt

Mariz Tadros

In early May 2009, the Egyptian government announced that it planned to cull all of the nation's estimated 300,000 pigs. This action was necessary, the government stated, in order to control the spread of so-called 'swine flu', which had recently been declared a 'public health emergency of international concern' by the WHO. The decision to cull the pigs, approved by parliament,[1] was taken to protect the country from the pandemic even though there was not yet a single confirmed case of novel H1N1 influenza in the country. In fact, as this chapter will describe, the culling of the pigs would threaten the health of the Egyptian people, as well as the livelihoods of a marginalized group of garbage collectors.

Commonly referred to as 'swine flu', the H1N1 influenza virus is a novel strain of influenza that first emerged in Mexico and the US. The virus contains a mixture of genes from humans, birds and pigs. Despite this mixture of genetic material, it appears to spread only between humans and no cases of animal-to-human transmission have been reported. 'Swine flu' has proved to be a catchy but misleading nickname for the new virus. Since its initial appearance in March 2009, the virus has spread globally. While it appears to cause a relatively mild form of influenza, it has infected large numbers of people and, by October 2009, had killed nearly 5000 people worldwide. In June 2009, the WHO declared a global pandemic of H1N1 as a result of sustained human-to-human transmission in multiple countries.

This chapter will explore the events that have occurred in Egypt in response to H1N1. The global outbreak narrative, which has driven much of the response to H1N1 at the international level, played out in a very particular way in Egypt, which had been criticized for its slow response to avian influenza in 2006 (more than 20 people died in the country of the disease). This case study reveals how serious unintended consequences of a rigid and heavy-handed action taken in response to an epidemic can be justified on health and scientific grounds but in essence be politically motivated. Interlinked social, environmental and technological dynamics, still at play in this as yet unfolding situation, had long provided a sustainable if largely informal means of managing garbage in the vast area of Cairo and its surrounds. With the pig culling, these interlinked dynamics, which had helped keep the streets clear of garbage and maintained the livelihood of a marginalized minority group, became dramatically disengaged. The consequences have been both surprising to those in power and highly damaging.

This chapter examines how the government narrative in favour of culling of the pigs became so dominant as to be hegemonic, ordering nearly all responses according to its prescribed pathways of response and ignoring alternative framings. It examines how institutional and governance structures allowed for its implementation with almost no accountability. It also documents the use of scientific arguments about the transmission of the virus to legitimize a response largely grounded in a religious abhorrence of pigs and a deep-seated sectarian antipathy towards the Christian minority who breed them and eat their meat. This case study also purposely seeks to capture the counter-narrative of the Zabaleen, the Christian garbage collectors,[2] who were directly affected by the culling decision. The Zabaleen have a long tradition of using pigs to consume the organic waste that is collected, which allows them to then extract valuable recyclable material from the garbage which can be sold. This system allows the Zabaleen to deal with a large amount of waste in a cost-effective way. The Zabaleen's narrative reveals the perspectives and priorities of a minority group with a long history of marginalization. Their understanding of the reasons for the cull, and its effects, is grounded in their long experience of subjugation at the hands of the government and their trans-generational tradition of being garbage collectors. Their counter-narrative sheds light on many of the problematic assumptions in the government narrative.

The chapter is divided into three parts. In the first part, the government narrative on public health and hygiene is examined against a backdrop of Islamist politicking and public hysteria. It describes the processes and events that led to the culling decision and the key actors who influenced the framing and implementation of the policies on various levels of governance: international, national and local. The chapter identifies some key critical elements of the narrative that shed light on the dynamics that influenced how the disease was understood as well as the recommended pathways of response. These key elements are the sectarian dynamics of the Egyptian context; the use of 'scientific arguments' to justify government policy and to prove the soundness of the religious position on pigs; and the national security threat emanating from having pigs and their owners abide in the midst of residential areas.

The second part of the chapter describes the counter-narrative of the Zabaleen who have lost their livelihoods. Their narrative presents their own perspective on the motives behind the framing of H1N1 by the government in terms of a threat from the pigs and their owners. Central to their narrative are three recurring themes:

- first, how the culling policy can only be understood against the historical background of government discrimination and exclusion of the Zabaleen;
- second, how the process of implementing the culling policy betrays the claims and justifications made by officials;
- third, how the mainstream narrative showed no understanding of their livelihoods or the nature of the disruption that the culling policy has caused and the kind of survival strategies they have had to consequently consider.

The final part of the chapter describes the unfolding waste disposal crisis in Cairo as a direct outcome of the culling policy. It discusses how the very policy that was advocated as a measure to protect Egyptian citizens' health was directly responsible for creating a major health hazard. It discusses how the garbage collectors' narrative spoke of their agency and how their marginalization not only had implications for themselves but for the entire city of Cairo.

Introduction

One well-established communal response to epidemics is to blame a scapegoat, most often a marginalized social group with little or no power (Markell, 2007, p51; McNeill, 2009). At the outset of the H1N1 outbreak, for example, Mexicans were vilified and there were voices in the US calling for the closure of the border between the two countries (McNeill, 2009). In the case of Egypt, when reports emerged about an international outbreak of 'swine flu', public attention immediately focused on Egypt's pig population. The undesirability of the pigs extended to three levels. The first level was the stigma of the pigs themselves: in Islam, the pig is seen as an unclean animal, and there are clear injunctions in the Koran prohibiting Muslims from breeding or eating pigs. The second is the religious undesirability of the social group raising the pigs: the garbage collectors are overwhelmingly members of the indigenous Coptic Christian minority, who number roughly 10 per cent of the population. The third is the social undesirability of a group whose profession is associated with garbage disposal. The Zabaleen have thus been doubly marginalized by virtue of their religion and, by both Muslims and Christians, by virtue of their profession.

As Markel notes, the scapegoating of a vulnerable or socially undesirable group may be one easy measure to take in response to a crisis, but understandings of the cause of a pandemic also help determine how it is addressed (Markel, 2007, p48). The narrative conveyed by the government and public opinion in the media and on the street constructing pigs and their breeders as responsible for swine flu became the mainstream narrative. Alternative narratives formulated by those who were sceptical about the logic of the mainstream narrative were either absent or vigorously marginalized. Those who have attempted to voice an alternative narrative include a few outspoken critics of the culling policy writing in the press, the garbage collectors themselves, whose narrative was largely ignored, and the Christian Copts living in the diaspora, who deplored the sectarian nature of the culling.

Ultimately, narratives tell the story of power relations which are influenced by historical and political trajectories. The government narrative is no different. The Egyptian government's response to the H1N1 pandemic is a conspicuous example of how a dominant narrative can engender far-reaching pathways of response, which in this case were implemented with unusual fervour, thoroughness and speed, with significant negative effects. There has still not been a serious questioning of this failed policy. This perhaps testifies to how deep-seated and entrenched are the values that have influenced the framing of this narrative. Even when H1N1 cases continued to spread in the population at large, despite the cull, government policy was not questioned. And when a public hygiene threat occurred as a consequence of the accumulating garbage, there were still no calls for holding the government accountable.

In order to capture the mainstream narrative, the Zabaleen's counter-narrative, and the events leading up to and following the culling of the pigs, field visits were conducted in Cairo in April, May and July 2009. Several interviews were conducted with Marie Assaad, who has over 40 years of experience working directly with garbage collectors in Muqattam and Torah el Maadi. Assaad is also a board member of the Association for the Protection of the Environment (APE), an NGO engaged in development interventions in Muqattam. Interviews were also conducted with Leila Iskander, board member of the Association of Spirit of Youth and director of the Centre for Community and Institutional Development, a consultancy firm. During more than 25 years of work in the Muqattam, she pioneered an innovative recycling initiative to generate sustainable livelihoods for many Zabaleen.

In addition to interviews with members of the Zabaleen in general, 15 in-depth case studies were undertaken in the three largest garbage collector communities[3] in Cairo.[4] Egypt has recently contracted private international companies to assist in the disposal of garbage in the main governorates of Cairo and Alexandria; however, their efficiency and scale of operation have been questioned. In 2002 the Giza governorate signed an agreement with two private companies (one Spanish and one Italian) to collect the

3000 tonnes of garbage produced daily by the governorate and dispose of it ('Dumping', 2002). In 2002, the garbage collectors protested that their role was being totally neglected in the contractual agreements and that they were against being governed by the Italian company. A spokesman from the company had said: 'I don't know what all the fuss is about; we are ready to accept the experienced labour in our business, but we are against the old fashioned non-environmental technique of garbage collection.' Instead, the Zabaleen have, over decades, developed a largely unregulated and informal system of garbage collection, sorting and recycling, which is provided in return for a small fee. The garbage collectors predominantly earn their living from recovering recyclable material from the garbage and selling it.

The largest Zabaleen community, Mansheyet Nasser, is situated in the Muqattam mountains, once a geographical area on the outskirts of the city, now very much part of it. Mansheyet Nasser is part of Cairo governorate. The community is estimated to be around 30,000 people. The second community is based in Ard el Lewa, a haphazard squatter settlement sandwiched between Dokki and Mohandessein, two of the city's upper class and upper middle class suburbs, and Bulaq el Dakrour, another squatter settlement. The population of Ard el Lewa is estimated to be around 7000 people. The community partly lies under Giza governorate, and partly the 6th of October governorate. The third site was the garbage collectors' community in Ezbet el Nakhl, a highly populated urban squatter and slum settlement, north of Cairo. The community is part of the Qalubiyya governorate. One of the common features of the garbage collectors in all three settlements is that the majority belong to Egypt's 10 per cent Christian minority. While all three communities are part of Greater Cairo, their affiliation to different governorates is significant in that they are subject to different governors' policies which may vary greatly. Interviews were deliberately conducted with garbage collectors who had recently lost their livelihoods to the cull in all three settlements in order to capture any differences between them. To protect them against possible political reprisals, garbage collectors' names have been omitted.

A review and analysis of how the subject was broached in both pro-government and opposition press, as well as those considered independent, was undertaken from the outset of the announcement of the H1N1 outbreak, at the end of August 2009, through September 2009. This was complemented by an analysis of various media programmes that have tackled the subject. In addition, an analysis of the parliamentary discussions as well as the Muslim Brotherhood's own interpretation of the events, as available on their website, has been undertaken. Finally, the research relied on secondary sources on the garbage collectors' communities in Egypt and background material collected during personal engagements and research in garbage collectors' communities since 1997.

Part One: The mainstream narrative

The lives of the pigs or the lives of Egyptians?

In response to the WHO's warnings of an imminent H1N1 pandemic in the spring of 2009, the Egyptian government's immediate reaction was to assure the population that there were no cases of H1N1 in the country and that all possible measures were going to be taken to prevent the pandemic from reaching domestic shores. It was keen to do so especially in the light of the public's criticism of its handling of the avian flu outbreak. Egypt was the country worst affected by that outbreak outside Asia and almost all of the people who contracted avian flu did so after either direct or indirect contact with infected household birds. The government's response to avian flu – which included sporadic rather than comprehensive bird culling, a public health awareness campaign on the dangers of handling live or dead poultry, and a limited bird vaccination initiative – was criticized for being slow and ineffective. The death toll from avian influenza, however, continues to rise.

The government response to the WHO's announcement *vis-à-vis* the H1N1 virus developed in stages. The first stage was the government emphasizing that it was in control, that all necessary precautionary measures would be taken to prevent the pandemic and that the country was currently free from any infection. The next stage of the narrative primarily focused on the pigs. First, the government assured its people that the pigs in Egypt were not infected with the 'swine flu'. This phase was short lived, and was followed by another fairly short-lived phase debating what to do with the pigs. The main thrust was that all pigs must be relocated urgently from the city's quarters to the outskirts of a satellite city in the desert where land had been allocated for their recycling activities. Within a short time space at the end of April, however, the story changed again: 'We have pigs, we can't move them; we must kill them. Do we slaughter or cull them?' Soon culling began, but even then – and without a single case of H1N1 being identified in Egypt – the anxiety about pigs remained: what if their slaughtered meat ended up being sold as beef? When cases of H1N1 began to appear (all traceable to overseas travel), the focus on the pigs continued: have we made sure that none of the pigs has escaped? Has the government killed every single pig in the country? The development of this narrative and the power relations it embodies will be discussed at length below.

The fact that H1N1 was commonly referred to as swine flu meant that from the outset rumours linked pigs with the pandemic: in this the WHO's regional office is not entirely free from blame. They were aware that the Arab-Muslim context in which they operated would be extremely sensitive to anything swine related. Yet there was no regional agenda implemented to inform governments and the public about the nature of H1N1, namely, the lack of risk of swine-to-human transmission. When the government narrative developed into one revolving around pigs, the WHO did not respond sensitively or decisively to these regional concerns. When the WHO finally made an international appeal against naming H1N1 'swine flu', the association between the pandemic and pigs had already become quite entrenched both in Egypt and in the Middle East more generally.

On the Egyptian national front, the immediate question became: if the flu is transmitted by swine, what about Egypt's pig population? The first articles flagging the swine flu threat in Egypt began to appear around 27 April 2009. An article titled 'Pigs ... ticking bombs ... 300,000 pigs in the governorates and fears for their infection with influenza' was published in the pro-government daily newspaper. It quoted veterinarians saying that the potential blend of the H5N1 (already widespread in Egypt) and H1N1 (if caught by pigs in Egypt) could result in a deadly new viral strain that might be passed on to humans. In the same issue of the newspaper the Ministry of Environment announced the immediate resettlement of the pigsties situated in Cairo to the outskirts of the 15th of May City, one of the new satellite cities established in the desert ('Pigs', 2009). From the outset, the discussion of H1N1 was linked to discussion of the country's pig population: this is where the virus appears, and is transmitted to humans, the reasoning went, so do something about the pigs.

Culling was not immediately decided upon as the best course of action, however. Presidential decree No 238, issued in 2008, had already set aside 238 feddans (roughly equivalent to the same number of acres) of desert land on the outskirts of the 15th of May City for garbage sorting and recycling. The Ministry of Environment called for the immediate relocation to this new settlement of all nine Cairo locations where pigs were bred. Yet if this represented the political preference of the Ministry of Environment, the Ministry of Agriculture saw things differently: they argued that an immediate relocation was not possible since resettling all these pigsties would be a lengthy process due to missing infrastructure. From this point onwards, it was clear that if various government ministries were deliberating between culling and resettling, the former looked increasingly attractive. Opposition to relocation came from another circle as well: the residents of the 15th of May City protested to the governor of Helwan that they did not want the garbage collectors to settle in their city, arguing that they would be a source of pollution and rubbish ('Cairo', 2009).

Consensus in favour of culling the pigs occurred very rapidly. The next day, 28 April 2009, it was announced that two governors (of the Delta governorate of Kafr el Sheikh and of the Upper Egyptian governorate of Minya) had unilaterally taken action: the first ordered the culling of all 100 pigs bred by the garbage collectors there and the second had ordered that the pigsties be relocated to outside the city of Abou Qorqas ('Culling', 2009). Yet if these were essentially trial runs for a national response, they revealed one important fact: there were no voices of protest against the measure, no questioning, no calls for accountability, and no campaign on behalf of the garbage collectors or the pigs. The hysterical treatment of the swine flu scare was predominant on all levels: the press, both the opposition and the national, as well as the national media and the satellite channels. There was talk of a plague that would sweep the country, and how the pigs represented a biological bomb about to be detonated, infecting Egyptians with its disease.[5] These voices calling for the culling of the pigs prevailed with no counter voices to challenge them.

The narrative further developed during the parliamentary discussions that took place on 28 April 2009. The growing consensus was that pigs were responsible for the transmission of H1N1, as well as many other viruses, and they must be killed immediately. Any delay was considered to be a risk to the health of Egyptian citizens. Besides, the pigs were not an important source of national wealth or a main feature of Egyptians' diets.[6] The religious inferences were striking – how could pigs be bred in the land of Al Azhar in the first place[7] one MP asked. Hussein Ibrahim, an MP with the Muslim Brotherhood, asked whether the pigs had 'special immunity' and that was why they were being spared the culling while the poultry was not. The implication of these questions, as one of the Coptic[8] MPs, Ibtessam Habib, pointed out, was that the government was reluctant to take action against the pigs because of their association with Christians. The comment was sufficiently inflammatory to propel the handful of Coptic MPs in the 554-member parliament to react. Another Coptic Christian MP, Georgette Kaleeny, made two interesting points. The first is that few Christians eat pork and that she personally does not, and second, that most of those who own pigsties are Muslims.[9] Although factually incorrect, these ideas were used to support the mainstream narrative about the culling of the pigs having nothing to do with Christians. Ibtessam Habib also spoke about there being nothing in the Bible to support the eating of pork ('The Coptic [women]', 2009).

Kaleeny made pleas that in case of slaughter, the garbage collectors needed to be adequately compensated and provided with alternative employment. Yet any attempt at making the livelihoods of the garbage collectors central to the debates was shunned: the matter was considered inconsequential since the lives of Egyptians were at risk. Besides, many argued 'if we culled a million poultry in the avian flu crisis, what is the problem with culling the pigs for a disease far worse?' Another asked 'what will happen if we live another fifteen years without pigs?' ('The People's Assembly decides', 2009). As one critic pointed out, the NDP (the ruling National Democratic Party) and the Muslim Brotherhood MPs were united against a common enemy, an enemy against both religion (Islam) and health ('O ye Ummah,' 2009). In addition to the vilification of pigs, attention also turned to the Zabaleen. An MP from the Muslim Brotherhood, Akram el Sha'er, called for all the garbage collectors in the country to be given a health check-up to ensure that they were not transmitters of the virus ('The People's Assembly obliges', 2009).[10] Exactly the same demands were made by the ruling party MPs: Magdy Allam, a member of the ruling party, called for a strict separation of the garbage collectors and the residents, in order to prevent the spread of the disease, especially since the former mingled closely with pigs.

Hamdy el Sayed, head of the Physicians' Syndicate and head of the health committee at the People's Assembly (and known for his pro-Islamist sympathies though not a formal member of the Muslim Brotherhood) said that the disease can spread in an hour or two and that it would be unwise even to wait for a week before commencing the culling. Some members of parliament urged more deliberation. Mofeid Shehab, a Minister of State, urged that the government be given 24 hours to study the matter and present it to parliament before a policy decision was made. During the parliamentary discussions, Amin Abaza of the Ministry of Agriculture argued that if the virus were coming from overseas, then culling the pigs would not solve the problem. He also pointed out that the pigs had been under veterinary surveillance for the past two years (that is, that the government had taken the necessary precautions to ensure that the pigs were not infected with any viruses), but his call fell on deaf ears. The Minister of Health also tried similar reasoning to no avail. In response, members of both the ruling party and the opposition argued for an even more urgent intervention. Eventually, all members of the government would publicly announce their support for the measure, possibly in order not to be on the wrong side of public opinion. Both the ministries of State and of Agriculture would release statements that fed into the mass hysteria that gripped the country. For example, the Ministry of Health predicted that 7.2 million Egyptians could die from the pandemic and consequently sought a *fatwa* (religious ruling) from the concerned religious authorities on whether it was possible to have mass burials in the desert, should the need arise ('The Ministry', 2009).

The hegemonic narrative that developed sheds light on how H1N1 was understood and interpreted. The first element of this narrative was its religious character; the second was the use of science to legitimize the religious stance; and the third was a critique of the pig itself and the conditions in which it was raised. Each is briefly discussed below.

Sitting on a sectarian volcano

The government was keen to publicly stress that the culling of the pigs was non-sectarian. Its announcements came at a period in history (roughly for the previous decade) when the country had been experiencing heightened incidence of communal violence, involving attacks on individuals, property or churches almost on a weekly basis. It is also a context where sectarian issues were being more openly discussed than perhaps at any other time in the history of the country. The culling of the pigs is no exception. For example, many prominent Islamist thinkers, such as Ihsan Abd el Kodous, a writer and active member of the press syndicate, objected to compensation being given to those whose pigs were culled, pointing to Egypt's status as a Muslim country under Shariah law, which prohibits the breeding or consumption of pigs in its territory.

Renowned writer Ibrahim Issa, editor in chief of prominent opposition newspaper *Al Distour*, was among the few critics who challenged both the government and the prevailing public opinion in favour of the culling. He sharply criticized the sectarian basis for the policy, pointing to the coalition between the ruling party and the Muslim Brotherhood 'in an Islamic campaign against the pigs' which he interpreted as a 'humorous exaggeration in line with the religious hypocrisy prevailing in our lives in Egypt' ('A very piggish', 2009). He argued that the hysterical, panic-stricken mood in the country was an exceptional response to a health issue, and must be understood in those exceptional terms. Why, he asked, did the people react so dramatically to the threat of H1N1, when the same people did not rise in anger against the contamination of their drinking water with sewage, the contamination of food, the rising rates of kidney and liver disease, or the air pollution that has caused respiratory disease in large numbers of children? The cause of this unexpected obsession with the health risks of H1N1, Issa suggested, is that 'Muslims deliberately or spontaneously found this an opportunity to despise the Copts, since the pig is forbidden in the Muslim religion and a symbol of filth in populist thought: hence the Coptic Christian was transformed into a source of infection (and harm) – since they come into contact with pigs and eat pork as opposed to Muslims who have no dealings with pigs and not the Muslim – who deals with pigs!' What the reaction to H1N1 also revealed, wrote Issa, was that the Copts act as if they consider themselves a second-class minority and not as citizens with equal rights. As a result of their own awareness of their diminished status, he argued, they neither defended their right to eat pork nor to breed pigs nor did they seek to correct the mistaken association between pigs and H1N1.

Certainly, the position adopted by the leadership of the Coptic Orthodox Church, the (spiritual) representative of the Coptic community in Egypt,[11] strongly supports Issa's scathing critique of the Christians' response to the crisis. Despite the refutations, the government must have been concerned about the impact that culling might have on the Christian Zabaleen because the Minister of Health paid their spiritual leader, Pope Shenouda, a visit. Following the visit Pope Shenouda made several remarks, quoted in the press, emphasizing that that the majority of Egyptians do not eat pork and that those who do tend to be either Westerners or local Christians who associate with them ('The pig fitna', 2009). In his weekly sermon on Wednesday, he warned parishioners not to go to places where pigs were raised. The implications of his statements were far-reaching: first, by making reference to the pork-eating Westerners, he reinforced a sense of Egyptian unity and attempted to disassociate Copts from the rest of the Christians. Second, the warning to avoid places where pigs are bred strengthened the myth that it is pigs that communicate the disease to humans, and further ostracized the garbage collectors who associated with them. Widely quoted in the press and in the media was Father Samaan, the local parish priest working among the garbage collectors of Mansheyet Nasser, who did not express any opposition to the government's decision to cull the pigs. The only Copts to express opposition to the culling of the pigs on account of its sectarian nature were those now living outside Egypt in the diaspora who have long lobbied against religious discrimination in their home country. Their protests were met with the conventional response that such claims of religious discrimination are inspired by a Western imperialist agenda in line with the former British colonialist policy of divide and rule ('Warning', 2009; 'Enlightened', 2009). In the narrative, the evidence that the culling of the pigs is not sectarian is that both the Coptic Orthodox Church leadership as well as Coptic MPs endorsed the decision.[12]

The intensity of the sectarian sentiment in the Egyptian street was far greater than in parliament or the media. Marie Assaad recounts that in the period preceding the decision to cull the pigs, 'Egypt was sitting on a sectarian volcano about to erupt in the most violent way. People were saying "the Christians are going to kill us. This is part of the West's plan to eradicate Muslims. We have to kill the pigs before they kill us".' Assaad said that the garbage collectors had legitimate reason to fear a mob taking things into their own hands and attacking them.

However, counter-arguments suggest that while the narrative may have been sectarian, the government's adoption of a pig culling policy was in fact more a result of poor governance than religious discrimination. The government's record in handling natural or man-made disasters and in particular health issues, such as avian influenza, certainly indicates poorly established and implemented policy responses which are lacking in transparency and accountability. The institutional processes for engaging with crises are characterized by a top-down, inconsistent and sporadic implementation of policy, with no regard for the socio-cultural context in which it is applied (Arram, 2009). No doubt the government's responses to H1N1, which along with the culling included the closing of schools and universities for a month, strict medical surveillance in airports and quarantine of identified cases in hospital, are symptomatic of these long-standing institutional dynamics which are themselves not necessarily motivated by sectarian concerns. Nevertheless, the actual implementation of the culling, as described later in this paper, suggests sectarian underpinnings in three ways:

- the inhumane manner of killing the pigs;
- the unjust compensation received by the Zabaleen;
- the persecution to which they were subjected.

Science and religion at a conjuncture

One of the salient features of the mainstream narrative endorsing the culling of the pigs was the use of scientific reasoning. All parties – the government, the Islamists, the press and others – resorted to science to justify their response. Interestingly, scientific evidence on the undesirability of pigs was used to directly support the religious narrative. Veterinarians acting as expert advisers to government described how pigs and pork carry numerous diseases, many of which are communicable to humans. According to one veterinarian, of the 57 diseases that pigs can carry, 37 are infectious diseases ('Slaughter', 2009). This veterinarian is a member of the parliament who attended a conference organized by the Physicians' Syndicate in which there was a consensus that pigs were too dangerous to slaughter so they must be culled. At the Muslim Brotherhood's salon,[13] one of the speakers commented that the impact of the imminent pandemic would be worse than a hydraulic bomb since the pig is a carrier of so many diseases ('The Coalition's', 2009). Mohammed Seif, a member of the Guidance Bureau (the governing body of the Muslim Brotherhood) emphasized that the pig is the only animal through which a mutation of the virus can take place, while Hamed Attiya, a professor of veterinary science, claimed that the WHO had been urging Egypt to adopt measures against its pig population since 2008, and warned against the dire implications of a mixed viral strain emerging if pigs came into contact with the avian flu. He then went on to reveal the numbers of pigs in different regions in Egypt and followed through by quoting the Koranic verses prohibiting the eating of and association with pigs. Many arguments in favour of the culling were made on the basis of a scientific premise: Hamdy Hassan, the leader of the Muslim Brotherhood, pointed out that the gravity of the current situation is that even if pigs test positive for infection with the virus, they still show no symptoms. Dr Mohammed Badei, a professor of pathology and member of the Guidance Bureau of the Muslim Brotherhood, highlighted that the pig carries 493 diseases and that it is the most dangerous of animals carrying the virus, because they act like a kitchen, mixing and mingling different viruses ('Dr Mohammed', 2009). The fact that scientific opinions rejecting these so-called 'expert' opinions were conspicuously absent from press accounts is testament to the strength of the mainstream narrative, and the way alternative views were excluded from public discussion.

Scientific evidence on the undesirability of pigs was woven into the religious narrative. Historically, notes Markell, there was a dichotomy in understanding deadly disease, with religion offering its accounts on the one hand and science on the other. The role of religious, spiritual or cultural beliefs in mitigating, containing or inflaming an epidemic in our own era, he warns, cannot be overlooked (Markell, 2007, p46). In more recent history, this dichotomy in engaging with health issues seems to have become blurred on many fronts. In the case of H1N1, the association of the virus with swine, and the implication that pigs were responsible in part for the transmission of the disease, gave support to those espousing the wisdom of Islam in prohibiting the breeding of pigs or the eating of pork. Sheikh El Sayed Askar, a leading member of the Muslim Brotherhood and an MP, emphasized that it is thanks to God that the Islamic Shariah sanctioned 'all that is good for us and prohibited all that is detestable' ('Dr Mohammed', 2009). Another MP said that Muslim scholars and the Organization of the Islamic Conference must unite to stand against the threatened harm and emphasized the catastrophes affecting the world such as AIDS and swine flu, and that Islam provides clear and truthful articles to prohibit them ('Dr Mohammed', 2009). The fact that the swine flu emerged in the Christian Western world, so the narrative goes, is because of the pig factor, while the Muslim world has been spared thanks to Islam's prescriptions.

This is not the first time that 'experts' have adopted a scientific discourse, to illustrate the wisdom and rightness of Islam. For example, doctors and, in particular, gynaecologists, were among the most vocal supporters of female genital mutilation in Egypt on 'scientific grounds'. They argued that the hadith (the saying of the Prophet) in support of 'circumcision' justifies the practice which also has medical or scientific justification, namely that it prevents the transmission of HIV/AIDS as well as cervical cancer (here too there is a pitting of the West against the Muslim world, with the former supposedly suffering from higher prevalence rates of the aforementioned illnesses).

There are pigs living in our midst!

International organizations such as the FAO openly criticized the government's pig culling decision. Joseph Domenech, the FAO's chief veterinary officer, said pig culling is 'a real mistake. There is no reason to do that. It's not a swine influenza, it's a human influenza', adding that the FAO had been trying to reach Egyptian officials but had so far been unsuccessful (Stewart, 2009). The reaction from the Egyptian ministries of Health and Agriculture was to announce that the culling of pigs was not a measure against H1N1 but a general health measure ('Egypt's pig', 2009). Further statements insisted that the measure was intended to protect public hygiene given the unacceptable environmental conditions in which the pigs were bred. This is very much in line with the government narrative that developed in response to the H1N1 virus in which there was a 'sudden' awakening to the existence of Zabaleen communities situated in the middle of Cairo. Revulsion, horror and condemnation characterized the public responses. The lack of sanitary hygiene was very much part of a narrative of naming and shaming all the Zabaleen communities.[14] From the start of the H1N1 pandemic scare, a deluge of articles in both pro-government and opposition press as well as in the independent media vilified the pig. In particular, the pig's physical and behavioural characteristics were a favourite subject for many writers, who described them as dirty disease carriers who thrived on rotten food and were just plain ugly. The obsession with the filthiness of the pig was so deeply seated that the press and media were still obsessed with them even after the culling: the public scare over the possible vending of pork as if it were beef lasted for several months, during which time citizens were advised not to purchase minced meat because it could be pork.

Government officials also contributed to the vilification of the Zabaleen. For example, Minister of Health El Gebally, speaking to both the upper and lower houses, advised on a series of measures to protect against H1N1 (such as hand washing) that included 'keeping away from pigs and *those who are in contact with them*' (emphasis added) ('Killing', 2009). The Zabaleen, it was also argued, had formed powerful mafias who had earlier resisted the implementation of the relocation orders made by the government. Their concern for their livelihoods came at the expense of the welfare of Egyptians.

There was much media and press focus on the squalor, the smell and the sight of humans living with animals and garbage, all of which was seen as an affront to the city's modern image. Writers argued that the continued presence of these Zabaleen settlements in the city constituted a health hazard and that an imminent plague was about to happen if something was not done about it. A typical commentary read as follows: 'When we [the writer and his family] saw the image of the Egyptian pigs on the satellite channels, we all screamed at the same time "how disgusting!" The image of the pig is filthiness itself working in all of this rot. I have one question: do you need a presidential decree for swine flu to remove this filth from the middle of the city to any hell hole?' He asked officials 'how did your conscience allow you to leave this rot to grow in the middle of the city, and in the heart of the residential area, being a source of infection to us all and our children?' ('The victory', 2009). The use of the term 'ticking bomb' to refer to the harsh (read: filthy) conditions in which the Zabaleen lived was reminiscent of the language that was used in the 1990s when the government and pro-government press suddenly 'discovered' the squatter settlements and shanty towns where many of the Islamist militants who undertook terrorist operations came from. Then too, there was much descriptive focus on how 'those people' lived, and how it was 'unacceptable' to continue to allow them to live in such conditions. The narrative decrying the conditions in which the Zabaleen live is revealing: certainly the garbage sorting process occurs in close proximity to the pigsties where the organic food is disbursed to the pigs. The piled up garbage bags waiting to be sorted do smell. However, the situation in many squatter settlements is not much better. Yet it seems the fact that the Zabaleen breed pigs is the qualifying differentiating factor.

In short, the pigs and those who raise them were considered filthy and a 'ticking bomb' about to transmit all kinds of infections to the rest of the Egyptian population ('The pigsties', 2009). The matter was so serious that it was deemed one of 'national security'. Writers urged that what was required was no less than the intervention of the Ministry of Health, the Ministry of Agriculture and the security forces in order to remove these settlements ('A national security', 2009). Deeming it a national security issue and calling for the physical intervention of the security forces elevated the issue of the pigs to a level where disputing the logic of these claims and policies would be tantamount to an act of national treason. It also meant that the 'price' to be paid – up to 300,000 pigs – seemed inconsequential in comparison to a national cause ('Kill the one', 2009). The securitization of the issue gave it a sense of urgency very much akin to preparing for a war.

Part two: Alternatives to the mainstream narrative

One of the most striking features of the way in which the mainstream narrative in favour of culling the pigs became hegemonic is the absence of alternative narratives before, during or after the decision was implemented. Certainly there were voices such as those of Ibrahim Issa, who decried in no uncertain terms the government, opposition and public response to H1N1. However, these writers were a minority. It might have been expected, for

example, that some human-rights-based narrative would develop, emphasizing the human rights abuses, social stigmatization and livelihood losses
that the Zabaleen suffered. It might also have been expected that the development NGOs working among the Zabaleen would voice their concerns.
Both were conspicuously absent. The human rights proponents, social
activists and development practitioners did not claim a narrative of their
own. For the human rights activists, it is possible that their failure to advocate on behalf of the Zabaleen was political: human rights organizations
lack support in the Egyptian context, and they may have feared that they
would antagonize everyone by speaking on behalf of a despised group.
Their allegiance and identity would be put in question. As for the development NGOs, they chose backdoor strategies of seeking to negotiate better
terms for the Zabaleen, yet because they only work in one community
(Mansheyet Nasser in Muqattam), Zabaleen elsewhere did not even have
a party to mediate their interests. The Zabaleen tell a very different narrative to the mainstream one, and it is one that has gone largely unheard and
unremarked. Their narrative is important in several respects:

- the historical narrative of how they came to settle in Cairo and how
  they entered their profession shows the extent to which the mainstream
  narrative failed to acknowledge their political and social marginalization;
- second, their suffering as a result of the culling policy exposed many of
  the underlying power dynamics;
- third, their narrative shows how the mainstream narrative misunder-
  stood the nature and complexity of their role. The way in which the
  mainstream narrative framed the pig solely in terms of the value of its
  meat contrasts sharply with the Zabaleen's narrative where pigs are inte-
  gral for their livelihoods.

'All we want is the government to leave us alone'

The Zabaleen communities are most heavily concentrated in Cairo (where
there is the most garbage) and are almost all Christians who migrated from
Upper Egypt in the past century. The neglect of Upper Egypt under the
centralized government of Nasser in the 1950s, which pursued an intensive
industrialization policy, led to a growing population and an increase in the
number of poor landless peasants who migrated to Cairo in search of work.
The narratives of the first garbage collectors who came to settle in Cairo
from other areas, whether from Ezbet el Nakhl (north of Cairo), Mansheyet
Nasser, Muqattam (south of Cairo) or Ard el Lewa (central Cairo) is almost
the same. Lacking in jobs, they came to Cairo in search of work. They met
with members of Al Wahat (Oasis) (namely members who originated from

Egypt's oasis and who came to Cairo) who were engaged in garbage-related work and who introduced them to the garbage collection profession. Subsequently they were introduced to the idea of breeding pigs in order to expand their work from garbage collection to garbage sorting. Once settled, other members of the family migrated to Cairo. Extended families belonging to the same tribe settled in close proximity to each other. Inter-marriage was usual and the social norms and traditions of the original rural community were maintained. Their experience was one of dispossession. They settled in obscure areas out of the eye of the government or on the fringes of the city (Muqattam and Ezbet el Nakhl). As the population of the city increased their settlement sites became attractive to a new governor, and they would be evicted, moving to a new settlement until the same events recurred. In most instances, the difficulty in obtaining formal ownership of the land obstructed their access to infrastructure. Many Zabaleen recount at least four different relocations before settling in their present community. For example, a migrant who would eventually work in the garbage profession might arrive at Imbaba, then relocate to Arab el Tawayla, before moving to Arab el Hessn, and then finally settling at Ezbet el Nakhl. Many of the Zabaleen at Ard el Lewa also tell a similar story: 'The government evicted us from one place to another. They say we are polluters of the environment. We arrived at Imbaba then moved to Ain el Seera, then to Hodn el Gabal (Batn el Baqqara), and then Mazalakn Ard el Lewa, where again, the government came to level us with the bulldozers, so we went to Shafi and then were evicted to Ard el Lewa'. With each move, the families would move their pigs and belongings and establish a new pigsty with an adjoining area for both the storage of garbage and for living.

There are hierarchies in the profession: at the bottom of the rung are the garbage scavengers who would wander the streets of Cairo with their donkey carts in search of any recyclable materials thrown in garbage bins or on the sides of the roads. Slightly better off are the garbage collectors who collect the garbage from the residential homes. The fees paid to the garbage collectors are a pittance, often amounting to less than LE5 (less than £1) a month per residential home. The prospects of earning a livelihood from garbage collection lie in the district covered – the better off the area, the more likely is its garbage to be rich in recyclable material, which is where the real opportunity for income generation lies. Garbage collectors collecting garbage from urban centres of Upper Egyptian towns or from the villages tend to be the poorest because the recyclable material is very limited. Garbage collectors based in Muqattam and Ezbet el Nakhl tend to be better off because of their collection of garbage from the upper class districts of Cairo. Garbage collectors who exclusively rely on the collection of garbage without owning pigsties have fewer income-generating prospects. The collected garbage is transferred to the garbage collectors who run pigsties.

The pigs, which consume the equivalent of their weight every day (a 90kg pig would consume 90kg of organic waste), relieved the Zabaleen in a cost-efficient way of the need to process an enormous amount of garbage every day. While the men were responsible for gathering the waste from locations around the city, the women were tasked with taking care of the pigs. After the pigs had removed the organic waste from the garbage, it was left to the women to complete the most tedious, and hazardous, job of all: sorting the remaining garbage in their homes.

In Ezbet el Nakhl, many of the garbage collectors own their own pigs and pigsties making them financially better off than other Zabaleen. The most economically stable are those in Ezbet el Nakhl and more so in Muqattam who have established micro and meso recycling industries. They purchase the recyclable material from the middle men who collect it from the pigsties, or from the pigsties directly. Raw recycled carton, metals, plastic and other elements are sold to exporters to China and elsewhere. The wealthiest members of the garbage collectors community are those who have well-established recycling industries, which are both capital and machine-intensive, with several paid labourers working for them. They are the least likely to be affected by the culling of the pigs. Running a pigsty, however, does not necessarily generate a good income for the Zabaleen. In Ard el Lewa, Israe'eel Ayad, a wealthy tycoon in the garbage industry, owns shares in both the pigs and the pigsties, leaving the Zabaleen raising pigs with minimal profit, a scenario very much reminiscent of a feudal order. In addition, very few recycling industries are established in that community, further limiting the Zabaleen's ability to generate additional income.

Social and political exclusion have meant that health and educational opportunities have been often compromized. Those better off in Ezbet el Nakhl, Ard el Lewa, and virtually all the inhabitants of Muqattam, have a work area separate from the living area. Yet the poorer garbage collectors often use the space for garbage sorting as also the space for living. Women in Ard el Lewa talk about giving birth in the pigsties amidst the pigs and garbage. Yet the narrative of the garbage collectors who owned pigsties is neither about the hardship of their lives nor of the daily exposure to hazard. It is not their livelihood that is a source of agony: it is the government's persecution of them.

'They attacked us as if we were criminals'

The story of the day the pigs were confiscated remains largely untold. The press and media were often not allowed in the areas. In Muqattam, the youth formed a human shield to prevent the authorities from entering the area or tried individually to prevent them entering their pigsties. Confrontations with the police ensued, and eyewitnesses from the Zabaleen said tear gas and rubber bullets were used to disperse the youth. The entire area was cordoned off by security forces with military vehicles. The Zabaleen believe the heavy militarized security forces and the arrest of many youths were intended to intimidate anyone from opposing the authorities. In Ezbet el Nakhl and Ard el Lewa, the majority of the Zabaleen did not show any opposition to the confiscation of their pigs 'because we saw on television what happened to our brothers in Muqattam and we did not want it to happen to us', as one pointed out. It is rare for images of police brutality (which is prevalent) to be broadcast on national television. However, perhaps the images of the garbage collectors being arrested were meant to act as a warning against forming opposition by garbage collectors in other communities. The stories are familiar: those who objected to the compensation or to the way the security barged into their homes were threatened and beaten and sometimes arrested. None of the communities knew when the security forces would arrive, a fact that was probably purposely kept secret in order to prevent the pigs being smuggled to another venue.

The scale of the operation was immense: national and local security forces, accompanied by members of the local council and veterinarians from the Ministry of Agriculture took control of the area, often advancing with large trucks and bulldozers to remove the pigs and raze the pigsties. They often stormed into houses with full force. 'They attacked us as if we were criminals', said one garbage collector from Ard el Lewa. The culling of the pigs went on for over two months and while the government claimed that the country became free from the animals, there is no way to verify whether this is the case.

The culling process reveals the extent to which religious motives influenced the actions of public officials. Following parliament's decision to cull the pigs, a presidential decree was issued recommending that the pigs be slaughtered according to agreed-upon standards rather than being simply killed. By slaughtering the pigs, the garbage collectors would then be able to sell the meat. But while many pigs belonging to the garbage collectors of Mansheyet Nasser were slaughtered, those belonging to Ard el Lewa and Ezbet el Nakhl were not. The experience of the garbage collectors from both communities is strikingly similar: in the case of the pigs bred in Ard el Lewa, some of the Zabaleen followed the government trucks to see where they would be taken: 'They took them alive and put them in a pit in the mountain and poured acid over them, covered them with sand and left them to die. It was a really barbarous way to treat them,' reported one member of the Zabaleen. In Ezbet el Nakhl, the Zabaleen tell a similar story: 'They lifted the pigs on trucks and they sprayed acid on them, then two men would hit the pigs with a heavy rod on their heads and then they would take the pigs to a burial place and cover them with acid…I witnessed this myself.'

These eyewitness accounts from the garbage collectors are corroborated by a journalist's filming of the entire process (the video was later uploaded to YouTube).[15] The journalist, affiliated to the independent newspaper *Al-Masry al Youm*, was severely reprimanded by the governor of al Qalubbiyya. Even after the video became public, however, there were no calls by the public to hold the government accountable, nor were there protests about the inhumanity of the way the cull was carried out. What protest there was came from international animal rights activists.

'They have taken away our livelihoods'

When the culling of the pigs was announced and implemented, the financial concerns of the Zabaleen were brushed aside: the government announced that it would compensate them. In line with the government's long history of granting compensation to politically and socially marginalized people (in particular the poor), the compensation given to the garbage collectors was less than what was announced. In all three communities, the Zabaleen told the same story: we were told we would be given LE250 for a pregnant sow (less than £25), LE150 for a grown pig (less than £15) and LE50 (less than £5) for a piglet but we were given LE250 for a pregnant sow and for all the other pigs we were given LE50. But for the Zabaleen, the evident injustice of the compensation is beside the point. 'What good is it to be given compensation when you have lost your livelihood?' asked many. Selling pork was only a marginal income-generating activity for most Zabaleen, who only sold their pigs in order to pay for exceptional expenses such as marriage or illness. The day-to-day survival of the Zabaleen and their families relied on their ability to extract recyclable material from the garbage which could then be sold to others in the recycling chain. The mainstream narrative completely ignored the complex dynamics of the garbage collecting and recycling arrangements that the Zabaleen had built up over time. As a result, the government and the media completely underestimated the scope of the devastation incurred by the Zabaleen, as well as the long-term implications for garbage collection in Egypt as a whole. Culling the pigs was the single greatest disincentive to collecting garbage that the government could have provided. The pigs enabled the Zabaleen to process in a cost-efficient way an enormous amount of garbage every day. Without the pigs, the entire recycling process was undermined.

The organic waste generated from the sorting process (and once consumed on site by the pigs) now needs to be transferred to the government garbage dump. There are three main obstacles to this:

- first, the poor garbage collectors who do not own trucks would need to hire them;

- second, even those who do own a vehicle must pay garbage dump fees;
- third, when the Zabeleen transfer the garbage after it has been sorted they risk incurring enormous fines from the traffic authorities on account of 'polluting the environment'. The latter is a particularly acute problem for the Zabaleen of Ezbet el Nakhl.

As a survival strategy, some Zabaleen hurriedly sort out the garbage in front of the residential homes at dawn, taking away only the recyclable material and leaving the organic waste there. Yet the men are not as experienced and efficient at sorting the garbage as the women, who could no longer be part of the process since they could not do the sorting in the streets. The result for the Zabaleen is that instead of 16 or 18 members of a household working in the garbage industry, there is scope for only one or two. The full implications for gender relations of the changes in the garbage collecting industry as a result of the cull need to be more thoroughly examined. What are the consequences of women now being excluded from this livelihood? What are the implications of women now pressing the men to 'go out and find a job to feed the family'? How has this affected their power to influence family decisions, such as whether the children get to go to school or stay at home?

Alternative livelihood options for the Zabaleen are currently difficult to see. Some of the Zabaleen expressed interest in raising goats, sheep or cattle instead of pigs. Yet according to Leila Iskander, goats and sheep cannot replace pigs in eating organic waste because they consume far less. As for cattle, this may have been a viable option in the rural areas from where the Zabaleen originally came, but is hardly viable in the much smaller pigsties where they hoped to raise them. The second most popular alternative expressed by the Zabaleen who have lost their pigsties is to work in different stages along the recycling chain. This would require figuring out how to dispose of large amounts of organic waste as well as protecting the Zabaleen from government harassment. To address the former, Marie Assaad and her organization have been lobbying the government to establish a compost plant, with no success to date. As for government harassment, Leila Iskander insists that unless the Zabaleen are given licenses and organize into a union with the power to negotiate for secure rights, they will continue to be vulnerable to daily arrests and exorbitant fines for simply collecting the garbage.

Part three: 'Let them rot in their own garbage'

When I first interviewed Leila Iskander in July, she predicted that during Ramadan, in late August and September,[16] when the garbage increases dramatically, and residents wake up to the absence of garbage collectors, they will ask to have the garbage collectors, and their pigs, back. The first part of her prediction came true: garbage waste increased to dangerous proportions. The second part, however, did not: the narrative justifying pig culling remained dominant and a nostalgic plea for the return of the garbage collectors did not materialize.[17] Following the stigmatization and culling of the pigs, many Zabaleen decided to leave the trade: 'Let them [the residents] rot in their own garbage', one explained. In many residential quarters the stigmatization predated culling. Many of the Zabaleen in Muqattam, Ezbet el Nakhl and Ard el Lewa tell a similar story: 'Suddenly from the beginning of the health scare regarding the "swine flu" at the end of April 2009, people began to treat us like a disease. People told us not to go up to their apartments to pick up the garbage, instead they would throw their garbage from the balconies or windows so we wouldn't contaminate them,' said one garbage collector bitterly. Such experiences may have been particularly painful in the light of the many years of contact between the residents and the Zabaleen, sometimes across generations. In Ard el Lewa, one garbage collector said that the local health clinic refused to treat his nephew 'because we are infected as we breed pigs'. In another Zabaleen community, children were expelled from school and told never to return because they were carriers of disease. Many garbage collectors left the profession following the cull. Others returned after the residents saw the accumulating piles of garbage and begged them to return.

The Zabaleen's narrative about both H1N1 and public hygiene is understandably very different from the mainstream narrative. They do not have their own scientific theory about the pathway of transmission but they are definitive about one thing: it is neither transmitted through their pigs nor through them. 'The pigs are perfectly healthy, there is nothing wrong with them. When the bird flu started, the government got worried that our pigs would be sick, and they took samples which showed they are perfectly healthy,' said one garbage collector. Some referred to scientific evidence to show that they themselves were perfectly healthy. 'In Ezbet el Nakhl they took blood samples from us and it proved we were not carrying an infection,' reported one garbage collector. Science features in their narratives, but to support the fact that they are healthy and to support the implicit interpretation of the mainstream narrative and the motives behind it: namely, that the move to cull the pigs and clamp down on them has nothing to do with H1N1 and everything to do with seizing an opportunity to strike them down, which they view as consistent with the government's historical engagement with them.

Yet the prediction of a garbage disaster that the Zabaleen had so confidently articulated became a reality in only a few months after the culling. By September, Cairo's streets and alleys and even motorways were piling up with garbage. Egypt's 26 governorates produce 25,000 tonnes of garbage daily, with Cairo, not surprisingly, providing the heaviest load: more than 12,000–15,000 tonnes a day. Giza is the next largest producer, with 3000 tonnes daily, while Alexandria and Qalyobiya governorates offer up another 2000 tonnes each. Included in this solid waste are medical, construction and demolition garbage ('Capital collection', 2002). In both wealthy and poor residential quarters, near schools[18] and hospitals, literal mountains of garbage piled up: empty spots in the middle of residential areas were converted into informal garbage dumps. As this chapter was being finalized in late 2009, the garbage problem remained acute. Residents spoke of the rotting garbage that was piling in front of their apartment buildings, while many observed the rise in rats, mice and snakes being detected.

What compounded the problem of garbage collection in Greater Cairo was the sudden discontinuance, due to a disagreement with local authorities, of the Italian company that the government had contracted to remove the garbage from the governorate of Giza. With neither the Zabaleen nor the Italian company functioning, by the beginning of September, 15,000 tonnes of garbage had piled up in the Giza governorate alone ('The crisis', 2009).

In response to the crisis there were calls to hire Egyptian as opposed to foreign companies to clean up the city. There were calls for 'the government to do something about it'. Exactly what, nobody was quite sure. The irony of the situation was evident but was not captured in the ensuing debates. The mainstream narrative had called for the culling of the pigs on grounds of protecting the health of Egyptians, yet by removing the pigs and marginalizing the garbage collectors, the government had in effect created a real health hazard for its citizens. This time, there was no 'scientific' evidence needed to show a health hazard: the images of garbage piled up everywhere and citizen testimonies of its implications said it all. The way in which the government has historically responded to policy failures suggests it is not likely to respond differently to this one by admitting misjudgement. Yet what is astounding is that the mainstream narrative, articulated and adhered to by intellectuals, the press and much of the general public, did not reflect on any of the potential environmental, sanitary and livelihood consequences of the cull.

Conclusions

This chapter began with the premise that in response to the H1N1 pandemic health scare, a mainstream narrative developed that described the virus as being transmitted from pigs to humans, and justified the mass culling of Egyptian pigs on this basis. When the scientific evidence used to prop up the argument was internationally refuted, the government reframed the justification of its policy decision on the basis of 'public hygiene'. The pathway of response – large-scale culling of pigs – emanating from the mainstream narrative went largely uncontested.

In the mainstream narrative, the understanding of the disease problem was conspicuously influenced by the Muslim prohibition against breeding and eating pigs as well as by the more generalized sectarian antipathy towards the Coptic Christian minority. Furthermore, the government has a long history of mismanagement of diseases and of heavy-handed imposition of top-down policies that disregard social realities on the ground. However, the intensity, speed and manner in which the culling was justified and implemented suggest a stronger religious and political animus at work.

An analysis of the governance of the H1N1 scare reveals existing power hierarchies; the Zabaleen have long been subject to social exclusion and marginalization. An analysis of how these power relations played out in this context reveals the following results. First, the government gained credence for espousing what was widely considered to be a pro-Islamic policy, playing up to populist sentiment and allowing for an alliance with Egypt's largest Islamist movement, the Muslim Brotherhood. Second, the Coptic Orthodox church leadership, represented by Pope Shenouda, was also able to gain political brownie points: by supporting the cull they were able to appear to take a 'nationalist' stance which, given the marginalization of the Zabaleen within the Christian minority, the Church was able to do without major internal political cost. Third, given the long-standing stigmatization of the garbage collectors, the risk of social protest in favour of the Zabaleen was minimal. Moreover, the power hierarchy within the Zabaleen community itself worked against those whose entire livelihood rested on the pigsties. The wealthier garbage collectors, whose livelihood was diversified or who relied on predominantly capital-intensive recycling industries, had the power to sit at the negotiating table with government officials in order to minimize government harassment after the culling ended, while the poorer ones were entirely excluded and their interests sidelined.

The counter-narrative of the poorer garbage collectors whose livelihood revolved around the pigsties was conspicuously absent from any discussion of the nature or consequences of the pig culling policy. The outcome was a continued perpetuation of myths and stereotypes largely based on ignorance and religious bigotry. Thanks to the government narrative and press coverage, the garbage collectors were treated like lepers. Certainly, there are health issues associated with their livelihood, particularly among the poorer Zabaleen. While the wealthier garbage collectors were able to separate the garbage sorting operations from their residential homes, the poorer Zabaleen had no option but to use the same space for breeding pigs, housing donkeys, and storing and sorting the garbage as well as working, cooking, sleeping and raising children (in particular in Ard el Lewa and Ezbet el Nakhl). However, there have been successful cases of engagement with garbage collectors to encourage them to keep work and home space separate. The case of the Zabaleen of Torah el Maadi where pigsties are kept distant from residential homes highlights some crucial issues. The intervention was successful because land titles were given to the garbage collectors, measures were instituted to ensure the security of the private pigsties and access to infrastructure (water, electricity, etc.) was secured. In other words, practical incentives associated with maintaining their livelihoods catalysed a process of social change in lifestyle. So far the government has not provided the garbage collectors with secure land titles for any proposed settlement.

The pre- and post-culling realities for Cairo indicate that although their methods of garbage sorting and recycling were traditional and largely informal, the Zabaleen had efficiently gathered and disposed of garbage in a way that the residents of Cairo both understood and had come to expect. According to Assaad, the Zabaleen recycled more than 90 per cent of all garbage, thus doing the environment a favour by minimizing the waste that needed to be dumped, buried or burnt. Ironically, the main losers behind the culling policy are the citizens of greater Cairo. The full scope of the health impact caused by the disposal of the dead pigs, as well as the accumulating garbage across the city, has yet to be fully gauged.

Notes

1   In this chapter parliament and People's Assembly are used interchangeably.

2   'Zabaleen' is a literal translation of garbage collector. However, the term is not without contention because the Zabaleen interpret their profession to include anyone engaged in garbage including those who sort the garbage and those who are involved in any part of its recycling process. The mainstream narrative has tended to use the word to refer only to those who collect the garbage from residential homes, thus undermining their wider role in environmental protection as well as excluding the considerable numbers of women and children who are primarily responsible for garbage sorting.

3   In Cairo, there are nine Zabaleen settlements. In addition to Mansheyet Nasser, Ard el Lewa and Ezbet el Nakhl, there are Torah el Maadi, Helwan, El Barageel, Wadi el Giza, Batn el Baqqara and Gattamiyya.

4   I am grateful to Mansour Kedeis and Ragaa Bekheet, two researchers and development practitioners from within the Zabaleen community of Muqattam, for conducting these interviews and for sharing with me their perspectives and insights on how the data should be interpreted.

5   The examples of highly inflammatory press articles of this nature are too many to quote here; however, they featured in both the national and oppositional newspapers from 28 April 2009 and for the next month.

6   What follows is a synthesis of the most important arguments and counter-arguments raised, not necessarily in the same chronological order in which they took place in parliament.

7   Al-Azhar being one of the oldest and largest places for Islamic teaching in the Muslim world.

8   A literal translation of the word is 'Egyptian'; however, it is commonly used to refer to Egyptian Christians.

9   An interesting statement though factually incorrect.

10   It is exactly this measure that the Minister of Health would publicly announce pursuing in response to the pandemic.

11   Although in the past half-century it has also sought to assume the political representation of Copts as well (though not always successfully).

12   This section discusses the narrative. An analysis of the implementation of the policies is offered later in the chapter.

13   A forum for discussion of contemporary issues among members of the movement.

14   See, for example, 'Pigs in government' (2009) which specifically named some of the communities in which pigs are bred such as the village of Al Bayadeya in Minya, and strongly urged that the pigs be immediately removed.

15   www.youtube.com/watch?v=jwMIlw7rCSc, accessed 10 October 2009.

16   Holy month of fasting for Muslims. In 2009 it began at the end of August and ended 20 September.

17   Except for a few marginal exceptions which have remained on the fringes (for example, a handful of press articles).

18   Which had yet to open in September 2009.

Chapter 11

Towards Conclusions: Science, Politics and Social Justice in Epidemic Accounts and Responses

Sarah Dry and Melissa Leach

The voices of those who suffer from epidemics are notably absent from much writing on the subject. Many of our contributors have noted the relative silence of the people who experience epidemics most directly: those who are infected, those who live close to an area of infection and those who are involved in responding. This silence is not simply metaphorical but actual. It is reflected even here, in a collection of accounts committed to presenting neglected and marginal accounts. We hear second-hand from those who live in areas where Lassa fever is endemic and avoid going to get injections because they fear they will contract the disease. We hear, from the perspective of a WHO epidemiologist, how he inspired terror in an old woman dying of Ebola, to whom he appeared, in his white isolation suit, as 'either God or the devil'. We hear from an HIV-positive woman in South Africa who describes how it 'depends on the heart of the doctor sometimes' whether she gets an extension of her disability grant: 'If the doctor has got your sympathy then he can do that.' On the other side of the equation, we hear from a doctor in the same setting that deciding who gets these grants is 'like you are God; you just have to look at the person's face and decide about whether they qualify or not'. Finally, we hear from the garbage collectors in Egypt who were stigmatized and whose pigs were slaughtered in response to H1N1 that 'they attacked us as if we were criminals'. But beyond these brief snatches, it is hard to hear the voices of those who are experiencing epidemics directly.

This paucity of first-hand accounts is instructive. Like microbes, words can be made to seem to travel with effortless ease, costing little to nothing to transport and reproduce. In fact, like microbes, words require an initial point of contact between the speaker and the outside world: a conversation, an interview, a letter, an announcement, a publication. Reaching across multiple scales of time and place to the place where these encounters can finally occur takes time, money, expertise and care, just as responding to epidemics themselves does. We begin our conclusion with this observation to bring our attention to the ultimate goal of this volume, and the research that has gone into it: to help ensure that our understandings of and responses to epidemic diseases are more like conversations and less like directives. This means listening closely to those who suffer, in order to better understand the diverse dynamics involved in epidemics and the specific circumstances that make each outbreak, and each infection, different. It then means continuing the conversation by responding with programmes that are adaptive to the particular circumstances of a given outbreak.

This final chapter presents some cross-cutting themes and conclusions about epidemics based on this book's engagement with science and knowledge, policy and politics, and equity and social justice. These themes, drawn from our case studies, also follow on from multidisciplinary discussions at the Epidemics project workshop, held at the STEPS Centre at the University of Sussex, in December 2008. They include the effects of disease exceptionalism on interventions, myths of the local and the global, and the shaping of – and shaping effects of – narratives. Throughout, we consider what factors tend to cluster together in dominant narratives, and which have acquired pre-eminence and power in scientific, policy and popular debate, using examples from our case studies. We also address what issues and questions emerge from alternative narratives, and why both scientists and policy-makers might need to pay these more attention. In this light, we draw our conclusion to a close by considering what is missing from the volume and what directions future research and research/policy engagements might take.

Disease exceptionalism

A striking feature of the dominant narrative in several of our case studies is that of disease exceptionalism. Labelling an epidemic disease exceptional serves to justify unusual or especially forceful interventions that might otherwise be considered wasteful, overly intrusive, or too expensive and complicated. This tactic provides a rebuttal to any potential querying of a response: this disease is so deadly, infectious or novel, the argument goes, that we must respond as we have not before. There is an interesting and seemingly paradoxical twist here: in several cases, diseases that have been labelled exceptional have helped to shape pathways of response that remain in place in global and national health institutions where they are then applied to subsequent outbreaks. In effect, these diseases become foundational, generating the grooves and ruts that global health policy will follow in years to come. We first discuss exemplar diseases that have been particularly strongly labelled as exceptional in dominant narratives, before reflecting on the effects that this pathway shaping has on global health responses more generally.

With its long history and powerful tradition of activism, AIDS is the grandfather of 'exceptional' epidemic diseases prominent today. Taken together, the global scale of HIV infection, the incurability of the infection, a long latency period that facilitates the spread of the virus, and the existence of hyperendemic areas with very high prevalence conspire to create a perfect epidemic storm that makes AIDS, the argument goes, unlike any other disease we are facing (see MacGregor and Edström, this volume, for a fuller discussion). This exceptionalist account has co-evolved with the epidemic over time. Organized and well-funded patient activists, initially based in the United States but subsequently present globally, have played a prominent role in lobbying for funding and attention for the disease since its emergence in the 1980s. These activists were successful in mobilizing support for an AIDS response on an unprecedented scale. Drawing on human rights discourse, they argued that because of the danger of the disease and the stigma associated with the primary means of transmission of the disease – intravenous drug use and sex – special interventions were required to reach those most vulnerable to the disease and to ensure that their rights to privacy and treatment were not disregarded. Today, the exceptionalist account of AIDS is articulated forcefully by people such as Peter Piot, who until recently was Executive Director of UNAIDS. Piot has compared the severity of the threat from the epidemic to that of nuclear war or global climate change, arguing that similarly exceptional responses are therefore needed.[1] The challenge for people like Piot has been to maintain this sense of urgency over the nearly three decades that have elapsed since the disease was first recognized.

As both MacGregor and Edström have explored in their contributions, AIDS exceptionalism and the particular forms it has taken have meant that voluntary counselling and concerns over patients' rights have been prioritized over testing and medical interventions in some cases. For reasons both of them discuss, the needs of many people infected with HIV or suffering with AIDS may not be best met by these approaches, which were developed in resource-rich countries with robust health systems.

While AIDS remains the disease for which the exceptionalist narrative is most prominent, other diseases considered in this book also demonstrate the tendency. The Ebola virus has often been described as exceptional in its infectiousness and its virulence. The high mortality it inflicts on sufferers, who often experience horrific deaths, make it exceptionally frightening in a more direct way than the slow deaths of AIDS patients. That Ebola virus seems to emerge at random intervals from the forests of Central Africa, where its animal reservoir remains a mystery, adds to its aura of special danger; the enigmatic virus seems to stand for the next great pandemic disease, lurking in dense undergrowth, ready to strike at any random moment. This image of the Ebola virus has accompanied most outbreaks of the disease but the 1995 Kikwit outbreak has special salience (see Leach and Hewlett, this volume). That outbreak, where 252 out of a suspected 316 people infected with the disease died, proved an important milestone in the careers of many leading figures in the field of infectious disease policy today, many of whom contributed to response efforts (Hall et al, 2008). It also helped determine the structure of GOARN, the WHO's rapid response network, as well as giving impetus to the revision of the WHO's International Health Regulations (Heymann et al, 1999; Leach and Hewlett, this volume). In both cases, the unpredictable emergence of the virus, its contagiousness and high mortality rates, and the speed of death in those who succumbed to it, served as implicit models for a system of monitoring and surveillance tuned to just such 'fast-twitch' events.

The importance of the outbreak at Kikwit shows how institutional pathways, such as GOARN and the revised IHR, depend partly on historical contingency – certain actors who happened to be at the outbreak proved influential in the subsequent shaping of policy – as well as on a longstanding tendency to fear such unpredictable, fast and bloody diseases more than slower, less dramatic outbreaks. Lassa fever, which shares many of the same virological features as Ebola, does not kill as many of those who become infected. Locally, however, it infects, and therefore kills, many more people than Ebola. And yet Lassa fever does not register with the same urgency as Ebola, since its case fatality rate is much lower and its animal reservoir is known. As understanding of the virological and biomedical profile of Ebola grows, it may prove to be less threatening and this strand of exceptionalism may peter out. Yet early experiences with Ebola continue to fuel cycles of fear, with both scientific and policy priority granted to rapidly identifying and responding to unpredictable zoonotic outbreaks with potentially devastating consequences.

A third, and very different, example of disease exceptionalism is to be found with SARS. While HIV/AIDS and Ebola are made to seem exceptionally dangerous or devastating, SARS has been described as an exceptional test for a transformed international health governance structure, a test which was successfully passed. SARS, then, is exceptional in that it both tested new governance structures, such as GOARN, and showed them to be working well, thus helping to justify the vision of global health that they instantiated. This thesis, articulated forcefully by David Fidler, has also, perhaps unsurprisingly, been part of the story that the WHO tells about itself (Fidler, 2004). 'The international response to the SARS outbreak', write David Heymann and Guénaël Rodier of the WHO, 'tested the assumption that a new and emerging infection ... could be prevented from becoming epidemic.' They conclude that, while it is early to tell at the time of writing, the answer is most likely 'yes', since 'all known chains of transmission' of the disease had been interrupted within four months of the first global alert about the new disease (Heymann and Rodier, 2004).

As Bloom writes in his chapter, SARS galvanized the community of international health experts to lobby for a shared global response, designed and led by scientists. The global threat that SARS seemed to pose provided a justification for a unified response, with scientists from the WHO at the helm. In the face of a disease like SARS, which travelled the international jet ways along with millions of air passengers, national sovereignty concerns over trade or control of biological samples were made to seem at best irrelevant and at worst dangerous. Such concerns threatened to limit sharing of information and access to samples that could slow the response or even help fan the epidemic. Because they were instrumental in helping to control the SARS outbreak, transnational institutional arrangements and procedures such as GOARN and unified, multilateral top-down responses came to be seen as best practice for identifying and responding to outbreaks. But, as should now be clear, not all epidemics will unfold in the same way as SARS. Will the current arrangements be flexible enough to respond to outbreaks of different kinds?

Such a question can be asked of all three cases just described. The exceptionalist elements in the dominant narratives about AIDS, Ebola and SARS have affected not only the responses to these diseases but subsequent responses to diseases – both epidemic and endemic, acute and chronic – more generally. In many ways, the tendency for exceptionalist narratives to shape enduring pathways of response makes sense. These narratives have a great persuasive force, often mobilizing vast amounts of money and energy, which inevitably help to re-make the institutional, social and political landscape in which health interventions of all kinds occur. Even when exceptionalist rhetoric leads to the creation of stand-alone institutions, such as UNAIDS, which does not have direct connections with responses to influenza epidemics, for example, this patterning applies. It is the very idea of a stand-alone institution, named after the disease it is meant to address, that leaves its mark in the minds of policy-makers. Similarly, the exceptionalist account of Ebola contributed to the creation of institutions such as GOARN, which then serve to privilege emergency-oriented short-term interventions while neglecting longer-term social and ecological factors.

In this way, dominant narratives tend to cluster together a set of related concepts. For example, disease exceptionalism goes hand-in-hand with disease eradication as a goal. If a disease is so uniquely dangerous, the argument goes, it is not enough merely to control it: it must be eradicated.

And, as previously discussed, global responses tend to accompany disease exceptionalism as well, since nothing short of such a broad response will be effective against such a special threat. Short-term, emergency-oriented solutions also accompany this approach. It is much easier to mobilize a response to an exceptional threat if there is a perception of both urgency and the potential for a relatively quick solution. Long wars – against diseases as well as nations – are unpopular. Finally, dominant versions of the concept of health security, with their emphasis on securing borders and protecting a putative global community against highly mobile and highly infectious pathogens, also contribute to exceptionalist approaches, as the cases of SARS, haemorrhagic fevers and avian influenza described in previous chapters demonstrate. We can begin, therefore, to build a picture of the complementarities between different framings of and responses to epidemic diseases. Exceptionalism, eradication, security and uniform global responses to short-term, explosive outbreaks travel together through the policy juggernaut.

These remarks on disease exceptionalism could be met with the response that it is inevitable that certain diseases become foundational for future policy: to wish otherwise would be to deny the force of history itself. In fact, we would argue that a greater historical memory is needed to fully understand the effects of previous claims to exceptionalism and the responses thereby engendered. The aim is not to deny the past but to recognize its contours and count the differences, as well as similarities, between previous outbreaks and present or anticipated outbreaks. This sensitivity might lead us to question whether diseases must compete to be the next exception – or the next emergency – in order to win the money and energy needed to mount an effective response. A valuable topic for future research and policy reflection, therefore, might be which kind of diseases, lobbied for by which actors, are most likely to win such a contest? If many boys cry wolf, who gets heard? From another perspective, who and what gets left out when such powerful organizing ideas as exceptionalism, eradication and emergency alertness travel together?

One indication of what may be missed is given by the growing importance of co-infection in shaping health and disease prevalence. As MacGregor, Edström and Nightingale describe in this volume, co-infection of HIV and TB represents a growing phenomenon of major significance. As Calain and Fidler have demonstrated, a recent episode of XDR-TB in South Africa reveals the limitations of the current privileging of acute rather than chronic diseases in the revised IHR (Calain and Fidler, 2007; see also Dry, this volume). If drug-resistant strains of TB are allowed to develop in HIV-positive patients because the IHR do not recognize the disease as the 'right kind' of outbreak, then the system needs to be re-evaluated. In a related vein, Loevinsohn (2009) has demonstrated in Malawi how multiple health problems co-exist and interact to shape the ways that sufferers and their families think about and deal with a disease such as AIDS. As several of our contributors also observe, people's experiences of health and illness are rarely driven by a single disease, meaning that the priorities of sufferers, their families and communities rarely map neatly onto exceptionalist disease-focused priority goals. As a result, policies can easily miss key interactions, or be locally perceived – and perhaps resisted – as inappropriate. To be sure, it is neither realistic nor appropriate to expect international agencies such as the WHO to manage and respond to all outbreaks of disease, or to address all diseases in a given setting. But what is crucial is recognizing the boundaries of our epidemic response mechanisms – and making explicit any favouring of acute versus chronic diseases. This is especially important in situations where the boundary line between the two is murky. It also clears a path towards recognizing where complementary, health-system or livelihood-focused responses are required to address the multiple health needs of communities affected by epidemics.

Another and related example of what may be missed by disease exceptionalism are disease events that do not count as outbreaks and thus do not register so strongly on the global radar, despite causing potentially more deaths and more disruption to livelihoods and communities than the blockbuster diseases. Diarrhoeal diseases and pneumonia clearly exemplify diseases in this category which this book, with its overt focus on epidemics, has not addressed directly. Amongst our cases, we have already noted the tendency for Ebola to eclipse more endemic haemorrhagic fevers such as Lassa fever. Obesity may provide an even more striking example of this phenomenon. Despite a relatively high profile in policy circles and media outlets, as Millstone points out, there are very few examples of successful responses to obesity. One reason may be that despite resembling a 'classic' epidemic in the rapid rise in prevalence, obesity is still considered to be chronic. Less urgency and importance is therefore attached to obesity interventions, despite the evident scale of the problem and the severity of its impact on health (and the work of those calling attention to the obesity 'epidemic'). Similarly, TB does not conform to the model of a disease with discrete and sudden outbreaks. With an estimated one-third of the world's population a carrier of the bacillus, this old disease strains the ability of the global health system to respond. As these cases make clear, the determination of whether a disease counts as epidemic or endemic matters greatly to the kinds of responses that are mounted. Recognizing that this process is partly socially constructed, and that diseases can cross the line between epidemic and endemic multiple times, should point to the importance of designing responses that cover both phases. We can thus begin to move away from an implicit paradigm of eradication, which may not be realistic for many diseases, and towards a sustainable programme of disease management, in 'good' times and bad.

Myths of the local and the global

Another blurry boundary that many of our case studies have explored is that separating the global and the local. While commentators have grown increasingly critical of easy separations between supposedly global and local realms, this binary framing remains tenacious, even as much analysis – and some policy attention – focuses on building bridges from local to global and vice versa (what has been referred to as 'the instantiation of global assemblages in local social arenas' (Janes and Corbett, 2009, p169)). We admit that such categories are hard habits to kick. In this section, we consider some of the myths that enliven both halves of this equation and consider how the narratives in our case study represent their relation. Finally, we highlight some narratives and pathways from our case studies that offer a way to transcend this pairing.

The first thing to note is that there are opposing myths for both the global and the local. To begin with the global: there is, on the one hand, the notion that Western biomedical and techno-scientific tools (such as surveillance systems, drugs and vaccines), in combination with international institutions, such as the WHO in general and GOARN in particular, can control and limit the risk of outbreaks to maintain the achievements of the post-war, antibiotic age. This myth, which has much in common with a health security narrative, animates many of the dominant narratives in our case studies: in particular, the first 'global' narrative described by Leach and Hewlett in relation to Ebola; the dominant 'scientific' narrative in relation to SARS; the cluster of dominant outbreak narratives that Scoones argues have mobilized the international response to avian influenza with its emphasis on risk management and top-down surveillance; the security narrative that Nightingale describes with respect to TB; and, in a form that is inflected with Islamic propaganda, the mainstream narrative used to justify the massive pig culling in Egypt described by Tadros.

In these accounts, the global is presented as powerful, scientific and 'modern' (for which read: Western). It is constituted primarily by expertise that can be mobilized quickly to protect global populations (which, as our case studies have explored, is often a code for inhabitants of industrialized nations). The flipside of this presentation of the global as a positive, protective force is the notion that modernity – constituted by the global systems of transport, communication, and science and technology referenced above – has created a unique contemporary vulnerability to novel threats that have the potential to create unprecedented systemic failures at the global level. Climate change, the global financial crisis, terrorism and pandemic disease are all presented as manifestations of this side of the global. The links between these two versions of the global have been eloquently discussed by, among others, Ulrich Beck, who coined the phrase reflexive modernity to capture the way that one aspect of the global modern – our techno-scientific prowess – has led to another aspect, our vulnerability to novel threats (Beck, 1998, 2008). Our case studies also contain accounts of this aspect of the global. Obesity can be seen as a side effect of industrialization, becoming global as sedentary lifestyles and unhealthy eating spread with other aspects of 'modernization'. AIDS is another disease whose spread seems to capture the downsides of the increased mobility and sexual freedom that is seen to accompany 'modernization'. Likewise, the high visibility of the response to SARS at airports cemented its image as a disease of modern travel.

In contrast to the dangers of globalization, there are two myths of the local that can be discerned in our case studies. In the first, there is a notion of communities who are living 'in balance' with a disease ecosystem through a combination of cultural and ecological adaptations developed over a long time frame. This myth of the local can be seen in aspects of the third narrative described in the Ebola chapter, where haemorrhagic fevers (both Ebola and Lassa) are accommodated and managed by local populations using cultural practices developed over a long period of cohabitation with the virus. Cases of Ebola are thus not considered as precursors to outbreaks with the potential to 'go global'. Instead, the Ebola and Lassa viruses are simply part of the fabric of life – albeit a hard life – in a given community, claiming lives occasionally before subsiding once more into quiescence. At their extreme – although notably not in the versions that have animated arguments to engage local knowledge and practices in disease responses – versions of this narrative can present a static notion of both 'traditional' culture and ecology, in which disease events are no more troubling than the occasional thunderstorm. While such a narrative accepts the unpredictability of such events, it remains blithe about the potential for systemic effects resulting from such outbreaks.

Rather than an image of a traditional society living in balance with its environment, a second myth of the local presents communities flexibly adapting to change, which enables them to mount a more robust and resilient response to disease threats. This response incorporates traditional knowledge about flora and fauna, as well as the agricultural, economic and social needs and realities of people living in an area subject to outbreaks. The local community's ability to draw on this complex knowledge accrued over generations makes them more resilient, and adaptable, in the face of unpredictable and potentially dramatic changes. Part of what enables local communities to be resilient is that they retain 'traditional' knowledge and remain to some extent outside the global system. This myth of the local can be seen in an alternative narrative that Scoones discusses in relation to avian flu. Here, a focus on the socio-ecological dynamics of the disease and local responses is seen to provide a more flexible, adaptive set of responses to avian influenza than the risk management-driven 'outbreak' narrative that has been dominant.

This version of the local can also be discerned in MacGregor's description of the way in which formal requirements for providing 'voluntary HIV counselling' are interpreted in local settings in Cape Town, where resources are extremely scarce. In this case, local counsellors with little training may reduce requirements to 'counsel' patients to mere information giving or the running through of a checklist. In this way, counsellors effectively circumvent the rights-based directive, which emanates from national and ultimately global sources of authority, in favour of a locally pragmatic, adapted response. The effect is that more people are tested, and find out their HIV status, in a region of very high prevalence. Rather than drawing on so-called 'traditional' knowledge, as in the avian flu example, these counsellors are making pragmatic decisions based on their level of training and local perceptions of the relative importance of rights to 'dignity' versus a more immediate goal of controlling the epidemic. While the context is very different, both examples point to the importance of the agency and knowledge of local people in responding to disease events in a flexible way. In as much as the concept of health security is relevant in such examples, it is redefined in localized, 'human security' terms, referring to secure community and individual livelihoods and well-being.

Having outlined these opposing pairs of myths – some positive and some negative – we now consider some examples from our cases of how we might transcend the limiting framing offered by simplistic divisions between global and local and start to describe the true complexity of disease outbreaks. As this last example suggests, one way forward is to consider how the rhetoric of a given response may not be as potent as we think. In a volume that uses narratives as a key conceptual tool, it is important to remind ourselves that official language and justifications, which appear frequently in dominant narratives, may not find much traction in the so-called 'real world' where policies are ultimately enacted. Dry makes this point in her chapter on global health governance, noting that while changes to the WHO's International Health Regulations make unofficial information technically equal to official sources, in practice, there are still expert judgements, made by those in positions of power, about what kinds of information, and knowledge, count. This is a necessary feature of any information gathering system. What requires our attention – and perhaps some healthy fresh air – is the way in which statements about the importance of local (another way of

saying unofficial) knowledge in the new IHR may conceal the true pathways by which information, and decision-making, travel.

Conversely, in MacGregor's work on HIV, we see the limits of a global
emphasis on rights in a local context of high disease prevalence and scarce
human and financial resources. Though these cases describe opposite
effects – on the one hand, we see a potential strengthening of official sources
while on the other we see local counsellors taking control – they both demonstrate how the relations between global and local cannot be reduced to a
question of either language or politics alone. This understanding can help
us to avoid a potential pitfall of relying on a narrative approach: reifying
accounts by themselves without attending to the question of which people,
operating from within which institutions, are responsible for formulating
and promulgating a given narrative.

A third way forward is to acknowledge and explore the myriad 'inter-
mediary' processes and practices through which global and local myths
come together in particular social and political settings. Several of our
cases begin to do this. Thus in Bloom's chapter, we see how global ideas
and imperatives around SARS became grounded and interpreted in China
amidst the concerns and priorities of early 21st century Chinese state
institutions. In the account by Tadros of H1N1 influenza in Egypt, we see
governmental and religious organizations jostling to capture global myths
and put them to work for long-standing strategic ends. In work extending
his contribution to this book, Scoones (2010) shows how global narratives and responses to H5N1 avian influenza have come to mean very
different things amidst the diverse political economies, histories and social
contexts of Indonesia, Thailand, Cambodia and Vietnam. As these cases
suggest, the process of assemblage (Ong and Collier, 2005; Li, 2007)
through which ideas, policies, personnel, practices, technologies, images,
and architectures of governance and resources are brought together,
constantly crosses spatial scales, confounding any separation between the
local and the global, and implicating national institutions – including those
of the state – in new ways.

Not all myths are created equal, and these so-called global and local
myths are not equally represented in our case studies. Representations of
epidemic diseases tend to draw on and perpetuate global myths, especially
in the dominant narratives our contributors have outlined, while the local
framings described in several of the alternative narratives seem to be more
comfortable with accepting a level of endemism. While we feel it is critical
to foster improved attention to local concerns, we are wary of falling into the
trap of simply exchanging global myths for local ones. As our case studies
demonstrate, it is impossible to separate local from global concerns, at the
level of microbes, or politics, or intervention. How might disease narratives

that take a multi-scale perspective, drawing together the near and the far, the fast and the slow, be fostered and put into circulation?

Shaping of narratives and their shaping effects

Recognizing that not all myths and narratives are created equal focuses attention on the processes that shape such inequality. What kinds of pressures enable some narratives to become and remain dominant – to grab scientific, public and policy attention – while others remain marginalized and even hidden? In this section, we briefly consider some of the key processes which the cases have identified as important in shaping narratives, especially dominant ones. We then address how some of the disease narratives in our case studies have shaped responses to diseases (and what the unintended consequences of this have been), as well as the paths described in other narratives that have not been taken.

In part, the relative power of epidemic narratives reflects the position and status of their proponents on an international stage. However, the case studies also indicate how a range of political, institutional and cognitive pressures may interlock in processes of governmentality (Burchell et al, 1991, p2) so that certain views become linked with more diffuse power relations. As Dry's chapter explored, today these relations implicate complex architectures extending across international and local scales, and encompassing public, private and hybrid institutions. Power dynamics, perhaps inevitably, encourage and enable powerful institutions to pursue strategies that maintain the status quo. Eradicating a disease or controlling an epidemic – or at least claiming to do so – is a powerful way of asserting political authority, whether this is the authority of an international health regime or of a national political one. Bloom's discussion of the SARS case alludes to this, where the Chinese government was initially reluctant to acknowledge the epidemic because of the implied threats to national authority and sovereignty. Yet once the disease was in the open, interests in maintaining strong state authority and social control, and disease eradication, have gone hand-in-hand – and reports suggest that this has continued in the tough state-orchestrated response to H1N1 influenza (Wong, 2009).

Political-economic interests are also at stake in the shaping of narratives, and in their relative power. The case of obesity illustrates this particularly starkly. Millstone shows how the junk food industry has actively constructed and promoted narratives that portray obesity as an individual lifestyle problem, unrelated to the 'obesogenic' food and advertising environment that the industry has helped create, to avoid blame and protect its commercial interests. The political economy of international funding flows also emerges as key, if not in the initial shaping of narratives, then certainly in sustaining them. Thus in the case of avian influenza, Scoones notes the huge amounts of public cash which have been invested in the standard, global surveillance, early warning and rapid response repertoires of the main agencies. As Calain (2007b) has argued of global public health and surveillance more generally, there are strong financial and economic pressures in play to maintain certain styles of response and their associated funding streams.

Institutional pressures are also at work, whether in international agencies, government or civil society organizations. Thus in exploring narratives produced and perpetuated by international agencies, for instance, our case studies have shown the 'institutional fit' between global outbreak narratives around various diseases and the WHO, and AIDS exceptionalist narratives and UNAIDS. The remits, structures and practices of particular institutions make certain kinds of narrative and response logical and feasible, while closing out others. As Scoones argues in the case of avian influenza, for example, the organizational mandates of international agencies such as the WHO and FAO are not geared up to deal with ignorance and surprise; the very existence and status of the agencies is dependent on the idea that outbreaks and their effects can be known about and thus rendered amenable to management. In these circumstances, planning procedures that are oriented towards risk management through outbreak containment at source are appealing and come to dominate. Bureaucratic procedures – in the way that outbreak alert and response programmes are organized – interlock with and support such framings. Over time, such responses and their supporting narratives can become routinized, as the 'repeated practices and behaviours' that constitute institutions (North, 1990).

Added to these political, economic and institutional pressures are professional, disciplinary and cognitive ones. In several of the case studies, we have seen how particular disciplinary cultures shape narratives – with those centred around biomedicine and epidemiology, and their emphasis on disease-focused, often quantitative assessments, coming to dominate. Understandings from ecology, history, social sciences and local knowledge are thus squeezed out. Yet different disciplinary and professional traditions inspire alternative narratives. In the case of Ebola, for example, Leach and Hewlett's contribution shows how anthropological perspectives have been key in shaping narratives about the integration of local knowledge, and environmental and ecological sciences are helping to generate a fourth narrative centred on disease–ecological dynamics. Several of our cases have addressed the interplay between professionalized knowledge and expertise, and the unofficial knowledge held by members of the public, including people living with diseases and the frontline health staff who interact with them. The relatively weak power of unofficial expertise in shaping those disease narratives which become dominant, and yet their value – especially in contributing to alternative narratives which acknowledge longer-term social–disease–ecological dynamics and social justice concerns – has been a recurring theme. Finally, as the cases of Ebola, SARS, H1N1 influenza and obesity have illustrated in different ways, the media often plays key roles in constructing and amplifying powerful narratives and associated public fears. In turn, this can help support the claims of powerful agencies to control the threat (see Wald, 2008). In short, the case studies begin to indicate how clusters of political, institutional and knowledge–power processes – which together constitute 'governance' in its broadest sense – help to produce and maintain particular narratives, while marginalizing others.

Just as it is easy to fall into the trap of treating narratives as actors, it is important to resist the temptation to assume that these 'actor narratives', even in their dominant form, have automatic effects. Narratives, because they shape understanding, define the framing of a relevant system and the key dynamics of interest (including the priority given to global or local scales, and the key question of whether a disease outbreak even counts as an epidemic) and suggest appropriate responses, do have the power to shape policy and action. But this is not automatic, nor is it equally true of all narratives.

In his chapter on HIV/AIDS, Edström highlights the limits of a vulnerability-based response to the epidemic. Edström describes how this approach, with its preoccupation with protecting vulnerable populations has led to policies that are too general in their focus, missing 'key populations' who act as super-spreaders of the disease. In her case study on grants, MacGregor analyses how a rights-based and exceptionalist narrative implicitly prioritizes the rights of healthy people infected with HIV ahead of those who are merely poor or unemployed. Though equity issues are arguably as significant in post-apartheid South Africa as the rights of HIV-positive citizens, the exceptionalist narrative has proved to be successful in promulgating policies that support the infected first. Bloom's study of the SARS outbreak suggests that a powerful shaping narrative assuming international consensus about the need for a coordinated global response missed the ongoing importance of national sovereignty concerns. Millstone's analysis of debates over obesity in Europe and America shows how powerful food lobbies urged government, with some success, not to intervene in the lives of citizens. Both Scoones, and Leach and Hewlett, emphasize the way in which certain narratives can limit the resilience and robustness of our responses. In the case of both Ebola and avian influenza, they show how dominant narratives for those diseases tend to foster pathways of response that rely on external scientific expertise and top-down (so-called global) interventions, such as large-scale culling of poultry, that may be unnecessary or counter-productive.

As discussed above, these global responses tend to privilege virulence and novelty above ongoing challenges to livelihoods and well-being posed both by disease dynamics and by intrusive interventions. The virulent Ebola virus receives much more attention than the low-level, quasi-endemic occurrences of Lassa fever. The effects of narratives can be even more dramatic, leading to negative unintended consequences. The case of H1N1 influenza in Egypt, described by Tadros, shows dramatically how a rapid and total approach can lead to a public health emergency. Similarly, Nightingale describes how misguided treatment of TB can make things worse by causing antibacterial resistance to frontline drugs. Such cases exemplify how certain pathways of response can generate effects which 'kick back' to shape the dynamics of disease themselves, bringing new implications for social justice – and who gains or loses – in their wake.

Looking forward – directions for future research and dialogue

As varied as our case studies are, there is inevitably much that we have missed. Much more could be said about the causes and effects of antibacterial resistance, a serious and growing problem. Antiviral resistance is also a concern, with one study showing 25 per cent of H1N1 viruses in Europe resistant to oseltamivir, a frontline response drug (Fleming et al, 2009). Waterborne and foodborne diseases are also highly significant sources of infection and sickness, and have received relatively little attention – certainly relative to the health damage they wreak. There are, of course, many other epidemic diseases that we could have included. Malaria, in particular, is a key disease, with over 1 million deaths annually, most of them young children in Africa. New tools such as insecticide-impregnated bednets and new antimalarial drugs have raised the hopes of some that malaria could even be eradicated. Increasing temperatures due to climate change, however, are expanding the range of the mosquito vector that spreads the disease, and weak health systems and the scale of the problem present serious challenges – along with growing evidence of emergent resistance to even the latest drug treatments. Case studies investigating the role of narratives in shaping responses to malaria at the global, national and local levels would be very welcome.

Other significant infectious diseases include:

- Chagas disease, spread by beetles that hide in the cracks of poorly built houses in regions of Latin America with high poverty;
- West Nile Virus, first identified in the US in 1999, and now present in all but three states;

- dengue fever, currently present in areas where 2.5 billion people live, and causing an estimated 50 to 100 million infections annually;
- lyssavirus infection and henipavirus infections, carried by fruit bats in many parts of Asia and Africa and causing encephalitis in humans.

This list could be much longer. Emerging and re-emerging infectious diseases continue to increase and case studies on their social–ecological–political dynamics, and the effects of narratives and policy responses, are thin on the ground.

In taking forward such case studies, more collaboration between natural and social scientists is clearly warranted. This will be important to overcome the cognitive divides that have pervaded so much analysis of epidemics, whereby particular disciplines end up shaping particular narratives that 'speak past' each other. The biology, ecology and virology of infectious diseases matter greatly to the nature of the epidemics they cause, and the responses they require. Social science brings tools for analysing how human behaviours contribute to the spread of disease, as well as more critical tools such as the narratives approach we have been developing, which can show the power of different understandings of the causes of diseases to shape pathways of response. But the vision suggested by this book is not just of a new generation of truly interdisciplinary, collaborative research activities, difficult as even these can be to mount. It is also of new styles of research–policy engagement, in which scientists, those in the hot seat of epidemics policy-making and prac-titioners dealing with these issues on the ground, can work together to explore particular narratives and their effects, and perhaps construct and implement new ones. Forms of participatory and action-oriented research, of delibera-tive dialogue, and of reflexive interaction through which both researchers and policy-makers make explicit and debate their particular framings may all find a place in such an agenda (see Leach et al, 2010).

There are several broad areas where such research–policy dialogue could make a difference to pathways of epidemic response, their effects and their consequences for social justice. The relationship between narratives and institutions deserves more attention. While, as the last section reviewed, our case studies have addressed elements of this relationship, they have not done so systematically and this is clearly an area warranting further research and discussion. Throughout our case studies, the importance of institutions such as the WHO and, to a lesser extent, FAO, has been emphasized. Often, we have been quite critical of the role of the WHO in helping to construct a certain type of 'global' emergency-oriented response. A potential rebuttal to this critique, however, is to say that the WHO is only as strong as the contri-butions and commitments of its member states. Are we asking too much of this organization? Answering this question requires taking a broad view that encompasses and involves a range of institutional actors (at the local, national and international level) in reflecting on the ways in which they either cooperate, ignore each other or work at cross-purposes in responding to a range of diseases, epidemic and endemic, chronic and acute. Much more work is needed that attempts to trace the relationship between which narratives become dominant for a given disease, and which institutions are key in formulating those narratives or implementing the responses they engender. This type of research, which could be termed political epidemiology, will require tracing flows of money and power from both large and smaller institutions to their endpoints. The outlook needs to broaden to explore not only the effect of centralized institutions such as the WHO, but also the relations between these institutions, state institutions and their combined effects on local populations. Conducted in a research-policy, or deliberative dialogue mode, it would involve people in those institutions reflecting on the flows which shape their own work – and what is thus excluded.

Another area for research and research-policy dialogue is the effectiveness of new forms of surveillance, such as event-based and information and communication technology (ICT) driven systems, in relation to broader systems of risk management-based surveillance (discussed in Dry and Scoones, this volume). There has been very little analysis or reflection on how these interventions have affected the kinds of outbreaks that are noted, and whether the information gathered is of any ongoing use to local populations. One might apply a similar political, research-policy lens to projects aimed at discovering future diseases before they emerge. How do these projects, exemplified by the 'origins' initiative focusing on populations exposed to wild animal populations that may act as reservoirs for disease (Wolfe et al, 2007), feed into a broader culture of precise forecasting? What kinds of dynamics and uncertainties are excluded from these approaches, and what kinds of interventions would be needed to address them?

Identifying truly interdisciplinary and integrated research-policy questions, which draw on the strengths of varied approaches, is not easy. Taking forward the work to address these is harder still, challenging as it is to the many disciplinary, policy and institutional silos that characterize understandings of and responses to epidemics. The first step, however, is recognizing there is a need. We hope that this volume can serve as an initial move towards a shared agenda for research and action, in which concerns with science, politics and social justice are integrated in new ways towards the building of sustainable, effective pathways of epidemics response.

Notes

1   http://data.unaids.org/Media/Speeches02/SP_Piot_LSE_08Feb05_en.pdf, accessed 6 December 2009.

References

'A national security issue' (2009) *Al Ahram*, 5 May, p4

'A very piggish affair' (2009) *Al Distour*, 7 May, p1

'Cairo under the pigsties' siege' (2009) *Al Masry AlYoum*, 27 April, p1

'Capital collection' (2002) *Al Ahram*, 28 February–6 March 2002, features page, http://weekly.ahram.org.eg/2002/575/sc3.htm, accessed 9 October 2009

'Culling of 100 pigs in Kafr el Sheikh' (2009) *Ros al Youssef*, 28 April, p3

'Dr Mohammed Badei: The pig carries 493 diseases' (2009) *Ikhwan* online, 29 April, available at www.ikhwanonline.com/Article.asp?ArtID=48352&SecID=250, accessed 18 August 2009

'Dumping the Zabaleen' (2002) *Al Ahram Weekly*, 11–17 July, http://weekly.ahram.org.eg/2002/594/eg7.htm, accessed 9 September 2009

'Egypt's pig cull not a swine flu measure' (2009) 1 May, www.medicalnewstoday.com/articles/148430.php, accessed 26 November 2009

'Enlightened Copts and sectarian lies' (2009) *AlWatany al Youm*, 12 May

'Insect study provokes questions over obesity causes' (2006) 21 September, available at www.obesitydiscussion.com/forums/miscellaneous-obesity-studies/insect-study-provokes-questions-obesity-2350.html, accessed 21 November 2009

'Kill the one whose religion you know' (2009) *Al Akhbar*, 3 May, p17

'Killing and not relocating [pigs]' (2009) *Al Ahram al Araby*, 2 May, p4

'North Karelia Project' (undated) available at www.ktl.fi/portal/english/research_people_programs/health_promotion_and_chronic_disease_prevention/projects/cindi/north_karelia_project/accessed 22 November 2009

'O ye Ummah' (2009) *Al Distour*, 2 May, p6

'Pigs in government refrigerators' (2009) *Al Ahrar*, 1 May, p3

'Pigs ... the ticking bomb' (2009) *Al Ahram*, 27 April, p3

'Slaughter or culling' (2009) *Al Wafd*, 1 May, p3

'Specific protein the answer to rising obesity' (2005) www.foodnavigator.com/Science-Nutrition/Specific-protein-the-answer-to-rising-obesity, issued 19 August 2005, accessed 22 Sept 2008

'The Coalition's Salon: The Swine Flu is more dangerous than the hydraulic bomb!' (2009) *Ikhwan* online, 29 April, available at www.ikhwanonline.com/Article.asp?ArtID=48318&SecID=250, accessed 6 October 2009

'The Coptic [women] MPs give the Muslim Brotherhood a lesson in civicness' (2009) *Al Musawer*, 6 May

'The crisis of Giza's garbage heightens' (2009) *Al Masry al Youm*, 3 September, p5

'The Ministry of Health's pessimistic plan for the spread of the virus to Egypt' (2009) *Al Distour*, 2 May, p2

'The People's Assembly decides to cull pigs immediately' (2009) *Al Ahrar*, 2 April, p1

'The People's Assembly obliges the government to kill the pigs in situ' (2009) *Ikhwan online*, 28 April, available at www.ikhwanonline.com/Article.asp?ArtID=48291&SecID=250, accessed 19 August 2009

'The pig fitna and the wisdom of the Pope' (2009) *Al Moussawer*, 6 May, p8

'The pigsties a ticking bomb' (2009) *Nisf el Donya*, 3 May, p22

'The victory of the pigs over the Minister of Health' (2009) *Al Distour*, 7 May, p6

'Warning against transforming the influenza into sectarianism' (2009) *Al Gomhorriyya*, 3 May

Abou Zahr, C., Cleland, J., Coullare, F., Macfarlane, S., Notzon, F., Setel, P. and Szreter, S. (2007) 'Who counts? 4', *Lancet*, vol 370, no 9601, pp1791–1799

Abraham, T. (2005) *Twenty-First Century Plague: The Story of SARS*, Johns Hopkins University Press, Baltimore, MD

Abuja Declaration (2001) available at www.wwan.cn/ga/aids/pdf/abuja_declaration.pdf, accessed 21 May 2009

Achmat, Z. and Roberts, R. (2005) *Steering the Storm: TB and HIV in South Africa. A policy paper of the Treatment Action Campaign*, available at www.tac.org.za/Documents/TBPaperForConference-1.pdf, accessed 3 December 2009

Ahmed, Y., Mwaba, P., Chintu, C., Grange, J., Ustianowski, A. and Zumla, A. (1999) 'A study of maternal mortality at the University Teaching Hospital, Lusaka, Zambia', *The International Journal of Tuberculosis and Lung Disease*, vol 3, pp675–680

AIDSCAP (1996) 'Behaviour change: A summary of four major theories', Behavioural Research Unit, Family Health International, available at ww2.fhi.org/en/aids/aidscap/aidspubs/behres/bcr4theo.html, accessed 3 December 2009

Aldis, W. (2008) 'Health security as a public health concept: A critical analysis', *Health Policy and Planning*, vol 23, no 6, pp369–375

Altman, D. (2001) *Global Sex*, University of Chicago Press, Chicago, IL

Arram, S. (2009) Unpublished MA Thesis, American University in Cairo

Baker, M. and Fidler, D. (2006) 'Global public health surveillance under new international health regulations', *Emerging Infectious Diseases*, vol 12, pp1058–1065

Balee, W. (ed) (2002) *Advances in Historical Ecology*, Columbia University Press, New York

Barnett, T. and Blaikie, P. (1992) *AIDS in Africa: Its Present and Future Impact*, Belhaven Press, London

Barnett, T. and Whiteside, A. (2002) *AIDS in the Twenty-First Century: Disease and Globalisation*, Palgrave Macmillan, Basingstoke

Barrett, R., Kuzawa, C., McDade, T. and Armelagos, G. (1998) 'Emerging and re-emerging infectious diseases: The third epidemiologic transition', *Annual Review of Anthropology*, vol 27, pp247–271

Bartlett, C., Kickbusch, I. and Coulombier, D. (2006) *Cultural and Governance Influence on Detection, Identification and Monitoring of Human Disease*, Infectious Diseases: Preparing for the Future, Foresight Project, UK Department of Trade and Industry, London

Bashford, A. (ed) (2006) *Medicine at the Border: Disease, Globalization and Security, 1850 to the Present*, Palgrave Macmillan, Basingstoke

Bhattacharya, S. (2006) 'WHO-led or WHO-managed? Re-assessing the smallpox eradication programme in India, 1960-1980', in Bashford, A. (ed.) *Medicine at the Border: Disease, Globalization and Security, 1850 to the Present*, Palgrave Macmillan, London, pp60–75

Bates, I., Fenton, C., Gruber, J., Lalloo, D., Lara, A. M., Squire, S. B., Theobald, S., Thomson, R. and Tolhurst, R. (2004) 'Vulnerability to malaria, tuberculosis and HIV/AIDS infection and disease. Part 1: Determinants operating at individual and household level', *Lancet, Infectious Diseases*, vol 4, no 6, pp368–375

Bates, J. and Stead, W. (1993) 'The history of tuberculosis as a global epidemic', *Medical Clinics of North America*, vol 77, pp1205–1217

Bausch, D., Feldmann, H., Geisbert, T., Bray, M., Sprecher, A., Boumandouki, P., Rollin, P., Roth, C. and the Winnipeg Filovirus Clinical Working Group (2007) 'Outbreaks of filovirus hemorrhagic fever: Time to refocus on the patient', *Journal of Infectious Diseases*, vol 196, suppl 2, ppS136–S141

Bayer, R. and Wilkinson, D. (1995) 'Directly observed therapy for tuberculosis: History of an idea', *Lancet*, vol 345, no 8964, pp1545–1548

Beck, U. (1998) *World Risk Society*, Polity Press, Cambridge

Beck, U. (2008) *World at Risk*, Polity Press, Cambridge

Beck, U., Giddens, A. and Lash, S. (1994) *Reflexive Modernization: Politics and Tradition in the Modern Social Order*, Polity Press, Cambridge

Bhatti, N., Law, M., Morris, J., Halliday, R. and Moore-Gillon, J. (1995) 'Increasing incidence of tuberculosis in England and Wales: A study of the likely causes', *British Medical Journal*, vol 310, pp967–969

Birmingham, K. and Kenyon, G. (2001) 'Lassa fever is unheralded problem in West Africa', *Nature Medicine*, vol 8, p878

Bloom, G., Edström, J., Leach, M., Lucas, H., MacGregor, H., Standing, H. and Waldman, L. (2007) *Health in a Dynamic World*, STEPS Working Paper 5, STEPS Centre, Institute of Development Studies, Brighton

Bloom, G., Kanjlal, B. and Peters, D. (2008a) 'Regulating health care markets in China and India', *Health Affairs*, vol 27, no 4, p952

Bloom, G., Standing, H. and Lloyd, R. (2008b) 'Markets, information asymmetry and health care: Towards new social contracts', *Social Science and Medicine*, vol 66, no 10, pp2076–2087

Bloom, G., Fang, L., Jonsson, K., Rithy Men, C., Bounfeng, P., Xeuatyongsa, A., Wang, Y. and Zhao, H. (2008c) 'Health policy processes in Asian transitional economies', in Meessen, B., Pei, X., Criel, B. and Bloom, G. (eds) *Health and Social Protection: Experiences from China, Cambodia and Lao PDR*, Institute of Tropical Medicine, Antwerp, available at www.povill.com/enjkw/emeetcont.aspx?id=5, accessed 3 December 2009

Bloom, G., Liu, Y. and Qiao, J. (2009) 'A partnership for health in China', *IDS Practice Paper*, vol 2009, no 2, Institute of Development Studies, Brighton

Blower, S., McLean, A., Porco, T., Small, P., Hopwell, P., Sanchez, M. and Moss, A. (1995) 'The intrinsic transmission dynamics of tuberculosis epidemics', *Nature Medicine*, vol 1, pp815–821

Blume, S. and Zanders, M. (2006) 'Vaccine independence, local competences and globalisation: Lessons from the history of pertussis vaccines', *Social Science and Medicine*, vol 63, no 7, pp1825–1835

Booth, P. and Silber, G. (2008) 'A draft briefing document for the establishment of a chronic diseases grant', SANAC Treatment, Care and Support Technical Task Team, available at http://alp.immedia.co.za/research/TTT%20CDG%20Position%20Paper%20FINAL.pdf, accessed 25 February 2010

Borchert, M., Boelaert, M., Sleurs, H., Muyembe-Tamfum, J. J., Pirard, P., Colebunders, R., Van der Stuyft, P. and Van der Groen, G. (2000) 'Viewpoint – Filovirus haemorrhagic fever outbreaks: Much ado about nothing?', *Tropical Medicine and International Health*, vol 5, no 5, pp318–324

Borg, P. and Fogelholm, M. (2007) 'Stakeholder appraisal of policy options for responding to obesity in Finland', *Obesity Reviews*, vol 8, supp 2, pp47–52

Boyce, P. (2007) '"Conceiving Kothis": Men who have sex with men in India and the cultural subject of HIV prevention', *Medical Anthropology*, vol 26, no 2, pp175–203

Brody, J. (1985) 'Panel terms obesity a major US killer needing top priority', *New York Times*, 14 February, pA1

Brown, D. (2003) 'Bushmeat and poverty alleviation: Implications for development policy', *ODI Wildlife Policy Briefing*, November, No 2, ODI, London

Brown, G. (2008) 'Preface' to the UK Department of Health's *Healthy Weight, Healthy Lives: A Cross-Government Strategy for England*, 23 January, piv, Department of Health, London

Brown, P. (2000) 'Drug resistant tuberculosis can be controlled, says WHO', *British Medical Journal*, vol 320, p821

Brown, S. and Eisenhardt, K. (1997) 'The art of continuous change: Linking complexity theory and time-paced evolution in relentlessly shifting organizations', *Administrative Science Quarterly*, vol 42, no 1, pp1–34

Brown, T., Cueto, T. and Fee, E. (2006) 'The World Health Organization and the transition from "International" to "Global" Health', in Bashford, A. (ed) *Medicine at the Border: Disease, Globalization and Security, 1850 to the Present*, Palgrave Macmillan, Basingstoke

Brownstein, J., Freifeld, C., Reis, B. and Mandl, K. (2008) 'Surveillance sans frontières: Internet-based emerging infectious disease intelligence and the HealthMap Project', *PLoS Medicine*, vol 5, no 7, pp1019–1024

Brownstein, J., Freifeld, C. and Madoff, L. (2009) 'Digital disease detection: Harnessing the web for public health surveillance', *New England Journal of Medicine*, vol 360, no 21, pp2153–2157

Buehler, J., Berkelman, R., Hartley, D. and Peters, C. (2003) 'Syndromic surveillance and bioterrorism-related epidemics', *Emerging Infectious Diseases*, vol 9, pp1197–1204

Burchell, P., Gordon, C. and Miller, P. (eds) (1991) *The Foucault Effect: Studies in Governmentality*, University of Chicago Press, Chicago, IL

Bureau of Tuberculosis Control (1991) *Tuberculosis in New York City*, Bureau of Tuberculosis Control, New York

Burns, A., Van der Mensbrugghe, D. and Timmer, H. (2006) *Evaluating the Economic Consequences of Avian Influenza*, World Bank, Washington, DC, available at http://siteresources.worldbank.org/INTTOPAVIFLU/Resources/EvaluatingAIeconomics.pdf, accessed 1 October 2009

Burton, B., Foster, W., Hirsch, J. and Van Itallie, T. (1985) 'Health implications of obesity: An NIH consensus development conference', *International Journal of Obesity*, vol 9, no 3, pp155–170

Butler, D. (2006) 'Disease surveillance needs a revolution', *Nature*, vol 440, pp6–7

Cahn, P., Perez, H., Ben, G. and Ochoa, C. (2003) 'Tuberculosis and HIV: A partnership against the most vulnerable', *Journal of the International Association of Physicians in AIDS Care*, vol 2, no 3, pp106–123

Calain, P. (2007a) 'Exploring the international arena of global public health surveillance', *Health Policy Plan*, vol 22, no 1, pp2–12

Calain, P. (2007b) 'From the field side of the binoculars: A different view on global public health surveillance', *Health Policy Plan*, vol 22, no 1, pp13–20

Calain, P. and Fidler, D. (2007) 'XDR tuberculosis, the new International Health Regulations, and human rights', *Global Health Governance*, vol 1, no 1, pp1–3

Calain, P., Fiore, N., Poncin, M. and Hurst, S. (2009) 'Research ethics and international epidemic response: The case of Ebola and Marburg hemorrhagic fevers', *Public Health Ethics*, vol 2, no 1, pp7–29

Campos, P. (2004) *The Obesity Myth: Why America's Obsession with Weight is Hazardous to your Health*, Gotham Books, New York

Castro, A. and Singer, M. (eds) (2004) *Unhealthy Health Policy: A Critical Anthropological Examination*, Alta Mira, Walnut Creek, CA

CDC (2006) *Extensively Drug-Resistant Tuberculosis (XDR TB) – Update*, Centers for Disease Control, Atlanta

Center for Consumer Freedom (2009) available at www.consumerfreedom.com/about.cfm, accessed 19 November 2009

Center for Science in the Public Interest (2009) available at www.cspinet.org/integrity/nonprofits/center_for_consumer_freedom_ccf_.html, accessed 19 November 2009

Chambers, R. (1989) 'Introduction' in *Vulnerability, Coping and Policy*, IDS Bulletin, vol 20, no 2

Chen, L., Leaning, J. and Narasimhan, V. (eds) (2003) *Global Health Challenges for Human Security*, Harvard University Press, Cambridge, MA

Chernin, E. (1988) 'Sir Ronald Ross, malaria and the rewards of research', *Medical History*, vol 32, pp119–141

Chiang, C. and Riley, L. (2005) 'Exogenous re-infection in tuberculosis', *Lancet Infectious Diseases*, vol 5, pp629–636

Chin, J. (2008) 'The myth of a general AIDS pandemic: How billions are wasted on unnecessary AIDS prevention programmes', *Campaign for Fighting Diseases Discussion Paper no 2*, School of Public Health, University of California, Berkeley, CA

Chintu, C. and Zumla, A. (1995) 'Childhood tuberculosis and infection with HIV', *Journal of the Royal College of Physicians of London*, vol 29, pp160–172

Chretien, J. (1990) 'Tuberculosis and HIV: The cursed duet', *Bulletin of the Union against Tuberculosis and Lung Disease*, vol 65, no 1, pp25–32

Christiakis, N. and Fowler, J. (2007) 'The spread of obesity in a large social network over 32 years', *The New England Journal of Medicine*, vol 357, pp370–379

Cobertt, E., Watt, C., Walker, N., Mahder, D., Williams, B., Raviglione, M. and Dye, C. (2003) 'The growing burden of tuberculosis: Global trends and interactions with the HIV epidemic', *Archives of Internal Medicine*, vol 163, pp1009–1021

Coburn, B., Wagner, B. and Blower, S. (2009) 'Modelling influenza epidemics and pandemics: Insights into the future of swine flu (H1N1)', *BMC Medicine*, vol 7, p30

Coetzee, D., Boulle, A., Hildebrand, K., Asselman, V., Van Cutsem, G. and Goemaere, E. (2004) 'Promoting adherence to antiretroviral therapy: The experience from a primary care setting in Khayelitsha, South Africa', *AIDS*, vol 18, suppl 3, ppS27–S31

Cohen, D. (1993) 'The economic impact of the HIV epidemic', *HIV and Development Programme*, Issues Papers no 2, UNDP, New York

Cohen-Cole, E. and Fletcher, J. (2008) 'Is obesity contagious? Social networks vs. environmental factors in the obesity epidemic', *Journal of Health Economics*, vol 27, pp1382–1387

Coker, R. (1998) 'Lessons from New York's tuberculosis epidemic', *British Medical Journal*, vol 317, p616

Colebunders, R., John, L., Huyst, V., Kambugu, A., Scano, F. and Lynen, L. (2006) 'Tuberculosis immune reconstitution inflammatory syndrome in countries with limited resources', *International Journal of Tuberculosis and Lung Disease*, vol 10, pp946–953

Collins, D. and Leibbrandt, M. (2007) 'The financial impact of HIV/AIDS on poor households in South Africa', *AIDS*, vol 21, suppl 7, ppS75–S81

Coninx, R., Maher, D., Reyes, H. and Grzemska, M. (2000) 'Tuberculosis in prisons in countries with high prevalence', *British Medical Journal*, vol 320, pp440–442

Cowen, J., Dembour, M. and Wilson, R. (eds) (2001) 'Introduction' in *Culture and Rights: Anthropological Perspectives,* Cambridge University Press, Cambridge

Cox, H., Morrow, M. and Deutschmann, P. (2008) 'Long term efficacy of DOTS regimens for tuberculosis: Systematic review', *British Medical Journal*, vol 336, pp484–487

Crawford, D. (2007) *Deadly Companions: How Microbes Shaped our History*, Oxford University Press, Oxford

Cross-Government Obesity Unit (2008) Department of Health and Department of Children, Schools and Families, *Healthy Weight, Healthy Lives: A Cross Government Strategy for England*, 23 January, available at www.dh.gov.uk/en/Publicationsandstatistics/Publications/PublicationsPolicyAndGuidance/DH_082378, accessed 21 November 2009

Cunningham, K. (2005) Oral presentation at 1st annual Obesity Europe Conference, Brussels, 14–15 June

Dahle, U. (2005) 'TB in immigrants is not public health risk, but uncontrolled epidemics are', *British Medical Journal*, vol 331, pp237–237

Daniel, T. (2006) 'The history of tuberculosis', *Respiratory Medicine*, vol 100, pp1862–1870

Davies, S. (2008) 'Securitizing infectious disease', *International Affairs*, vol 84, no 2, pp295–313

De Cock, K. and Chaisson, R. (1999) 'Will DOTS do it? A reappraisal of tuberculosis control in countries with high rates of HIV infection', *International Journal of Tuberculosis and Lung Disease*, vol 3, no 6, pp457–465

De Paoli, M., Mills, E. and Grønningsæter, A. (2008) '"It is about my life". AIDS, social grants and the HIV roll-out in South Africa: Is there a tension between health, economy and welfare?', Poster Presentation, XVII International AIDS Conference, Mexico City

De Waal, A. (2006), *AIDS and Power*, Polity Press, Cambridge

Del Amo, J., Malin, A., Pozniak, A. and De Cock, K. (1999) 'Does tuberculosis accelerate the progression of HIV disease? Evidence from basic science and epidemiology', *AIDS*, vol 13, no 10, pp1151–1158

Delpeuch, F., Maire, B., Minnier, E. and Holdsworth, M. (2009) *Globesity: A Planet Out of Control*, Earthscan, London

Denys, C., Lecompte, E., Calvet, E., Camara, M. D., Dore, A., Koulemou, K., Kourouma, F., Soropogui, B., Sylla, O., Allai-Kouadio, B., Kouassi-Kan, S., Akoua-Koffi, C., Ter

Meulen, J. and Koivogui, L. (2005) 'Community analysis of muridae (mammalia, rodentia) diversity in Guinea: A special emphasis on Mastomys species and Lassa fever distributions', in Huber, B. A. et al (eds) *African Biodiversity*, Springer, Dordrecht, The Netherlands, pp339–350

Department of Health (2007) *About Small Change, Big Difference*, 8 February, available at www.dh.gov.uk/en/Publichealth/Healthimprovement/Smallchangebigdifference/DH_4134038, accessed 21 November 2009

Devereux, S. (2001) 'Livelihood insecurity and social protection: A re-emerging issue in rural development', *Development Policy Review*, vol 19, no 4, pp507–519

Dionisio, D., Cao, Y., Hongzhou, L., Kraisintu, K. and Messeri, D. (2006) 'Affordable anti-retroviral drugs for the under-served markets: How to expand equitable access against the backdrop of challenging scenarios?' *Current HIV Research*, vol 4, no 1, pp3–20

Doak, C. (2002) 'Large-scale interventions and programmes addressing nutrition-related chronic diseases and obesity: Examples from 14 countries', *Public Health Nutrition*, vol 5(1A), pp275–277

Dondorp, A., Nosten, F., Yi, P., Das, D., Phyo, A. P., Tarning, J., Lwin, K. M., Ariey, F., Hanpithakpong, W., Lee, S. J., Ringwald, P., Silamut, K., Imwong, M., Chotivanich, K., Lim, P., Herdman, T., An, S., Yeung, S., Pratap, S., Day, N., Lindegardh, N., Socheat, D. and White, N. J. (2009) 'Artemisinin resistance in *Plasmodium falciparum* malaria', *New England Journal of Medicine*, vol 361, no 5, pp455–467

Dorrington, R. (2005) 'Population projections for the Western Cape 2001 to 2025', report prepared for PGWC (Provincial Government of Western Cape), Centre for Actuarial Research, Cape Town, available at www.capegateway.gov.za/Text/2006/10/western_cape_hiv_aids_infection_mortality_fertility_population_projections_report.doc, accessed 20 May 2009

DRC (Development Research Centre) (2005) 'An evaluation and recommendations on the reforms of the health system in China', *China Development Review*, Supplement, vol 7, no 1, pp1–259

Dye, C., Scheele, S., Dolin, P., Pathania, V. and Raviglione, M. (1999) 'Global burden of TB: Estimated incidence, prevalence and mortality by country', *JAMA*, vol 282, pp677–686

Dye, C., Williams, B., Espinal, M. and Raviglione, M. (2002) 'Erasing the world's slow stain: Strategies to beat multidrug-resistant tuberculosis', *Science*, vol 295, pp2042–2046

Edström, J. (2007) 'Rethinking "vulnerability" and social protection for children affected by AIDS', *IDS Bulletin*, vol 38, no 3, pp101–105, IDS, Brighton

Edström, J., with Turquet, L. and Young, I. (2006) 'AIDS: Questions for development', *IDS Policy Briefing*, Issue 32, July, IDS, Brighton

Egger, G. and Swinburn, B. (2002) 'An "ecological" approach to the obesity pandemic', in Marks, D. F. (ed) *The Health Psychology Reader*, pp186–194, Sage, London, cited by Giles, D., 'Narratives of obesity as presented in the context of a television talk show', *Journal of Health Psychology*, vol 8, no 3, pp317–326

Egger, G., Swinburn, B. and Rossner, S. (2003) 'Dusting off the epidemiological triad: Could it work with obesity', *Obesity Reviews*, vol 4, p115

Eggleston, K., Li, L., Meng, Q., Lindelow, M. and Wagstaff, A. (2006) 'Health service delivery in China: A literature review', World Bank Policy Research Working Paper 3978, World Bank, Washington, DC

Elbe, S. (2005) 'AIDS, security, biopolitics', *International Relations,* vol 19, no 4, pp403–419

Elbe, S. (2006) 'HIV/AIDS: A human security challenge', *The Whitehead Journal of Diplomacy and International Relations,* Winter/Spring, pp1–13

Elbe, S. (2009) *Virus Alert: Security, Governmentality and the AIDS Pandemic,* Columbia University Press, New York

Elzinga, G., Raviglione, M. C. and Maher, D. (2004) 'Scale up: Meeting targets in global tuberculosis control', *Lancet,* vol 363, pp814–819

England, R. (2007) 'Are we spending too much on HIV?', *British Medical Journal,* vol 334, no 7589, p344

England, R. (2008) 'The writing is on the wall for UNAIDS', *British Medical Journal,* vol 336, no 7652, p1072

Englund, H. (2006) *Prisoners of Freedom: Human Rights and the African Poor,* University of California Press, Berkeley, CA

Espinal, M. A. (2003) 'The global situation of MDR-TB', *Tuberculosis,* vol 83, pp44–51

Espinal, M. A. and Dye, C. (2005) 'Can DOTS control multidrug-resistant tuberculosis?', *Lancet,* vol 365, no 9466, pp1239–1245

Fairhead, J. (2008) 'Climate, history and emerging diseases in West African forests', Seminar presented to the Wellcome/WHO history series, Geneva, May

Fairhead, J. and Leach, M. (1996) *Misreading the African Landscape: Society and Ecology in a Forest-Savanna Mosaic,* Cambridge University Press, Cambridge

Fairhead, J. and Leach, M. (1998) *Reframing Deforestation: Global Analyses and Local Realities – Studies in West Africa,* Routledge, London

Fang, J. (2008) 'The Chinese health care regulatory institutions in an era of transition', *Social Science and Medicine,* vol 66, no 4, pp952–962

FAO (2009) 'The developing world's new burden: Obesity', available at www.fao.org/FOCUS/E/obesity/obes1.htm, accessed 6 December 2009

FAO and OIE (2008) 'The global strategy for prevention and control of H5N1 highly pathogenic avian influenza', FAO, Rome, www.fao.org/avianflu/en/index.html, accessed 1 October 2009

FAO, OIE, WHO, UNSIC, UNICEF and World Bank (2008) 'Contributing to One World, One Health. A strategic framework for reducing risks of infectious diseases at the animal–human–ecosystems interface', 14 October, consultation document, Sharm-el-Sheikh, Egypt

Farmer, P. (1992) *AIDS and Accusation: Haiti and the Geography of Blame,* University of California Press, Berkeley, CA

Farmer, P. (1995) 'Culture, poverty and the dynamics of HIV transmission in rural Haiti', in Brummelhuis, H. and Herdt, G. (eds) *Culture and Sexual Risk: Anthropological Perspectives on AIDS,* Gordon and Breach, Amsterdam

Farmer, P. (1996) 'Social inequalities and emerging infectious diseases', *Emerging Infectious Diseases,* vol 2, no 4, pp259–269

Farmer, P. (1999a) *Infections and Inequalities: The Modern Plagues,* University of California Press, Berkeley, CA

Farmer, P. (1999b) 'Cruel and unusual: Drug resistant tuberculosis as punishment', in Stern, V. and Jones, R. (eds) *Sentence to Die? The Problem of TB in Prisons in East and Central Europe and Central Asia,* International Centre for Prison Studies, London

Farmer, P. (2003) *Pathologies of Power: Health, Human Rights, and the New War on the Poor*, University of California Press, Berkeley, CA

Farmer, P. (2007) 'From "marvelous momentum" to health care for all: Success is possible with the right programs', response to L. Garrett, *Foreign Affairs*, vol 86, no 2, pp155–161

Farmer, P., Furin, J. J. and Shin, S. S. (2000) 'Managing multidrug-resistant tuberculosis', *Journal of Respiratory Diseases*, vol 21, pp53–56

Farmer, P., Nizeye, B., Stulac, S. and Keshavjee, S. (2006) 'Structural violence and clinical medicine', *PLoS Medicine*, vol 3, e449

Fassin, D. and Schneider, H. (2003) 'The politics of AIDS in South Africa: Beyond the controversies', *British Medical Journal*, vol 326, pp495–497

Ferguson, N. M., Cummings, D. A., Cauchemez, S., Fraser, C., Riley, S., Meeyai, A., Lamsirithaworn, S. and Burke, D. S. (2005) 'Strategies for containing an emerging influenza pandemic in Southeast Asia', *Nature*, vol 437, p209–214

Fidler, D. (1996) 'Globalization, international law, and emerging diseases', *Emerging Infectious Diseases*, vol 2, pp77–84

Fidler, D. (1997) 'Return of the fourth horseman: Emerging infectious diseases and international law', *Minnesota Law Review*, vol 8, pp771–868

Fidler, D. (2004) *SARS, Governance and the Globalization of Disease*, Palgrave Macmillan, Basingstoke

Fidler, D. (2005) 'From international sanitary conventions to global health security: The new International Health Regulations', *Chinese Journal of International Law*, vol 4, no 2, pp325–392

Fidler, D. (2007) 'Architecture amidst anarchy: Global health's quest for governance', *Global Health Governance*, vol 1, no 1, pp1–17

Fidler, D. (2008) 'Influenza virus samples, international law, and global health diplomacy', *Emerging Infectious Diseases*, vol 14, no 1, www.cdc.gov/EID/content/14/1/pdfs/88.pdf, accessed 3 August 2009

Fleming, D., Elliot, A., Meijer, A. and Paget, W. (2009) 'Influenza virus resistance to oseltamivir: What are the implications?', *The European Journal of Public Health*, vol 19, no 1, pp238–239

Foresight (2006) *Infectious Diseases: Preparing for the Future. Executive Summary*, Office of Science and Innovation, London

Foucault, M. (1997) 'The birth of biopolitics', in Rabinow, P. (ed) *Michel Foucault, Ethics: Subjectivity and Truth*, The New Press, New York

Freeman, M., Patel, V., Collins, P. and Bertolote, J. (2005) 'Integrating mental health in global initiatives for HIV/AIDS', *British Journal of Psychiatry*, vol 187, pp1–3

Frieden, T. R., Fujiwara, P. I., Washko, R. M. and Hamburg, M. A. (1995) 'Tuberculosis in New York City – turning the tide', *New England Journal of Medicine*, vol 333, pp229–233

Froguel, P. (2007) 'Influence of the genome on human obesity risk and associated phenotypes', paper presented to a conference organized by the Biotechnology Group and Chemical Biology Forum of the Royal Society of Chemistry, 9 July, London

Galaz, V., Crona, B., Daw, T., Nyström, M., Bodin, O., Olsson, P. (2009) 'Can web crawlers revolutionize ecological monitoring?', *Frontiers in Ecology and the Environment e-View*, www.esajournals.org/doi/abs/10.1890/070204?prevSearch=null&searchHistoryKey=, accessed 1 October 2009

Gandy, M. and Zumla, Z. (2002) 'The resurgence of disease: Social and historical perspectives on the "new" tuberculosis', *Social Science and Medicine*, vol 55, pp385–396

Gao, F., Bailes, E., Robertson, D., Chen, Y., Rodenburg, C., Michael, S., Cummins, L., Arthur, L., Peeters, M., Shaw, G., Sharp, P. and Hahn, B. (1999) 'Origin of HIV-1 in the chimpanzee *Pan troglodytes troglodytes*', *Nature*, vol 397, no 6718, pp436–441

Garrett, L. (1994) *The Coming Plague: Newly Emerging Diseases in a World out of Balance*, Penguin, New York

Garrett, L. (2000) *Betrayal of Trust: The Collapse of Global Public Health*, Hyperion, New York

Garrett, L. (2007) 'The challenge of global health', *Foreign Affairs*, vol 86, no 1, pp14–38

Ghandi, N. R., Moll, A., Sturm, A. W., Pawinski, R., Govender, T., Lalloo, U., Zeller, K., Andrews, J. and Friedland, G. (2006) 'Extensively drug-resistant tuberculosis as a cause of death in patients co-infected with tuberculosis and HIV in a rural area of South Africa', *Lancet*, vol 368, pp1575–1580

Gillespie, S. and Greener, R. (2006) 'Is poverty or wealth driving HIV transmission?', Working Paper for the UNAIDS Technical Consultation on Prevention of Sexual Transmission of HIV, UNAIDS, Geneva

Gillespie, S. and Loevinsohn, M. (2003) 'HIV/AIDS, food security and rural livelihoods: Understanding and responding', Food Consumption and Nutrition Division Discussion Paper 157, IFPRI, Washington, DC

Ginsberg, J., Mohebbi, M. H., Patel, R. S., Brammer, L., Smolinski, M. S. and Brilliant, L. (2009) 'Detecting influenza epidemics using search engine query data', *Nature*, vol 457, pp1012–1014

GMA (2008) www.gmabrands.com/publicpolicy/docs/Comment.cfm?docid=1348, accessed 4 November 2008

Goldgeir, J. (2003) 'Will SARS be the Chinese Chernobyl?', *Los Angeles Times* Op. Ed., 23 April

Grange, J. M. and Festenstein, F. (1993) 'The human dimension of tuberculosis control', *Tubercle and Lung Disease*, vol 74, pp219–222

Greger, M. (2007) 'The human/animal interface: Emergence and resurgence of zoonotic infectious diseases', *Critical reviews in microbiology*, vol 33, no 4, p243–299

Grein, T., Kamara K.-B. O., Rodier, G., Plant, A., Bovier, P., Ryan, M., Ohyama, T. and Heymann, D. (2000) 'Rumours of disease in the global village: Outbreak verification', *Emerging Infectious Diseases*, vol 6, pp97–102

Griffith, D. and Kerr, C. (1996) 'Tuberculosis: Disease of the past, disease of the present', *Journal of PeriAnesthesia Nursing*, vol 11, no 4, pp240–245

Groce, N. and Reeve, M. (1996) 'Traditional healers and global surveillance strategies for emerging diseases: Closing the gap', *Emerging Infectious Diseases*, vol 2, no 4, pp351–353

Haas, P. (1992) 'Epistemic communities and international policy coordination', *International Organization*, vol 46, no 1, pp1–35

Haines, A., Kovats, R., Campbell-Lendrum, D. and Corvalan, C. (2006) 'Climate change and human health: Impacts, vulnerability and public health', *Public Health*, vol 120, no 7, pp585–596

Hall, R., Hall, R. and Chapman, M. (2008) 'The 1995 Kikwit Ebola outbreak: Lessons hospitals and physicians can apply to future viral epidemics', *General Hospital Psychiatry*, vol 30, pp446–452

Hamel, G. and Välikangas, L. (2003) 'The quest for resilience', *Harvard Business Review,* vol 81, pp52–63

Hanefeld, J. (2009) 'The impact of global health initiatives on policy implementation processes of antiretroviral treatment (ART) roll-out in Zambia and South Africa', draft paper delivered at University of East Anglia conference 'Expanding anti-retroviral therapy provision in resource-limited settings: Social dynamics and policy challenges', 7–8 May

Haraway, D. (1988) 'Situated knowledges: The science question in feminism and the privilege of partial perspective', *Feminist Studies,* vol 14, pp575–609

Hardin, R. (ed) (forthcoming) *Socioemergence: Historical Ecology and Cultural Politics of Emergent Viral Diseases in Tropical Forests,* Duke University Press, Durham, NC

Hardin, R. and Froment, A. (forthcoming) 'From virgin forests to viral forests', in Hardin, R. (ed) (forthcoming) *Socioemergence: Historical Ecology and Cultural Politics of Emergent Viral Diseases in Tropical Forests,* Duke University Press, Durham, NC

Hardy, C. and Richter, M. (2006) 'Disability grants or antiretrovirals? A quandary for people with HIV/AIDS in South Africa', *African Journal of AIDS Research,* vol 5, no 1, pp85–96

Healthlink Bulletin (2009) 9 April, 'Funds running out for ARVs', http://lists.hst.org.za/pipermail/hlinfo-l/2009-April/000237.html, accessed 3 December 2009

Healy, M. (2003) 'Defoe's journal and the plague writing tradition', *Literature and Medicine,* vol 22, no 1, pp25–44

Hewlett, B. and Hewlett, B. (2008) *Ebola, Culture and Politics: The Anthropology of an Emerging Disease,* Wadsworth Books, Florence, KY

Heymann, D. and Rodier, G. (1998) 'Global surveillance of communicable diseases', *Emerging Infectious Diseases,* vol 4, pp362–365

Heymann, D. and Rodier, G. (2001) 'Hot spots in a wired world: WHO surveillance of emerging and re-emerging infectious diseases', *Lancet Infectious Diseases,* vol 1, pp345–353

Heymann, D. and Rodier, G. (2004) 'Global surveillance, national surveillance, and SARS', *Emerging Infectious Diseases,* vol 10, pp173–175

Heymann, D. L., Barakamfitiye, D., Szczeniowski, M., Muyembe-Tamfum, J. J., Bele, O. and Rodier, G. (1999) 'Ebola hemorrhagic fever: Lessons from Kikwit, Democratic Republic of the Congo', *Journal of Infectious Diseases,* vol 179, suppl 1, SS283–286

Heymann, D., de Gourville, E. and Aylward, R. (2004) 'Protecting investments in polio eradication: The past, present and future of surveillance for acute flaccid paralysis', *Epidemiology and Infection,* vol 132, pp779–780

HHS (2005) US Department of Health and Human Services, *HHS Launches African American Anti-Obesity Initiative,* 7 April, HHS Office of Minority Health, available at www.dhhs.gov/news/press/2007pres/11/20071127a.html, accessed 5 November 2008

Hogan, B. (2008) Address to the media by the Minister of Health Barbara Hogan at a Press Conference, Pretoria, www.info.gov.za/speeches/2008/08100612511002.htm, accessed 7 April 2010

Holbrooke, R. and Garrett, L. (2008) '"Sovereignty" that risks global health', *Washington Post,* 10 August

Holdsworth, M., Delpeuch, F., Kameli, Y., Lobstein, T. and Millstone, E. (forthcoming) 'The acceptability of mandatory nutritional labelling in two contrasting food cultures – findings from France and the UK', *Journal of Public Health Policy*

Horton, R. (2007) 'Chronic diseases: The call for urgent global action', *Lancet*, vol 370, no 9603, pp1881–1882

House of Commons Health Select Committee (2004) *Report on Obesity*, Third Report of Session 2003–2004, 23 May, p47, available at www.publications.parliament.uk/pa/cm200304/cmselect/cmhealth/23/23.pdf, accessed 3 December 2009

HPA (2008) *Tuberculosis in the UK: Annual Report on Tuberculosis Surveillance in the UK 2008*, Health Protection Agency, London

HSRC (2009) *South African National HIV Prevalence, Incidence, Behaviour and Communication Survey, 2008*, Human Sciences Research Council Press, Cape Town

Hunter, M. (2007) 'The changing political economy of sex in South Africa: The significance of unemployment and inequalities to the scale of the AIDS pandemic', *Social Science and Medicine*, vol 64, pp689–700

Hyde, M. (2008a) 'The war on obesity must be won round the cabinet table', *The Guardian*, 26 January

Hyde, R. (2008b) 'Europe battles with obesity', *Lancet*, vol 371, no 9631, pp2160–2161

Institute of Medicine (2003) *Microbial Threats to Health: Emergence, Detection, Response*, National Academy of Sciences, Washington, DC

Iseman, M. (1993) 'Treatment of multidrug-resistant tuberculosis', *New England Journal of Medicine*, vol 329, no 11, pp784–791

Jacobson, H. and Oksenberg, M. (1990) *China's Participation in the IMF, the World Bank and GATT*, University of Michigan Press, Ann Arbor, MI

Janes, C. and Corbett, K. (2009) 'Anthropology and global health', *Annual Review of Anthropology*, vol 38, pp167–183

Jasanoff, S. (2005) *Designs on Nature*, Princeton University Press, Princeton, NJ

Jasanoff, S. and Wynne, B. (1998) 'Scientific knowledge and decision making', in Rayner, S. and Malone, E. L. (eds) *Human Choice and Climate Change 1*, Battelle Press, Washington, DC, pp1–87

Jebb, S. and Prentice, A. (1995) 'Obesity in Britain: Gluttony or sloth?', *British Medical Journal*, vol 311, pp437–439

Jensen, S. (2001) 'The battlefield and the prize: ANC's bid to reform the South African state', in Hansen, T. and Stepputat, F. (eds) *States of Imagination: Ethnographic Explorations of the Postcolonial State*, Duke University Press, Durham, NC

Jeppsson, A. (2002) 'Defend the human rights of the Ebola victims!', *Tropical Doctor*, vol 32, no 3, pp181–182

Joffe, H. and Haarhoff, G. (2002) 'Representations of far-flung illnesses: The case of Ebola in Britain', *Social Science and Medicine*, vol 54, no 6, pp955–969

Johannessen, H. and Lázár, I. (2006) *Multiple Medical Realities: Patients and Healers in Biomedical, Alternative and Traditional Medicine*, Berghahn Books, Oxford

John, T., Samuel, R., Balraj, V. and John, R. (1998) 'Disease surveillance at district level: A model for developing countries', *Lancet*, vol 352, pp58–61

John, T., Rajappan, K. and Arjunan, K. (2004) 'Communicable diseases monitored by disease surveillance in Kottayam district, Kerala state, India', *Indian Journal of Medical Research*, vol 120, pp86–93

Jones, K. E., Patel, N. G., Levy, M. A., Storeygard, A., Balk, D., Gittleman, J. L. and Daszak, P. (2008) 'Global trends in emerging infectious diseases', *Nature*, vol 451, no 7181, pp990–993

Jost, C., Mariner, J., Roeder, P. and Sawitri, E. (2007) 'Participatory epidemiology in disease surveillance and research', *Revue Scientifique et Technique*, vol 26, no 3, pp537–549

Ka, H., Zhao, L., Daviglus, M., Dyer, A., Van Horn, L., Garside, D., Zhu, L., Guo, D., Wu, Y., Zhou, B. and Stamler, J. (2008) 'Association of monosodium glutamate intake with overweight in Chinese adults: The INTERMAP study', *Obesity*, vol 16, no 8, pp1875–1880

Kapan, D., Bennett, S., Ellis, B., Fox, J., Lewis, N., Spencer, J. H., Saksena, S. and Wilcox, B. (2006) 'Avian influenza (H5N1) and the evolutionary and social ecology of infectious disease emergence', *EcoHealth*, vol 3, no 3, pp1–8

Kaufman, J. (2006) 'SARS and China's health care response: Better to be both red and expert!', in Kleinman, A. and Watson, J. (eds) *SARS in China: Prelude to a Pandemic?* Stanford University Press, Stanford, CA

Kaufmann, S. (2004) 'New issues in tuberculosis', *Annals of the Rheumatic Diseases*, vol 63 (Supplement II), ii50–ii56

Kaufmann, S. H. E. (2007) 'Tuberculosis and AIDS – a devilish liaison', *Drug Discovery Today*, vol 12, pp891–893

Kaufmann, S. (2009) *The New Plagues: Pandemics and Poverty in a Globalized World*, Haus Publishing (The Sustainability Project), London

Kaul, I., Grunberg, I. and Stern, M. (eds) (1999) *Global Public Goods: International Cooperation in the 21st Century*, Oxford University Press, Oxford

Keller, M., Blench, M., Tolentino, H., Freifeld, C., Mandl, K., Mawadeku, A., Eysenbach, G. and Brownstein, J. (2009) 'Use of unstructured event-based reports for global infectious disease surveillance', *Emerging Infectious Diseases*, vol 15, no 5, pp689–695

Kersh, R. and Morone, J. (2002) 'The politics of obesity: Seven steps to government action', *Health Affairs*, vol 21, no 6, pp142ff

Khanna, A. (2007) 'The soft boy and her/his hard epidemiological fact: Or the meleichhele becomes MSM', paper presented at 'Politicising Masculinities: Beyond the Personal' – An international symposium linking lessons from HIV, sexuality and reproductive health with other areas for rethinking AIDS, gender and development, 15–18 October, Dakar

Kickbusch, I. (1999) 'Global + local: Glocal public health', *Journal of Epidemiology and Community Health*, vol 53, pp451–452

Kickbusch, I. (2003) 'Global health governance: Some theoretical considerations on the new political space', in Lee, K. (ed) *Health Impacts of Globalization: Towards Global Governance*, Palgrave Macmillan, London

Kilbourne, E. D. (1996) 'The emergence of "emerging diseases": A lesson in holistic epidemiology', *Mt Sinai Journal of Medicine*, vol 63, no 3–4, pp159–166

Kim, J., Shakow, A., Mate, K., Vanderwarker, C., Gupta, R. and Farmer, P. (2005) 'Limited good and limited vision: Multidrug resistant tuberculosis and global health policy', *Social Science and Medicine*, vol 61, no 4, pp847–859

Kimball, A., Moore, M., French, H., Arima, Y., Ungchusak, K., Wibulpolprasert, S., Taylor, T., Touch, S. and Leventhal, A. (2008) 'Regional infectious disease surveillance networks and their potential to facilitate the implementation of the International Health Regulations', *Medical Clinics of North America*, vol 92, no 6, pp1459–1471

Kimerling, M. E., Kluge, H., Vezhnina, N., Lacovazzi, T., Demeulenaere, T., Portaels, F. and Matthys, F. (1999) 'Inadequacy of the current WHO re-treatment regimen in a central Siberian prison: Treatment failure and MDR-TB', *The International Journal of Tuberculosis and Lung Disease*, vol 3, no 5, pp451–453

King, N. (2002) 'Security, disease, commerce: Ideologies of postcolonial global health', *Social Studies of Science*, vol 32, pp763–789

Kirby, D. (2008) 'The impact of abstinence and comprehensive sex and STD/HIV education programs on adolescent sexual behaviour', *Sexuality Research and Social Policy*, vol 5, no 3, pp6–17A

Kleinman, A. (1988) *The Illness Narratives: Suffering, Healing, and the Human Condition*, Basic Books, New York

Knobler, S., Mahmoud, A., Lemon, S. and Pray, L. (2006) *The Impact of Globalization on Infectious Disease Emergence and Control: Exploring the Consequences and Opportunities, Workshop Summary – Forum on Microbial Threats*, National Academies Press, Washington, DC

Kruk, M. (2008) 'Emergency preparedness and public health settings: Lessons for developing countries', *American Journal of Preventive Medicine*, vol 34, no 6, pp529–534

Kuiken, T., Fouchier, R., Rimmelzwaan, G. and Osterhaus, A. (2003) 'Emerging viral infections in a rapidly changing world', *Current Opinion in Biotechnology*, vol 14, no 6, pp641–646

Kunii, O., Kita, E. and Shibuya, K. (2001) 'Epidemics and related cultural factors for Ebola hemorrhagic fever in Gabon', *Nippon Koshu Eisei Zasshi*, vol 48, no 10, pp853–859

LA Times (2002) 'Annan urges US not to go it alone against Iraq', 12 September 2002, available at http://articles.latimes.com/2002/sep/12/world/fg-un12, accessed 3 December 2009

Lambin, E. (2008) paper presented at conference 'Resilience 2008', Stockholm, Sweden, 14–16 April

Lancet (2004) 'Avian influenza: The threat looms', *Lancet*, vol 363, no 9405, p257

Lawrence, R. (2004) 'Framing obesity: The evolution of news discourse on a public health issue', *The Harvard International Journal of Press/Politics*, vol 9, no 3, pp56–75

Lawson, S. and Mariner, J. (2008) 'Avian influenza H5N1 outbreaks in village poultry of West Java, Indonesia: A detailed investigation using participatory epidemiology', *International Journal of Infectious Diseases*, vol 12, ppE136–137

Lawther, P. J. and Aldridge, W. N. (1979) 'Epidemics of non-infectious disease', *Proceedings of the Royal Society of London. Series B, Biological Sciences*, vol 205, no 1158, pp63–75

Leach, M. and Fairhead, J. (2007) *Vaccine Anxieties: Global Science, Child Health and Society*, Earthscan, London

Leach, M. and Mearns, R. (1996) *The Lie of the Land: Challenging Received Wisdom on the African Environment*, James Currey, London

Leach, M., Scoones, I. and Stirling, A. (2007) 'Pathways to sustainability: An overview of the STEPS Centre approach', STEPS Approach Paper, STEPS Centre, Brighton

Leach, M., Scoones, I. and Stirling, A. (2010a) *Dynamic Sustainabilities: Technology, Environment, Social Justice*, Earthscan, London

Leach, M., Scoones, I. and Stirling, A. (2010b) 'Governing epidemics in an age of complexity: Narratives, politics and pathways to sustainability', *Global Environmental Change*, vol 20, no 3

Lebel, J. (2003) *Health: An Ecosystem Approach*, IDRC, Ottawa

Leclerc-Madlala, S. (2005) 'Popular responses to HIV/AIDS and policy', *Journal of Southern African Studies*, vol 31, no 4, pp845–856

Leclerc-Madlala, S. (2006) '"We will eat when I get the grant": Negotiating AIDS, poverty and antiretroviral treatment in South Africa', *African Journal of AIDS Research*, vol 5, pp249–256

Lee, K. (2000) 'Globalization and health policy: A review of the literature and proposed research and policy agenda', in Bambas, A. et al (eds) *Health and Human Development in the Global Economy*, Pan American Health Organization, Washington, DC, pp15–41

Lee, K. (2003a) *Globalization and Health: An Introduction*, Palgrave Macmillan, London

Lee, K. (2003b) *Health Impacts of Globalization: Toward Global Governance*, Palgrave Macmillan, New York

Lee, K. and Fidler, D. (2007) 'Avian and pandemic influenza: Progress and problems with global health governance', *Global Public Health*, vol 2, no 3, pp215–234

Lee, K., Fustukian, S. and Buse, K. (2002) 'An introduction to global health policy', in Lee, K., Buse, K. and Fustukian, S. (eds) *Health Policy in a Globalizing World*, Cambridge University Press, Cambridge

Lee, K., Chan, L. H. and Chan, G. (2009) 'China engages global health governance: Processes and dilemmas', *Global Public Health*, vol 4, no 1, pp1–30

Lerner, B. H. (1997) 'From careless consumptives to recalcitrant patients: The historical construction of non-compliance', *Social Science and Medicine*, vol 45, pp1423–1431

Li, P. (2009) 'Exponential growth, animal welfare, environmental and food safety impact: The case of China's livestock production', *Journal of Agricultural and Environmental Ethics*, vol 22, no 3, pp217–240

Li, T. (2007) 'Practices of assemblage and community forest management', *Economy and Society*, vol 36, no 2, pp263–293

Lillebaek, T., Andersen, A. B., Bauer, J., Dirksen, A., Glismann, S., De Haas, P. and Kok-Jensen, A. (2001) 'Risk of mycobacterium tuberculosis transmission in a low-incidence country due to immigration from high-incidence areas', *Journal of Clinical Microbiology*, vol 39, pp855–861

Lipsitch, M., Hayden, F., Cowling, B. and Leung, G. (2009) 'How to maintain surveillance for novel influenza A H1N1 when there are too many cases to count', *Lancet*, vol 374, no 9696, pp1209–1211

Lloyd, C. B. (2007) 'The role of schools in promoting sexual and reproductive health among adolescents in developing countries', *Poverty, Gender, and Youth Working Paper 6*, Population Council, New York

Lloyd, E. S., Zaki, S. R., Rollin, P. E., Tshioko, K., Bwaka, M. A., Ksiazek, T. G., Calain, P., Shieh, W. J., Konde, M. K., Verchueren, E., Perry, H. N., Manguindula, L., Kabwau, J., Ndambi, R. and Peters, C. J. (1999) 'Long-term disease surveillance in Bandundu region, Democratic Republic of Congo: A model for early detection and prevention of Ebola hemorrhagic fever', *Journal of Infectious Disease*, vol 179, suppl 1, pp274–280

Lloyd-Smith, J., Schreiber, S., Kopp, P. and Getz, W. (2005) 'Superspreading and the effect of individual variation on disease emergence', *Nature*, vol 438, no 7066, pp335–359

Lobstein, T. and Bauer, L. (2005) 'Policies to prevent childhood obesity in the European Union', *European Journal of Public Health*, vol 15, no 6, pp576–579

Lobstein, T. and Millstone, E. (2006) 'Policy options for responding to obesity: UK national report of the PorGrow project', SPRU, University of Sussex, available at: www.sussex.ac.uk/spru/documents/uk_english.pdf, accessed 21 November 2009

Lobstein, T., Baur, L. and Uauy, R. (2004) 'Obesity in children and young people: A crisis in public health', *Obesity Reviews*, vol 5, supp 1, pp4–85

Lobstein, T., Millstone, E. and the PorGrow Team (2007) 'The public health and policy context of the PorGrow project', *Obesity Reviews*, vol 8, pp7–16

Loevinsohn, M. (2009) 'Seasonal hunger, the 2001–03 famine and the dynamics of HIV in Malawi', paper presented at international conference on 'Seasonality Revisited', Institute of Development Studies, UK, 8–10 July

Longini, I. M. Jr., Nizam, A., Xu, S., Ungchusak, K., Hanshaoworakul, W., Cummings, D. A. T. and Halloran, E. (2005) 'Containing pandemic influenza at the source', *Science*, vol 309, no 5737, pp1083–1087

MacGregor, H. (2006) '"The grant is what I eat": The politics of disability and social security in the post-apartheid South African state', *Journal of Biosocial Science*, vol 38, pp43–55

Mack, E. (2006) 'The World Health Organization's new International Health Regulations: Incursions on state sovereignty and ill-fated response to global health issues', *Chicago Journal of International Law*, vol 7, no 1, pp365–377

Mahapatra, P., Shibuya, K., Lopez, A., Coullare, F., Notzon, F., Rao, C. and Szeter, S. (2007) 'Civil registration systems and vital statistics: Successes and missed opportunities', *Lancet*, vol 370, pp1653–1663

Maley, J. (2002) 'A catastrophic destruction of African forests about 2,500 years ago still exerts a major influence on present vegetation formations', *IDS Bulletin*, vol 33, no 1, pp13–30

Manderson, L. (1996) *Sickness and the State: Health and Illness in Colonial Malaya, 1870–1940*, Cambridge University Press, Cambridge

Mann, J. M. and Tarantola, D. (eds) (1996) *AIDS in the World II: Global Dimensions, Social Roots and Responses*, Oxford University Press, New York

Markell, H. (2007) 'Pandemic-mitigation strategies for the twenty-first century', in Lemon, S., Hamburg, M., Sparling, P. F., Choffnes, E. and Mack, A. (rapporteurs) *Ethical and Legal Considerations in Mitigating Pandemic Disease: Workshop Summary*, National Academy Press, Washington, DC, available at www.nap.edu/catalog/11917. html, accessed 20 July 2009

Marston, B. and Miller, B. (2006) 'Tuberculosis: The elephant in the AIDS clinic?', *AIDS*, vol 20, pp1323–1325

Mascolini, M. (2007) 'African study finds more HIV in women in discordant couples', *International AIDS Society*, 22 June

Mathema, B., Kurepina, N. E., Bifani, P. J. and Kreiswirth, B. N. (2006) 'Molecular epidemiology of tuberculosis: Current insights', *Clinical Microbiology Reviews*, vol 19, pp658–685

Matsuda, R. (2007) 'Midcourse review of "Health Japan 21"', Kinugasa Research Institute, Ritsumeikan University, Kyoto

McCurry, J. (2006) 'Japanese grab girdles as obesity crisis looms', *The Guardian*, 2 March

McInness, C. and Lee, K. (2006) 'Health, security and foreign policy', *Review of International Studies*, vol 32, no 1, pp5–23

McMichael, A. J. (2001) 'Human culture, ecological change and infectious disease: Are we experiencing history's fourth great transition?', *Ecosystem Health*, vol 7, pp107–115

McNeill, D. (2009) 'Finding a scapegoat when epidemics strike', *New York Times*, 1 September

Medical Research Council (1948) 'Streptomycin treatment of pulmonary tuberculosis. A Medical Research Council investigation', *British Medical Journal*, vol ii, pp790–791

Medical Research Council (1955) 'Various combinations of isoniazid with streptomycin or with PAS in the treatment of pulmonary tuberculosis', *British Medical Journal*, vol i, pp435–445

Meek, J. (1998) 'Killer TB threat to the world', *The Guardian*, 23 September

Meessen, B. and Bloom, G. (2007) 'Economic transition, institutional changes and the health system: Some lessons from rural China', *The Journal of Economic Policy Reform*, vol 10, no 3, pp209–232

Meng, Q., Shi, G., Yang, H., Gonzalez-Block, M. and Blas, E. (2004) *Health Policy and Systems Research in China*, Special Programme for Research and Training in Tropical Diseases, WHO, Geneva

Merlin (2002) '"Licking" Lassa fever: A strategic review', Merlin, London, available at www.merlin.org.uk, accessed 27 November 2009

Migliori, G. B., Ortmann, J., Girardi, E., Besozzi, G., Lange, C., Cirillo, D. M., Ferrarese, M., De Laco, G., Gori, A., Raviglione, M. C. and the SMIRA/TBNET Study Group (2007) 'Extensively drug-resistant tuberculosis, Italy and Germany', *Emerging Infectious Diseases*, vol 13, pp780–782

Milleliri, J. M., Tevi-Bennissan, C., Baize, S., Leroy, E. and Georges-Courbot, M. C. (2004) 'Epidemics of Ebola haemorrhagic fever in Gabon (1994–2002). Epidemiologic aspects and considerations on control measures', *Bulletin de la Société Pathologiques Exotiques*, vol 97, no 3, pp199–205

Mills, E. (2008) *Swimming in Confusion: A Qualitative Study of Factors Affecting Uptake and Adherence to Antiretroviral Treatment in South Africa*, Centre for Social Science Research, AIDS and Society Research Working Paper no 208, University of Cape Town, Cape Town

Millstone, E. and Lobstein, T. (2007) 'The PorGrow project: Overall cross-national results, comparisons and implications', *Obesity Reviews*, vol 8, suppl 2, pp29–38

Millstone, E., Mohebati, L., Lobstein, T. and Jacobs, M. (2007) 'Policy options for responding to the growing challenge from obesity in the United Kingdom', *Obesity Reviews*, vol 8, suppl 2, pp109–115

Morens, D., Folkers, G. and Fauci, A. (2004) 'The challenge of emerging and re-emerging infectious diseases', *Nature*, vol 430, pp242–249

Morgan, M. and Morrison, M. (1999) *Models as Mediators: Perspectives on Natural and Social Science*, Cambridge University Press, Cambridge

Morgenthau, H. J. (1948) *Politics among Nations: The Struggle for Power and Peace*, Knopf, New York

Morse, S. (1995) 'Factors in the emergence of infectious diseases', *Emerging Infectious Diseases*, vol 1, no 1, pp7–15

Morton, J. (2006) 'Conceptualising the links between HIV/AIDS and pastoralist livelihoods', *The European Journal of Development Research*, vol 18, no 2, pp235–254

Morvan, J. M., Nakoune, E., Deubel, V. and Colyn, M. (2000) 'Forest ecosystems and Ebola virus', *Bulletin de la Société Pathologie Exotique*, vol 93, no 3, pp172–175

Moszynski, P. (2006) 'Experts devise strategy to fight new TB strain', *British Medical Journal*, vol 333, p566

Moszynski, P. (2007) 'Doctors disagree over detention of patients with extensively drug resistant tuberculosis', *British Medical Journal*, vol 334, p228

MSF (2000) 'MSF calls for government action for TB treatment research', Press Release, MSF, Brussels, available at www.msfaccess.org/media-room/press-releases/press-release-detail/?tx_ttnews%5Btt_news%5D=152&cHash=d480071305, accessed 25 February 2010

MSF (2007) 'TB and HIV: The Failure to Act', MSF, Amsterdam, available at www.msfaccess.org/fileadmin/user_upload/diseases/tuberculosis/TB%20and%20HIV.%20The%20failure%20to%20act.pdf, accessed 25 February 2010

Mukherjee, J. S., Rich, M. L., Socci, A. R., Joseph, J. K., Virú, F. A., Shin, S. S., Furin, J. J., Becerra, M. C., Barry, D. J., Kim, J. Y., Bayona, J., Farmer, P., Smith Fawzi, M. C. and Seung, K. J. (2004) 'Programmes and principles of treatment of MDR TB', *Lancet*, vol 363, pp474–481

Muraskin, W. (2004) 'The global alliance for vaccines and immunization: Is it a new model for effective public–private cooperation in international public health?', *American Journal of Public Health*, vol 94, pp1922–1925

Murray, C. J. L., De Jonghe, E., Chum, H. J., Nyangulu, D. S., Salomao, A. and Styblo, K. (1991) 'Cost effectiveness of chemotherapy for pulmonary tuberculosis in three sub-Saharan African countries', *Lancet*, vol 338, pp1305–1308

Musgrave, A. and Brown, K. (2008) *'South Africa: Social Welfare System Revisited'*, 21 October, www.businessday.co.za/Articles/Content.aspx?id=55265, accessed 22 May 2009

Myers, J. and Naledi, T. M. (2007) *Western Cape Burden of Disease Reduction Project: Overview of the Report: Volume 1*, prepared for Provincial Government of the Western Cape, Department of Health, https://vula.uct.ac.za/access/content/group/91e9e9d8-39b6-4654-00ae-f4d74cba085f/CD%20Volume%201%20Overview%20and%20Executive%20Summaries180907.pdf, accessed 22 May 2009

Nagel, T. (1989) *The View from Nowhere*, Oxford University Press, Oxford

Naidoo, P. (2006) 'Scaling up VCT in Cape Town', presentation to the Joint Civil Society Monitoring Forum

National Centre for Social Research (2004) *Health Survey for England 2003*, commissioned by Department of Health, The Stationery Office, London

National Department of Health (2008) *Progress Report on Declaration of Commitment on HIV and AIDS, Republic of South Africa, January 2006–December 2007*, Third Report prepared for the United Nations General Assembly Special Session on HIV and AIDS, National Department of Health, Pretoria

National Intelligence Council (2002) 'The Next Wave of HIV/AIDS: Nigeria, Ethiopia, Russia, India, and China', ICA 2002-04D, September

Nattrass, N. (2006) 'Trading off income and health?: AIDS and the disability grant in South Africa', *Journal of Social Policy*, vol 35, pp3–19

Nature (2009) 'Patchy pig monitoring may hide flu threat', *Nature*, vol 459, pp894–895

Nguyen, V. K. (2005) 'Antiretroviral globalism, biopolitics, and therapeutic citizenship', in Ong, A. and Collier, S. J. (eds) *Global Assemblages: Technology, Politics, and Ethics as Anthropological Problems*, Blackwell Publishing, Malden, MA

Nichter, M. (2008) *Global Health: Why Cultural Perceptions, Social Representations, and Biopolitics Matter*, University of Arizona Press, Tucson, AZ

NIH (1985) 'Health implications of obesity', *NIH Consensus Statement Online*, vol 5, no 9, pp1–7, accessed 19 November 2009

Normile, D. (2007) 'Indonesia taps village wisdom to fight bird flu', *Science*, vol 315, no 5808, pp30–33

North, D. C. (1990) *Institutions, Institutional Change, and Economic Performance*, Cambridge University Press, New York

North, D. C. (2005) *Understanding the Process of Economic Change*, Princeton University Press, Princeton, NJ

Nunn, P., Williams, B., Floyd, K., Dye, C., Elzinga, G. and Raviglione, M. C. (2005) 'Tuberculosis control in the era of HIV', *Nature Reviews Immunology*, vol 5, pp819–826

OAG Review (2006) www.oag.com/oag/website/com/en/Press+Room/Press+Releases+2006/OAG+Review+of+2006+030606

Ong, A. and Collier, S. (2005) *Global Assemblages: Technology, Politics, and Ethics as Anthropological Problems*, Blackwell, Malden, MA

Parkes, M., Bienen, L., Breilh, J., Hsu, L.-N., McDonald, M., Patz, J., Rosenthal, J., Sahani, M., Sleigh, A., Waltner-Toews, D. and Yassi, A. (2004) 'All hands on deck: Transdisciplinary approaches to emerging infectious disease', *EcoHealth*, vol 2, no 4, pp258–272

Patel, R. (2007) *Stuffed and Starved*, Portobello Books, London

Patz, J. A., Campbell-Lendrum, D., Holloway, T. and Foley, J. A. (2005) 'Impact of regional climate change on human health', *Nature*, vol 438, pp310–317

Pepper, D. J., Meintjes, G. A., McIlleron, H. and Wilkinson, R. J. (2008) 'Combined therapy for tuberculosis and HIV-1: The challenge for drug discovery', *Drug Discovery Today*, vol 12, pp280–289

Perry, H., McDonnell, S., Alemu, W., Nsubuga, P., Chungong, S., Otten, M., Lusambadikassa, P. and Thacker, S. (2007) 'Planning an integrated disease surveillance and response system: A matrix of skills and activities', *BMC Medicine*, vol 5, p24

Pfuetze, K. H., Pyle, M. M., Hinshaw, H. C. and Feldman, W. H. (1955) 'The first clinical trial of streptomycin in human tuberculosis', *American Review of Tuberculosis*, vol 71, no 5, pp752–754

Pinzon, J. E., Wilson, J. M., Tucker, C. J., Arthur, R., Jahrling, P. B. and Formenty, P. (2004) 'Trigger events: Enviroclimatic coupling of Ebola hemorrhagic fever outbreaks', *American Journal of Tropical Medicine and Hygiene*, vol 71, no 5, pp664–674

Piot, P. (2005) 'Why AIDS is exceptional', lecture given at the London School of Economics, London, 8 February

Piot, P. and Seck, A. M. C. (2001) 'Policy and practice. International response to the HIV/AIDS epidemic: Planning for success', *Bulletin of the World Health Organization*, vol 79, no 12, pp1106–1112

Piot, P., Kazatchkine, M., Dybul, M. and Lob-Levyt, J. (2009) 'AIDS: Lessons learnt and myths dispelled', *Lancet*, vol 374, no 9685, pp260–263

Pisani, E., Garnett, G. P., Grassly, N. C., Brown, T., Stover, J., Hankins, C., Walker, N. and Ghys, P. D. (2003) 'Back to basics in HIV prevention: Focus on exposure', *British Medical Journal*, vol 326, pp1384–1387

PLoS Medicine Editors (2007) 'How is WHO responding to global public health threats?', *PLoS Medicine,* vol 4, no 5, e197

Plummer, F., Nagelkerke, N., Willbond, B., Ngugi, E., Moses, S., John, G., Nduati, R., MacDonald, K. S. and Berkley, S. (2001) 'The evidence base for interventions to prevent HIV infection in low and middle income countries', CMH Working Paper no WG5: 2, Commission on Macroeconomics and Health, WHO, Geneva

Polesky, A. and Bhatia, G. (2003) 'Ebola hemorrhagic fever in the era of bioterrorism', *Seminars in Respiratory Infections,* vol 18, no 3, pp206–215

Porter, D. and Porter, R. (1988) 'The enforcement of health: The British debate', in Fee, E. and Fox, D. (eds) *AIDS: The Burdens of History,* University of California Press, Berkeley, CA

Posel, D. (2004) 'Afterword: Vigilantism and the burden of rights: Reflections on the paradoxes of freedom in post-apartheid South Africa', *African Studies,* vol 63, no 2, pp231–236

Quan, T. (2006) 'The name of the pose: A sex worker by any other name', in Spector, J. (ed) *Prostitution and Pornography: Philosophical Debate about the Sex Industry,* Stanford University Press, Stanford, CA

Randerson, J. (2006) 'China's alarming increase in obesity blamed on more affluent lifestyles', *The Guardian,* 18 August, p19

Raviglione, M. and Pio, A. (2002) 'Evolution of WHO policies for tuberculosis control, 1948–2001', *Lancet,* vol 359, no 9308, pp775–780

Rayner, S. (2006) 'Clumsy solutions for a complex world', *Public Administration,* vol 84, pp817–843

Reid, E. (1993) 'The HIV epidemic and development: The unfolding of the epidemic', HIV and Development Programme, Issues Papers no 1, UNDP, New York

Reingold, A. (2003) 'If syndromic surveillance is the answer, what is the question?', *Biosecurity and Bioterrorism: Biodefense Strategy, Practice and Science,* vol 1, pp1–5

Ren, D., Li, M., Duan, C. and Rui, L. (2005) 'Identification of SH2-B as a key regulator of leptin sensitivity, energy balance, and body weight in mice', *Cell Metabolism,* vol 2, no 2, pp95–104

Richmond, J. K. and Baglole, D. J. (2003) 'Lassa fever: Epidemiology, clinical features, and social consequences', *British Medical Journal,* vol 327, no 29, pp1271–1275

Richter, M. (2006) 'Different models of HIV-testing: What are the considerations in South Africa?', AIDS Law Project Discussion Paper, AIDS Law Project, Johannesburg

Robins, S. (2004) '"Long live Zackie, long live": AIDS activism, science and citizenship after apartheid', *Journal of Southern African Studies,* vol 30, no 3, pp651–672

Robins, S. (2005) 'From "medical miracles" to normal(ised) medicine: AIDS treatment, activism and citizenship in the UK and South Africa', IDS Working Paper, no 252, IDS, Brighton

Robins, S. (2006) 'From "rights" to "ritual": AIDS activism in South Africa', *American Anthropologist,* vol 108, no 2, pp312–323

Roe, E. (1991) '"Development Narratives" or making the best of blueprint development', *World Development,* vol 19, pp287–300

Rohleder, P. and Swartz, L. (2005) '"What I've noticed what they need is the stats": Lay HIV counsellors' reports of working in a task-orientated health care system', *AIDS Care,* vol 17, no 3, pp397–406

Rose, N. (2006) *The Politics of Life Itself: Biomedicine, Power, and Subjectivity in the Twenty-First Century*, Princeton University Press, Princeton, NJ

Rosenberg, C. E. (1992) *Explaining Epidemics and Other Studies in the History of Medicine*, Cambridge University Press, Cambridge

Rosenberg, C. E. (2002) 'The tyranny of diagnosis: Specific entities and individual experience', *The Milbank Quarterly*, vol 80, no 2, pp237–260

Ryan, F. (1993) *The Forgotten Plague: How the Battle against Tuberculosis Was Won – and Lost*, Little Brown, Boston, MA

Saich, T. (2006) 'Is SARS China's Chernobyl or much ado about nothing?', in Kleinman, A. and Watson, J. (eds) *SARS in China: Prelude to a Pandemic?*, Stanford University Press, Stanford, CA

Saker, L., Lee, K., Cannito, B., Gilmore, A. and Campbell-Lendrum, D. (2004) *Globalization and Infectious Diseases: Special Topics in Social, Economic and Behavioural Research*, UNDP/World Bank/WHO/UNICEF Special Programme on Tropical Diseases Research, WHO, Geneva

Sarewitz, D. (1999) *Frontiers of Illusion*, Temple University Press, Philadelphia, PA

Schäfer Elinder, L. (2005) 'Obesity, hunger, and agriculture: The damaging role of subsidies', *British Medical Journal*, vol 331, pp1333–1336

Schaffer, H., Hunt, B. and Ray, D. (2007) 'US Agricultural Commodity Policy and its Relationship to Obesity', background paper developed for the Wingspread Conference on Childhood Obesity, Healthy Eating and Agriculture Policy, Racine, WI

Schneider, H. (2002) 'On the fault-line: The politics of AIDS policy in contemporary South Africa', *African Studies*, vol 61, no 1, pp146–167

Schneider, H. (2009) 'Lay health workers and HIV programmes: Implications for health systems', draft paper delivered at University of East Anglia conference 'Expanding anti-retroviral therapy provision in resource-limited settings: Social dynamics and policy challenges', 7–8 May

Schneider, M. and Goudge, J. (2007) 'Developing a policy response to provide social security benefits to people with chronic diseases', Report for Department of Social Development, Pretoria, 30 March

Schnur, A. (2006) 'The role of the World Health Organization in combating SARS, focusing on the efforts in China', in Kleinman, A. and Watson, J. (eds) *SARS in China: Prelude to a Pandemic?*, Stanford University Press, Stanford, CA

Scoones, I. (ed) (2010) *Avian Influenza: Science, Policy and Politics*, Earthscan, London

Scoones, I. and Forster, P. (2008) *The International Response to Highly Pathogenic Avian Influenza: Science, Policy and Politics*, STEPS Working Paper 10, STEPS Centre, Brighton

Scoones, I., Leach, M., Smith, A., Stagl, S., Stirling, A. and Thompson, J. (2007) *Dynamic Systems and the Challenge of Sustainability*, STEPS Working Paper 1, STEPS Centre, Brighton

Setel, P., Macfarlane, S., Szreter, S., Mikkelsen, L., Jha, P., Stout, S. and AbouZahr, C. (2007) 'Who Counts? 1 – A scandal of invisibility: Making everyone count by counting everyone', *Lancet*, vol 370, pp1569–1577

Shin, S., Furin, J., Bayona, J., Mate, K., Kim, J. Y. and Farmer, P. (2004) 'Community-based treatment of multidrug-resistant tuberculosis in Lima, Peru: 7 years of experience', *Social Science Medicine*, vol 59, pp1529–1539

Sidley, P. (2006) 'South Africa acts to curb spread of lethal strain of TB', *British Medical Journal*, vol 333, p825

Singer, M. (2009) 'Pathogens gone wild? Medical anthropology and the "Swine Flu" pandemic', *Medical Anthropology*, vol 28, no 3, pp199–206

Singh, J. A., Upshur, R. and Padayatchi, N. (2007) 'XDR-TB in South Africa: No time for denial or complacency', *PLoS Medicine*, vol 4, no 1, e5

Slingenbergh, J., Gilbert, M., De Balogh, K. and Wint, W. (2004) 'Ecological sources of zoonotic diseases', *Revue Scientifique et Technique – Office International des Épizooties*, vol 23, no 2, pp467–484

Slovic, P. (1989) 'Perception of risk', *Science*, vol 236, no 4799, p280

Smith, A. and Stirling, A. (2006) 'Moving inside or outside? Positioning the governance of socio-technical systems', SPRU Electronic Working Paper 148, SPRU, University of Sussex

Smith, G., Bahl, J., Vijaykrishna, D., Zhang, J., Poon, L., Chen, H., Webster, R., Pieris, M. and Guan, Y. (2009) 'Dating the emergence of pandemic influenza viruses', *PNAS*, vol 106, no 28, pp11709–11712

Smith, R. (2006) 'Responding to global infectious disease outbreaks: Lessons from SARS on the role of risk perception, communication and management', *Social Science and Medicine*, vol 63, pp3113–3123

Soon, G., Koh, Y., Wong, M. and Lam, P. (2008) 'Obesity prevention and control efforts in Singapore', 2008 Case Study, National Bureau of Asian Research, Seattle, WA

South African Mail and Guardian (2009) 'Zuma's top ministers: A thoroughly mixed bag', available at www.mg.co.za/article/2009-05-15-zumas-top-ministers-a-thoroughly-mixed-bag, accessed 22 May 2009

Standing, H., Mushtaque, A. and Chowdhury, R. (2008) 'Producing effective knowledge agents in a pluralistic environment: What future for community health workers', *Social Science and Medicine*, vol 66, no 10, pp2096–2107

State Council (1997) 'Decision of the Central Committee of the Chinese Communist Party and the State Council on Health Reform and Development', 15 January

Stewart, P. (2009) 'UN agency slams Egypt order to cull all pigs', Reuters, 29 April, www.reuters.com/article/idUSLT11Z50, accessed 7 April 2010

Stirling, A. (1999) '*On "science" and "precaution" in the management of technological risk*', report to the EU Forward Studies Unit, IPTS, Seville

Stirling, A. (2006) 'Precaution, foresight, and sustainability: Reflection and reflexivity in the governance of science and technology', in Voß, J. P., Bauknecht, D. and Kemp, R. (eds) *Reflexive Governance for Sustainable Development*, Edward Elgar, Cheltenham

Stirling, A. (2008) '"Opening up" and "closing down": Power, participation, and pluralism in the social appraisal of technology', *Science, Technology, and Human Values*, vol 33, no 2, pp262–294

Stirling, A. and Scoones, I. (2009) 'From risk assessment to knowledge mapping: Science, precaution and participation in disease ecology', *Ecology and Society*, vol 14, no 2, p14

Swartz, L. and MacGregor, H. (2002) 'Integrating services, marginalising patients: Psychiatric patients and primary health care in South Africa', *Transcultural Psychiatry*, vol 39, no 2, pp155–172

Swinburn, B., Egger, G. and Raza, F. (1999) 'Dissecting obesogenic environments: The development and application of a framework for identifying and prioritising environmental interventions for obesity', *Preventive Medicine*, vol 29, pp563–570

Szreter, S. (2006) 'The right of registration: Development, identity registration, and social security – A historical perspective', *World Development*, vol 35, no 1, pp67–86

Szreter, S. and Woolcock, M. (2004) 'Health by association? Social capital, social theory, and the political economy of health', *International Journal of Epidemiology*, vol 33, pp650–667

TAC (2008) 'TAC, ALP and ARASA demand better social assistance to protect the rights of people living with chronic illnesses', available at www.tac.org.za/community/node/2412, accessed 20 May 2009

Tang, S. and Squire, S. B. (2005) 'What lessons can be drawn from TB control in China in the 1990s? An analysis from a health system perspective', *Health Policy*, vol 72, pp93–104

Tanne, J. H. (1999) 'Drug resistant TB is spreading worldwide', *British Medical Journal*, vol 319, p1220

Taylor, C. (1992) 'Surveillance for equity in primary health care: Policy implications from international experience', *International Journal of Epidemiology*, vol 21, no 8, pp1043–1049

Thorpe, N. (2008) 'Breaking the strain', *Developments*, available at www.developments.org.uk/articles/breaking-the-strain/, accessed 5 December 2009

Tillotson, J. (2004) 'America's obesity: Conflicting public policies, industrial economic development and unintended human consequences', *Annual Review of Nutrition*, vol 24, pp617–643

Time Magazine (2003) 'The Truth About SARS', cover story, 5 May

Toh, C., Cutter, J. and Chew, S. (2002) 'School based intervention has reduced obesity in Singapore', *British Medical Journal*, vol 324, no 7334, p427

Tsai, K. (2007) *Capitalism without Democracy: The Private Sector in Contemporary China*, Cornell University Press, Ithaca, NY

Tuberculosis Prevention Trial (1979) 'Trial of BCG vaccines in south India for tuberculosis prevention', *Indian Journal of Medical Research*, vol 70, pp349–363

UN Wire (2002) 'Annan stresses "shades of grey" after Bush "axis of evil" speech', 11 February, available at www.unwire.org/unwire/20020211/23736_story.asp, accessed 6 December 2009

UNAIDS (2008) 'Report on the Global AIDS Epidemic', Geneva, UNAIDS, available at www.unaids.org/en/KnowledgeCentre/HIVData/GlobalReport/2008/2008_Global_report.asp, accessed 20 October 2008

UNAIDS/WHO (2008) 'UNAIDS/WHO Epidemiological Fact Sheets on HIV and AIDS', Update, South Africa, available at http://apps.who.int/globalatlas/predefined-Reports/EFS2008/full/EFS2008_ZA.pdf, accessed 6 December 2009

UNDP (1994) *Human Development Report*, United Nations Development Programme, New York

US Department of Health and Human Services (2006) 'Pandemic planning update: A report from Secretary Michael O. Leavitt', available at www.hhs.gov/panflu20060313.pdf, accessed 6 December 2009

Van Damme, W., Kober, K. and Kegels, G. (2008) 'Scaling up anti-retroviral treatment in southern African countries with human resource shortage: How will health systems adapt?', *Social Science and Medicine*, vol 66, no 10, pp2108–2121

Vaughan, M. (1991) *Curing their Ills: Colonial Power and African Illness*, Polity Press, Cambridge

Venkataramani, A. S., Maughan-Brown, B., Nattrass, N. and Prah Ruger, J. (2008) *Social Grants and the Incentive to Trade-Off Health for Income among Individuals on HAART in South Africa*, Centre for Social Science Research Working Paper, University of Cape Town, Cape Town

Wald, P. (2008) *Contagious: Cultures, Carriers, and the Outbreak Narrative*, Duke University Press, Durham, NC

Wallace, R., Wallace, D., Andres, H., Fullilove, R. and Fullilove, M. T. (1995) 'The spatiotemporal dynamics of AIDS and TB in the New York metropolitan region from a socio-geographic perspective. Understanding the linkages of central city and suburbs', *Environment and Planning A*, vol 27, pp1085–1108

Wallace, R., Wallace, D., Ullman, J. E. and Andrews, H. (1999) 'Deindustrialisation, inner-city decay and the hierarchical diffusion of AIDS in the USA: How neoliberal and cold war policies magnified the ecological niche for emerging infections and created a national security crisis', *Environment and Planning A*, vol 31, pp113–139

Walsh, P. D., Biek, R. and Real, L. A. (2005) 'Wave-like spread of Ebola Zaire', *PLoS Biol*, vol 3, no 11, p371

Wang, L., Wang, Y., Jin, S., Wu, Z., Chin, D. P., Koplan, J. and Wilson, M. E. (2008) 'Emergence and control of infectious diseases in China', *Lancet*, vol 372, pp1598–1605

Wang, Y. (2008) 'The policy process and context of the rural new cooperative medical scheme and medical financial assistance in China', in Meessen, B., Pei, X., Criel, B. and Bloom, G. (eds) *Health and Social Protection: Experiences from China, Cambodia and Lao PDR*, Institute of Tropical Medicine, Antwerp

Wanless, D. (2004) *Securing Good Health for the Whole Population*, HMSO, London

Wardlaw, T., Salama, P., Brocklehurst, C., Chopra, M. and Mason, E. (2009) 'Why children are still dying and what can be done', *Lancet*, published online 14 October

Wardle, J., Carnell, S., Haworth, C. and Plomin, R. (2008) 'Evidence for a strong genetic influence on childhood adiposity despite the force of the obesogenic environment', *American Journal of Clinical Nutrition*, vol 87, pp398–404

Washington Post (2007) 'Singapore to scrap anti-obesity program', available at www.washingtonpost.com/wp-dyn/content/article/2007/03/20/AR2007032001145.html, accessed 6 December 2009

Weick, K. (1987) 'Organizational culture as a source of high reliability', *California Management Review*, vol 29, pp112–127

Weick, K. (1993) 'The collapse of sensemaking in organizations: The Mann Gulch disaster', *Administrative Science Quarterly*, vol 38, no 4, pp628–652

Weick, K., Sutcliffe, K. and Obstfeld, D. (1999) 'Organizing for high reliability: Processes of collective mindfulness', *Research in Organizational Behavior*, vol 21, pp81–123

Weir, L. and Mykhalovskiy, E. (2006) 'The geopolitics of global public health surveillance in the 21st century', in Bashford, A. (ed) *Medicine at the Border: The History, Politics and Culture of Global Health*, Palgrave, Basingstoke, pp240–263

Weiss, R. (2001) 'The Leeuwenhoek Lecture 2001. Animal origins of human infectious disease', *Philosophical Transactions of the Royal Society, B Biological Sciences*, vol 356, no 1410, pp957–977

Weiss, R. and McMichael, A. (2004) 'Social and environmental risk factors in the emergence of infectious diseases', *Nature Medicine*, vol 10, ppS70–S76

Weldon, R. A. (2001) 'An "urban legend" of global proportion: An analysis of nonfiction accounts of the Ebola virus', *Journal of Health Communication*, vol 6, no 3, pp281–294

Wells, C. D., Cegielski, J. P., Nelson, L. J., Laserson, K. F., Holtz, T. H., Finlay, A., Castro, K. G. and Weyer, K. (2007) 'HIV infection and multidrug-resistant tuberculosis: The perfect storm', *Journal of Infectious Disease*, vol 15, no 196, supp 1, pp86–107

Wells, J. (2008) 'Obesity researchers must understand how capitalism works', SciDev Net, 23 July, available at www.scidev.net/en/opinions/obesity-researchers-must-understand-how-capitalism.html#, accessed 21 November 2009

Welshman, J. (2006) 'Compulsion, localism, and pragmatism: The micro-politics of tuberculosis screening in the United Kingdom, 1950–1965', *Social History Medicine*, vol 19, pp295–312

Whiteside, A. (2009) Oral presentation to International HIV/AIDS Alliance, Brighton, entitled 'Is Aids still exceptional?' 22 June 2009. Summarized on www.aidsalliance.org/sw59789.asp, accessed 27 June 2009

Whiteside, A., De Waal, A. and Gebre-Tensae, T. (2006) 'AIDS, security and the military in Africa: A sober appraisal', *African Affairs*, vol 105, no 419, pp201–218

WHO (1978) 'Declaration of Alma-Ata', International Conference on Primary Health Care, Alma-Ata, USSR, WHO, Geneva

WHO (1997) 'WHO recommended guidelines for epidemic preparedness and response: Ebola haemorrhagic fever (EHF)', WHO, Geneva

WHO (2000a) 'An integrated approach to communicable disease surveillance', *Weekly Epidemiological Record*, vol 75, pp1–8

WHO (2000b) 'Obesity: Preventing and managing the global epidemic', WHO Technical Report Series 894, Geneva

WHO (2001) *Macroeconomics and Health: Investing in Health for Economic Development*, WHO, Geneva

WHO (2003) 'Cumulative number of reported probable cases of SARS', 7 August, available at www.who.int/csr/sars/country/en/, accessed 6 December 2009

WHO (2004a) *The World Health Report 2004*, World Health Organization, Geneva

WHO (2004b) 'Acute flaccid paralysis surveillance: A global platform for detecting and responding to priority infectious diseases', *Weekly Epidemiological Record*, vol 27, pp232–240

WHO (2005) 'Global tuberculosis control: Surveillance, planning, financing', WHO/HTM/TB/2005.349, WHO, Geneva

WHO (2006) 'Global tuberculosis control: Surveillance, planning, financing', WHO/HTM/TB/2006.362, WHO, Geneva

WHO (2007a) *The World Health Report 2007 – A Safer Future: Global Public Health Security in the 21st Century*, WHO, Geneva

WHO (2007b) 'Global XDR-TB task force update – February 2007', available at www.who.int/tb/xdr/globaltaskforce_update_feb07.pdf, accessed 6 December 2009

WHO (2007c) Media interview with Guenal Rodier, Director of International Health Regulations Co-ordination, available at www.who.int/bulletin/volumes/85/6/07-100607/en/index.html, accessed July 2008

WHO (2008a) *World Health Report 2008 – Primary Health Care: Now More Than Ever*, WHO Publications, Geneva

WHO (2008b) 'World malaria report 2008', available at http://apps.who.int/malaria/wmr2008, accessed 3 November 2009

WHO (2008c) 'Framework and standards for country health information systems', *Health Metrics Network*, World Health Organization, Geneva

WHO (2008d) 'Guidelines for the programmatic management of drug-resistant tuberculosis: Emergency update 2008', WHO/HTM/TB/2008.402, Geneva

WHO (2009) 'Concern over flu pandemic justified', address by Margaret Chan to 62nd World Health Assembly, 18 May

WHO European Ministerial Conference on Counteracting Obesity (2006) *European Charter on Counteracting Obesity*, WHO, Istanbul and Copenhagen, available at www.euro.who.int/Document/E89567.pdf, accessed 20 October 2008

WHO European Ministerial Conference on Counteracting Obesity (2007) 'Conference report15–17 November 2006', WHO Regional Office, available at www.euro.who.int/obesity/conference2006, accessed 2 November 2009

Wilding, J. (2007) 'Obesity: Finding pharmacological solutions to a 21st century epidemic', presentation at Biotechnology Group Chemical Biology Forum conference, 'Obesity: Causes, Consequences, Prevention and Treatment', held at Institute of Physics Conference Centre, London

Williams, S. J. and Calnan, M. (1996) 'The "limits" of medicalization? Modern medicine and the lay populace in "late" modernity', *Social Science and Medicine*, vol 42, pp1609–1620

Wilson, K., Tigerstrom, B. and McDougall, C. (2008) 'Protecting global health security through the International Health Regulations: Requirements and challenges', *Canadian Medical Association Journal*, vol 179, no 1, pp44–48

Wilson, R. (2000) 'Reconciliation and revenge in post-apartheid South Africa: Rethinking legal pluralism and human rights', *Current Anthropology*, vol 41, no1, pp75–98

Wolfe, N. (2009a) 'How to prevent a pandemic', *New York Times*, 28 April

Wolfe, N. (2009b) 'Preventing the next pandemic', *Scientific American*, April, pp76–81

Wolfe, N., Switzer, W., Carr, J., Bhullar, V., Shanmugam, V., Tamoufe, U., Prosser, A., Torimoro, J., Wright, A., Mpoudi-Ngole, E., McCutchan, F., Birz, D., Folks, T., Burke, D. and Heneine, W. (2004) 'Naturally acquired simian retrovirus infections in central African hunters', *Lancet*, vol 363, no 9413, pp932–937

Wolfe, N., Daszak, P., Kilpatrick, A. and Burke, D. (2005) 'Bushmeat hunting, deforestation, and prediction of zoonotic disease emergence', *Emerging Infectious Diseases*, vol 11, no 12, pp1822–1827

Wolfe, N., Dunavan, C. and Diamond, J. (2007) 'Origins of major human infectious diseases', *Nature*, vol 447, pp279–283

Wong, E. (2009) 'China's tough policy seems to slow flu's spread', *The New York Times*, 22 November

Woolhouse, M. (2008) 'Epidemiology: Emerging diseases go global', *Nature*, vol 451, pp898–899

World Health Assembly (2005) 'Revision of the International Health Regulations, WHA58.3. 2005', available at www.who.int/gb/ebwha/pdf_files/WHA58-REC1/english/Resolutions.pdf, accessed 6 December 2009

Yahya, M. (2006) 'Polio vaccines – difficult to swallow: Story of a controversy in northern Nigeria', *IDS Working Paper 261*, Institute of Development Studies, Brighton

Yamey, G. (2003) 'Multidrug resistant tuberculosis', *British Medical Journal*, vol 326, no 7389, p606

Yang, D. (2004) *Remaking the Chinese Leviathan, Market Transition and the Politics of Governance in China*, Stanford University Press, Stanford, CA

Yong Kim, J., Shakow, A., Mate, K., Vanderwarker, C., Gupta, R. and Farmer, P. (2005) 'Limited good and limited vision: Multidrug-resistant tuberculosis and global health policy', *Social Science & Medicine*, vol 61, pp847–859

Young, R. M. and Meyer, I. H. (2005) 'The trouble with "MSM" and "WSW": Erasure of the sexual-minority person in public health discourse', *American Journal of Public Health*, vol 95, no 7, pp1144–1149

Zachariah, R., Teck, R., Harries, A. D. and Humblet, P. (2004) 'Implementing joint TB and HIV interventions in a rural district of Malawi: Is there a role for an international non-governmental organisation? (Unresolved issues)', *The International Journal of Tuberculosis and Lung Disease*, vol 8, no 9, pp1058–1064

Zhang, Z., Fang, L. and Bloom, G. (forthcoming) 'The rural health protection system in China', in Lin, V., Guo, Y., Legge, D. and Wu, Q. (eds) *Health Policy in Transition: The Challenges for China*, Peking University Medical Press, Beijing

Zinsstag, J., Schelling, E., Bonfoh, B., Fooks, A., Kasymbekov, J., Waltner-Toews, D. and Tanner, M. (2009) 'Towards a "One Health" research and application tool box', *Veterinaria Italiana*, vol 45, no 1, pp121–133

Index